T0275623

The development of drug-resistant canc... ...s considered to be the most significant obstacle to the cure of cancer today. Nearly half of all patients with cancer suffer from tumors that are intrinsically resistant to chemotherapy, and most of the remaining half develop drug resistance during the course of their treatment.

This book reviews the mechanisms and clinical implications of drug resistance in cancer with unrivalled authority. Chapters cover topics of current clinical concern, including multiple drug resistance and its reversal, topoisomerase drugs, apoptosis, dose intensity and escalation, gene therapy and hematopoietic support. The authors are among the leading clinicians and investigators in the field.

Volumes in this series are intended for a wide audience of clinicians and researchers with an interest in the applications of biomedical science to the understanding and management of cancer.

DRUG RESISTANCE IN THE TREATMENT OF CANCER

CANCER: CLINICAL SCIENCE IN PRACTICE

General Editor
Professor Karol Sikora
Department of Clinical Oncology
Royal Postgraduate Medical School
Hammersmith Hospital, London

A series of authoritative review volumes intended for a wide audience of clinicians and researchers with an interest in the application of biomedical science to the understanding and management of cancer.

Also in this series:
Molecular Endocrinology of Cancer
ISBN 0 521 473 670
Edited by Jonathan Waxman

Cell Therapy
ISBN 0 521 473 152
Edited by George Morstyn and William Sheridan

Tumor Immunology: Immunotherapy and Cancer Vaccines
ISBN 0 521 472 377
Edited by A. G. Dalgleish and M. Browning

DRUG RESISTANCE IN THE TREATMENT OF CANCER

Edited by
HERBERT M. PINEDO
and
GIUSEPPE GIACCONE
University Hospital Vrije Universiteit, Amsterdam, The Netherlands

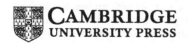

CAMBRIDGE
UNIVERSITY PRESS

CAMBRIDGE UNIVERSITY PRESS
Cambridge, New York, Melbourne, Madrid, Cape Town, Singapore, São Paulo

Cambridge University Press
The Edinburgh Building, Cambridge CB2 2RU, UK

Published in the United States of America by Cambridge University Press, New York

www.cambridge.org
Information on this title: www.cambridge.org/9780521473217

© Cambridge University Press 1998

First published 1998
This digitally printed first paperback version 2006

A catalogue record for this publication is available from the British Library

Library of Congress Cataloguing in Publication data
Drug resistance in the treatment of cancer / edited by Herbert M.
    Pinedo, Giuseppe Giaccone.
        p. cm. – (Cancer, clinical science in practice)
    ISBN 0 521 47321 7 (hb)
    1. Drug resistance in cancer cells. I. Pinedo, H. M.
II. Giaccone, Giuseppe. III. Series.
    [DNLM: 1. Drug Resistance, Neoplasm – physiology.
    2. Antineoplastic Agents – therapeutic use.   QV 269 D7945 1997]
    RC271.C5D7778   1997
    616.99'4061 – dc21
    DNLM/DLC
    for Library of Congress   97-6482 CIP

ISBN-13 978-0-521-47321-7 hardback
ISBN-10 0-521-47321-7 hardback

ISBN-13 978-0-521-03074-8 paperback
ISBN-10 0-521-03074-9 paperback

Contents

Contributors

Joseph R. Bertino, MD
Molecular Pharmacology Laboratories, Sloan-Kettering Institute, New York, USA

John P. A. Crown, MB
Memorial Sloan-Kettering Cancer Center, New York, USA

Elisabeth G. E. de Vries
Division of Medical Oncology, University Hospital Groningen, The Netherlands

William S. Dalton, MD PhD
H. Lee Moffitt Cancer Centre & Research Institute, University of South Florida, Tampa, Florida, USA

Wil Dolsma
Department of Radiotherapy, University Hospital Groningen, The Netherlands

David Fennelly, MB
St Vincent's Hospital, Dublin, Ireland

Antonio Tito Fojo
Medicine Branch, National Cancer Institute, Bethesda, Maryland, USA

Emil Frei III
Dana-Farber Cancer Institute, Boston, Massachusetts, USA

Giuseppe Giaccone, MD PhD
Department of Medical Oncology, University Hospital Vrije Universiteit, Amsterdam, The Netherlands

Erdem Göker
Memorial Sloan-Kettering Cancer Center, New York, USA

Richard Gorlick
Molecular Pharmacology Laboratories, Sloan-Kettering Institute, New York, USA

John A. Hickman
Cancer Research Campaign Molecular and Cellular Pharmacology Group, School of Biological Sciences, University of Manchester, UK

Geke A. P. Hospers
Department of Medical Oncology, University Hospital Groningen, The Netherlands

Lyn Mickley
Medicine Branch, National Cancer Institute, Bethesda, Maryland, USA

Nanno H. Mulder
Department of Medical Oncology, University Hospital Groningen, The Netherlands

Larry Norton, MD
Memorial Sloan-Kettering Cancer Center, New York, USA

Herbert M. Pinedo
Department of Medical Oncology, University Hospital Vrije Universiteit, Amsterdam, The Netherlands

George Raptis, MD
Memorial Sloan-Kettering Cancer Center, New York, USA

Karol Sikora, MB PhD FRCR FRCP
Imperial Cancer Research Fund Oncology Unity, Department of Clinical Oncology, Royal Postgraduate Medical School, Hammersmith Hospital, London, UK

Beverly A. Teicher, PhD
Lilly Research Laboratories, Indianapolis, USA

Henk M. W. Verheul
Department of Medical Oncology, University Hospital Vrije Universiteit, Amsterdam, The Netherlands

Series Editor's Preface

The last 40 years have brought tremendous advances in the management of several rare cancer types by chemotherapy. Unfortunately for most patients with one of the common cancers, progress has been less rapid. Impressive initial response rates to systemic therapy can often be achieved but drug resistance rapidly supervenes.

This volume examines the biochemical mechanisms of tumor drug resistance and their clinical relevance. Written by a group of internationally recognized clinicians and scientists, it provides an excellent synopsis of the current situation. Advances in molecular genetics will almost certainly lead to novel concepts that can be utilized in the clinic. During the next decade this area is likely to provide a focus for intense translational research activity.

Karol Sikora

Abbreviations

ABC	ATP-binding cassette
ABMT	allogeneic bone marrow transplantation
ABVD	doxorubicin/bleomycin/vinblastine/decarbazine
AC	doxorubicin/cyclophosphamide
ADEPT	antibody-dependent enzyme–prodrug therapy
AGAT	O^6-alkylguanine-DNA alkyltransferase
AFP	alpha fetoprotein
ALL	acute lymphocytic leukemia
AML	acute myeloid leukemia
AMSA	amsacrine
ANC	absolute neutrophil counts
ANLL	nonlymphoblastic leukemia
AP	alkaline phosphatase
AraC	cytosine arabinoside
AUC	area under the curve
BCNU	N,N-bis(2-chloroethyl)-N-nitrosourea, carmustine
BMT	bone marrow transplantation
BSO	buthionine sulfoxide
CAF	cyclophosphamide/doxorubicin/5-fluorouracil
CAM	chick choroallantoic membrane
CAT	chloramphenicol acetyltransferase
CCNU	1-(2-chloroethyl)-3-cyclohexyl-1-nitrosourea, lomustine
CD	cytosine deaminase
2-CdA	2-chlorodeoxyadenosine
CDDP	cisplatin, i.e. cis-diamminedichloroplatinum II

CEA	carcinoembryonic antigen
CENU	chloroethylnitrosourea
CFTR	cystic fibrosis gene product
CFU	colony-forming units
CHO	Chinese hamster ovary
CLL	chronic lymphocytic leukemia
CMF	cyclophosphamide/methotrexate/5-fluorouracil
CMFVP	CMF plus vincristine and prednisone
CML	chronic myeloid leukemia
CPB	cyclophosphamide/cisplatin/carmustine
CPT	camptothecin
CSF	colony stimulating factor
CT	computerized tomography
CTX	cyclophosphamide
dCK	deoxycytidine kinase
DHFR	dihydrofolate reductase
DOPA	dihydroxyphenylalanine
DOPA DC	DOPA decarboxylase
EGF	epidermal growth factor
EGFR	epidermal growth factor receptor
5-FC	5-fluorocytosine
FdUDP	fluorodeoxyuridine diphosphate
FdUMP	fluorodeoxyuridine monophosphate
FEC	5-fluorouracil/epirubicin/cyclophosphamide
FUDR	5'-deoxy-5-fluorouridine
FUTP	fluorouracil triphosphate
G-CSF	granulocyte colony-stimulating factor
GCV	gancyclovir
GDEPT	genetically directed enzyme prodrug therapy
GM-CSF	granulocyte–macrophage-colony stimulating factor
GPT	guanine phosphotransferase
GSH	glutathione
GST	glutathione-S-transferase
HA	hemagglutinin
HAI	hepatic arterial infusion

HD	high dose
HDC	high-dose chemotherapy
HGF	hepatocyte growth factor
HPLC	high-performance liquid chromatography
HSV	herpes simplex virus
IL	interleukin
IGF	insulin-like growth factor
IRF	interferon regulatory factor
L-PAM	melphalan
LRP	lung resistant-related protein
LTR	long terminal repeat
LV	leucovorin
MDR	multidrug resistance
MoAb	monoclonal antibody
MOPP	mechlorethamine/Oncovin/procarbazine/prednisone
6-MP	6-mercaptopurine
MRI	magnetic resonance imaging
MRP	multidrug resistance-associated protein
MTX	methotrexate
MUC	mucin
9-NC	9-nitro-camptothecin
NHL	non-Hodgkin's lymphoma
NSCLC	non-small-cell lung cancer
NSE	neuro-specific enolase
5-NT	5-nucleotidase
OPT	ortho-phthaldialdehyde
ORCC	outwardly rectifying chloride channels
ORDIC	outwardly rectifying depolarization induced chloride currents
PAI	plasminogen activator inhibitor
PBPC	peripheral blood-derived hematopoietic progenitor cells
PBSCG	peripheral blood stem cell grafting
PCR	polymerase chain reaction

PD	penicillin diamine
PDR	pleiotropic drug resistant
PEG	polyethylene glycol
PET	positron emission tomography
Pgp	P-glycoprotein
PKA	protein kinase activity
PLDB	protein-linked DNA breaks
PMN	peripheral mononuclear
PSA	prostate-specific antigen
Rb	retinoblastoma
RT-PCR	reverse transcriptase polymerase chain reaction
SAR	scaffold-associated region
scFv	single chain variable fragment
SCLC	small-cell lung cancer
SDS	sodium dodecyl sulfate
TAP	transporter associated with antigen processing
6-TG	6-thioguanine
TGF	transforming growth factor
tk	thymidine kinase
TMTX	trimetrexate
TNF	tumor necrosis factor
topo	topoisomerase
TS	thymidilate synthase
6-TX	6-thiouracil
VAD	vincristine/adriamycin/dexamethasone
VATH	vinblastine/doxorubicin/thiotepa/fluoxymesterone

1

Resistance mechanisms to antimetabolites

ERDEM GÖKER, RICHARD GORLICK
and JOSEPH R. BERTINO

Introduction

Antimetabolites are a class of chemotherapeutics that compete with biologic substrates and interfere with many biochemical reactions in the cell. Following the introduction of aminopterin, a 4-amino analog of folic acid, for the treatment of childhood acute lymphocytic leukemia (ALL) in 1948 (Farber et al.), a less toxic analog, methotrexate (MTX) subsequently replaced aminopterin in the clinic in 1956 (Li, Hertz and Spencer). One year later, 5-fluorouracil (5-FU) was synthesized as an analog of uracil by Duschinsky and Heidelberg et al. It was subsequently determined to demonstrate anticancer activity in human tumors. The development of 5-FU is an excellent example of rational drug design, based on the observation that uracil is salvaged more efficiently by tumor cells compared to normal cells (Rutman, Cantarow and Paschkis, 1954). Both MTX and 5-FU are used to treat many kinds of cancer including head and neck, breast, gastrointestinal and bladder cancers. MTX is also used for maintenance and central nervous system prophylaxis of acute lymphoblastic leukemia.

The development of other effective drugs and combinations of drugs with antimetabolites has markedly improved the therapy of certain malignancies. Cytosine arabinoside (AraC), thiopurines (6-thioguanine, 6-TG and 6-mercaptopurine, 6-MP) and 2-chlorodeoxyadenosine (2-CdA) are other important antimetabolites that have been found effective for the treatment of acute leukemia (Henderson, Hoelzer and Freeman, 1990).

In potentially curable tumors, drug resistance occurs rapidly if cure is not achieved, and is the reason for treatment failure. Beside acquired resistance, in some tumors treatment with antimetabolites is ineffective from the beginning because of inherent or intrinsic cellular resistance

1

to these drugs. A detailed understanding of mechanisms of intrinsic and acquired resistance to antimetabolites may allow development of new drugs and new chemotherapeutic approaches for treatment or strategies to prevent the occurrence of resistance. In this chapter we review the status of our information on resistance to antimetabolites, with emphasis on clinical resistance.

Methotrexate

MTX is a potent inhibitor of dihydrofolate reductase (DHFR), a key enzyme for intracellular folate metabolism (Figure 1.1). As a consequence of DHFR inhibition, intracellular levels of tetrahydrofolate coenzymes are rapidly depleted. Since reduced folates are required for thymidylate biosynthesis as well as purine biosynthesis, DNA synthesis is blocked (Schweitzer, Dicker and Bertino, 1990). Cell death follows depletion of thymidylate, and possibly from misincorporation of uridine nucleotides into DNA because of the change in the balance between purine and pyrimidine bases (Allegra, 1990).

Resistance mechanisms to MTX have been extensively studied both in vitro and in vivo including animal models and in patients (Gorlick et al., 1997). At least four different resistance mechanisms may occur after treatment of tumor cells in vitro: decreased intracellular accumulation of MTX due to decreased transport or impaired polyglutamylation of this drug; increased target enzyme activity via DHFR gene amplification; or dysregulation of transcriptional or translational control of this

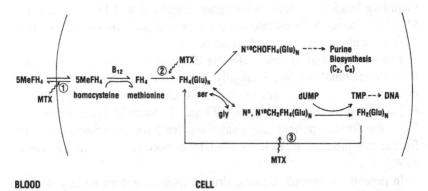

BLOOD   CELL

Figure 1.1. Mechanism of action and resistance mechanisms to MTX. MTX enters cells by the reduced folate carrier (1), is polyglutamylated (2) and MTX or its polyglutamylated forms are potent inhibitors of dihydrofolate reductase (3).

enzyme; and decreased inhibition of DHFR activity by MTX because of a mutation of the DHFR gene.

Decreased transport

Transport resistance is a common mechanism of acquired resistance to MTX in experimental tumors both in vitro and in vivo (Sirotnak, 1986). Recently the putative carrier for active MTX transport (the reduced folate transport carrier) has been isolated and the cDNA cloned (Dixon et al., 1994; Williams et al., 1994). The study of MTX transport in tumor samples from patients has limitations, such as limited sampling, lack of internal controls, and heterogeneity of tumors. An additional limiting factor to resistance assessment is the requirement of pre- and post-treatment samples for comparative analysis. A competitive displacement assay utilizing the fluorescent lysine analog of MTX (PT 430) was developed as a sensitive method of detection of transport resistance to MTX in cell lines as well as in blast cells from patients with leukemia (Trippett et al., 1992). After achievement of steady-state level of intracellular PT 430, subsequent incubation with the folate antagonists, MTX and trimetrexate (TMTX), which differ in the mode of carrier transport, produced characteristic displacement patterns of PT 430 (Trippett et al., 1992). We evaluated this assay for use in fresh blasts from patients with leukemia. Analysis of samples from 30 patients with untreated leukemia shows that 30% displacement of PT 430 was observed in all but two samples. In 35 relapsed patients that were considered to have acquired resistance to MTX, we found over half of the patient samples had less than 30% of displacement of PT 430 with MTX. Thus decreased transport is a common resistance mechanism to MTX in relapsed ALL. This finding has important implications for clinical use of this drug and new drug development. In acute non-lymphoblastic leukemia, a disease to be considered naturally resistant to MTX, we found that transport resistance is uncommon in blast cells from untreated patients, indicating that uptake of MTX is not the basis for natural resistance to this drug (Gorlick *et al.*, 1997).

Impaired polyglutamylation

Polyglutamylation of MTX is a metabolic process that has great pharmacologic importance. Long-chain polyglutamates of MTX ($n = 2$–5) have an equal affinity for the target enzyme, DHFR, as does MTX itself and exit the cell much more slowly than MTX monoglutamates. The intracellular content of polyglutamate derivatives of MTX are controlled by a balance between folylpolyglutamate synthetase and gamma-glutamyl hydrolase activities (Goldman and Matherly, 1986).

Patients with acute nonlymphoblastic leukemia (ANLL) and patients with sarcoma are considered to be naturally resistant to MTX with low clinical response. To explore the reasons for this natural resistance, we examined these tumors for mechanisms known to produce MTX resistance in vitro and compared these results to the results in a sensitive neoplasm, childhood acute lymphoblastic leukemia (ALL). Patient tumor samples were evaluated for formation of MTX polyglutamates after a 24 hour incubation with 10 μM [³H]-MTX and HPLC analysis. Although the total MTX (MTX plus MTX polyglutamate content) was almost the same in ANLL and ALL, we found lower levels of long-chain polyglutamates in ANLL blast cells as compared to ALL blasts (Göker et al., 1993). The amounts of long-chain polyglutamates formed by ANLL blasts were quite variable. Of interest, monoblastic ANLL (M5) cells formed as much MTX polyglutamates as the childhood ALL blasts (Goker *et al.*, 1995). We also evaluated adult ALL blasts for in vitro MTX polyglutamate accumulation. Adult pre-B ALL and T cell ALL blasts were found to accumulate less MTX polyglutamates as compared to childhood ALL blasts (Lin et al., 1991). A lower content of MTX polyglutamates could be due to decreased synthesis by FPGS or an increased catabolism of MTX polyglutamates by gamma-glutamyl hydrolase. We therefore are assessing activities of both of these enzymes in various leukemia blasts. A wide range of FPGS activity, proportion to FPGS mRNA levels, has been observed in leukemic blasts (Lenz et al., 1993b).

Increased DHFR enzyme activity

MTX is a tight-binding inhibitor of DHFR, and the concentration of MTX required to achieve inhibition of enzyme activity increases in direct proportion to the amount of the enzyme in the target cells. It is now well established that an important mechanism of resistance of cells to MTX is an increase in DHFR activity due to amplification of the DHFR gene (Carman et al., 1984). Mouse, hamster and human MTX-resistant cell lines have been described with increased levels of DHFR activity due to gene amplification (Schimke, 1988). Following reports indicating that gene amplification is a common mechanism of resistance in cell lines exposed to gradually increased doses of MTX, four case reports in the literature appeared, one from our laboratory, indicating that low-level gene amplification occurs in tumor cells from patients treated with MTX, consistent with the expectation that a low level of amplification would be sufficient to cause clinical resistance to this drug. In ALL, we assessed the frequency of DHFR gene amplification as an acquired resistance mechanism to MTX. DHFR gene amplification was determined with a DNA dot blot assay and confirmed by Southern and Northern analysis and DHFR enzyme activity. We found that low-level gene amplification was detected frequently in relapsed ALL blasts (9/29 samples) (Göker et al., 1995).

Mutant DHFR and transcriptional or translational control

Although mutations in the DHFR gene have been described in several MTX resistant cell lines, in our series of samples from leukemia patients, we have not detected any mutant DHFR enzymes using both enzymologic or molecular biology techniques, i.e. DNA SSPC (Fanin et al., 1993).

DHFR protein itself has a suppressive effect on translation of DHFR mRNA. When MTX binds to DHFR protein, this suppressive effect may be lost, allowing new enzyme synthesis (Chu et al., 1993; Ercikan et al., 1993). Thus far, limited data is available about the importance of these control mechanisms in clinical drug resistance.

Tumor suppressor genes and drug resistance

The effect of the retinoblastoma gene (*Rb*), a tumor suppressor gene, on DHFR expression is under active investigation in this laboratory. Lack of *Rb* may lead to MTX resistance as a consequence of increase DHFR mRNA expression and enzyme activity without gene amplification (Li et al., 1994).

Cell lines with mutated *p53*, a tumor suppressor gene, have the capacity to undergo gene amplification after antimetabolite exposure (Livingstone et al., 1992; Yin et al., 1992). We showed that low-level DHFR gene amplification in blasts from patients with ALL was associated with *p53* gene mutations (Göker et al., 1995). Association of low-level DHFR gene amplification with *p53* mutations in ALL blasts strengthens the concept that the loss of wild-type *p53* function results in the loss of the checkpoint at the G_1/S boundary (Harris and Hollstein,

1993) and permits cells to enter S phase without repair of DNA damage caused by MTX.

Strategies to treat tumor cells resistant to methotrexate

Understanding mechanisms of resistance to MTX in the clinic may allow us to develop new treatment modalities and new drugs. For example, the finding that defective transport of MTX is the most common resistance mechanism to MTX in relapsed ALL, has led to interest in drugs like trimetrexate (TMTX), which do not utilize the reduced folate transporter for uptake. TMTX has broad preclinical anti-tumor activity and it is very active in leukemia cells that are transport resistant to MTX (Lin and Bertino, 1987). However, clinical results with TMTX in relapsed ALL have been disappointing, as doses have been limited due to development of mucositis (Kheradpour et al., 1997).

The combination of TMTX and leucovorin (LV) is very active against *Pneumocystis carinii* infections in AIDS patients without serious side effects (Allegra et al., 1987). While TMTX is transported by passive diffusion in this parasite, LV cannot rescue this organism because of the absence of the reduced folate carrier that is necessary for LV transport. With this combination, the side effects of TMTX on the host are eliminated as normal host cells are protected by LV. In vitro cytotoxicity studies with CCRF/CEM cells showed that TMTX is not rescued by LV when the cells are resistant to MTX because of defective transport, but LV can rescue cytotoxic effects of TMTX in the MTX sensitive cells. We recently studied blast cells from patients with MTX-resistant ALL due to impaired uptake of this drug and found also that LV does not protect these resistant cells from TMTX cytotoxicity. We also showed that TMTX is still active in cells even with low-level DHFR gene amplification, because of the high intracellular concentration achieved. In view of these in vitro data, we plan to test TMTX with LV in relapsed ALL patients with transport resistance.

Pyrimidine antimetabolites

5-Fluorouracil (5-FU)

5-FU is an antimetabolite used for the treatment of gastrointestinal system malignancies, breast and head and neck cancers (Grem, 1990).

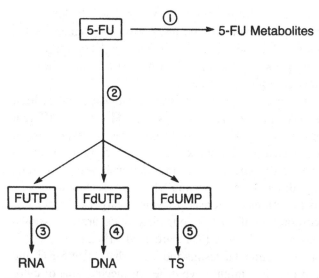

Figure 1.2. Mechanism of action of 5-FU. 5-FU is converted in cells to FUTP, which is incorporated into RNA; or to FdUTP, which can be incorporated into DNA. FdUMP is a potent inhibitor of TS in the presence of methylene tetrahydrofolate polyglutamylates. 5-FU may also be catabolyzed rapidly in cells, and increased catabolism may also play a role in intrinsic resistance to this drug.

5-FU produces its antitumor effect by inhibition of TS (thymidilate synthetase) and/or incorporation of 5-FU into RNA or DNA. 5-FU requires intracellular activation for its cytotoxicity (Figure 1.2). 5-FU rapidly enters into cells using the same transport system as uracil. After entering the cells, 5-FU may be anabolized either to fluorouracil triphosphate (FUTP) and incorporated to RNA at the ribonucleotide level, using phosphoribosylpyrophosphate as a ribophosphate source; or may be converted to fluorodeoxyuridine diphosphate (FdUDP) by ribonucleotide reductase and is consequently converted to fluorodeoxyuridine monophosphate (FdUMP), a potent inhibitor of TS (Spiegelman et al., 1980).

In the last several years, the addition of modulating agents, for example, leucovorin, MTX, or levamisole, to 5-FU have improved the treatment of colon cancer (Grogan, Sotos and Allegra, 1993). However, an objective clinical response is obtained in less than 40% of patients with advanced disease, and these responses are inevitably followed by the development of resistance to 5-FU. Mechanisms of resistance to 5-FU in tumor cells obtained from patients are more complex than found in cell lines in vitro. In the clinic, patients receive repetitive courses of the same dose of chemotherapy, which leads to low-grade resistance; but in experimental conditions, most investigators have studied resistant clones developed either by increasing the concentration of drug stepwise or by a single exposure to high doses, approaches that lead to development of highly resistant clones.

5-FU metabolism involves several activation pathways and at least three different targets (TS, RNA, and DNA), and several different resistance mechanisms to 5-FU have been described in experimental systems. Beside decreased cellular uptake of 5-FU, alterations in activation pathway enzymes (orotate phosphoribosyl transferase, thymidine phosphorylase, thymidine kinase, uridine phosphorylase and uridine kinase), as well as mutations or increased levels of target enzyme, TS, and decreased incorporation of 5-FU into nucleic acids, are well-known resistance mechanisms to this drug (Reichard et al., 1962).

Both clinical and experimental results indicated that pulse 5-FU and continuous infusion of 5-FU might have different mechanisms of cyto-toxicity (Seifert et al., 1975). Resistance mechanisms to these two differ-ent schedules of 5-FU were found to be different and tumor cells that are resistant to pulse 5-FU were found to be still sensitive to continuous exposure to this drug. Of interest is that cells resistant to 7-day exposure to 5-FU were partially cross-resistant to 4-hour pulse 5-FU, possibly indicating that both TS inhibition and 5-FU incorporation into RNA contribute to pulse cytotoxicity (Aschele et al., 1992).

Measurement of TS mRNA levels in colon cancer biopsies from patients using quantitative PCR showed that high TS mRNA levels are correlated with a low response rate in patients (Lenz et al., 1993a). Besides the level of intracellular TS activity, prolonged inhibition of this enzyme has been suggested to be another important determinant of 5-FU cytotoxicity (Sobrero et al., 1993).

Despite the large amount of experimental data relating to 5-FU resist-ance, mechanisms of acquired resistance to this drug in patients still remains to be elucidated.

Cytosine arabinoside

Cytosine arabinoside (AraC) is an important drug for the treatment of acute myeloid leukemia (AML) (Hiddemann, 1991). AraC produces its antitumor effect by incorporation into DNA and causing premature chain termination and slowing of chain elongation. This cytotoxic effect of AraC is mediated by its metabolite, ara-CTP, a product of first-step phosphorylation by deoxycytidine kinase (dCK) (Shewach, Reynolds and Hertel, 1992).

Resistance to AraC contributes to the short survival of patients with AML, despite the high percentage of complete remissions obtained in most centers that use this drug in combination with an anthracycline. The mechanisms of resistance to AraC and effect of dosing (high dose versus conventional doses) on occurrence of resistance are still under investigation. Decreased transport of AraC (Wiley et al., 1982), decreased or lack of dCK activity (Flasshove et al., 1994), increased cytidine deaminase activity (Steuart and Burke, 1971), an increased dCTP pool (Whelan et al., 1994), insensitivity of DNA polymerases to Ara-CTP inhibition and the presence of DNA repair enzyme(s) that removes AraC residues from DNA (Kufe et al., 1980) are possible causes for acquired AraC resistance. Previous studies showed that decreased transport of AraC is not frequent in clinical samples as a resistance mechanism (Wiley et al., 1982). Increased dCTP levels in blast cells were found in some blast samples from patients who were clinically resistant to AraC treatment. Intracellular dCTP levels are crucial for the metabolic activation of AraC as dCTP regulates the Ara-CTP biosynthetic pathway at two key reactions; by feedback inhibition of dCK and by allosteric activation of the catabolic enzyme, deoxycytidylate deaminase. Less commonly, decreased or lack of activity of dCK has been found as a mechanism to AraC resistance. The frequency and importance of this resistance mechanism to AraC in the clinic needs to be further investigated.

Purine antimetabolites

6-Mercaptopurine and 6-thioguanine

6-Mercaptopurine (6-MP) and 6-thioguanine (6-TG) are used in the treatment of both adult and childhood leukemia (Creaven and Rustum, 1990). They cause cytotoxic effects by incorporation into DNA after conversion via purine salvage pathways to thio-dGTP (McCormack and Johns, 1990). Although resistance mechanisms to these drugs have been investigated for a long time, the information as to the mechanisms of resistance in human tumors is limited. Decreased levels of the anabolic enzyme (hypoxanthine–guanine phosphoribosyl transferase), which is necessary for activation of these drugs, is the most common mechanism of resistance found in nonhuman tumors but was not found to be a major cause of resistance in human leukemia blasts (Rosman et al., 1974). 5-Nucleotidase (5-NT) and alkaline phosphatase (AP) were found to be increased in some resistant ALL blasts. Increased levels of these enzymes may result in decreased thiopurine nucleotide levels in the cell. Levels of the catabolic enzymes, thiopurine methyltransferase for 6-MP and xanthine oxidase for 6-TG, play an important role for the inactivation of these drugs.

2-Chlorodeoxyadenosine

The adenosine analog, 2-chlorodeoxyadenosine (2-CdA) has shown promise in the treatment of acute leukemia. 2-CdA accumulates selectively as the 5'-triphosphate metabolite form in cells that are rich in dCK (Seto et al., 1985). Since the cytotoxic activity of 2-CdA is independent of cell division and cell cycle, it is active in the treatment of low-grade malignancies of the lymphatic system including chronic lymphocytic leukemia, non-Hodgkin's lymphoma and hairy cell leukemia (Cheson, 1992). Further studies are needed to define its pharmacologic properties and mechanism(s) of resistance to this drug.

Conclusions

A detailed understanding of drug resistance mechanisms in human tumors is essential for the more effective use of antimetabolites, as well as for new strategies to prevent, overcome, or take advantage of the drug resistant phenotype. Improved methodology for isolation and propagation of tumor cells in vitro, as well as development of sensitive assays for biochemical as well as genetic changes that occur in drug resistant cells, is now allowing an assessment of resistance mechanisms in various types of human tumors.

References

Allegra, C. J. (1990). Antifolates. In *Cancer Chemotherapy. Principles and Practice* (ed. B. A. Chabner and J. M. Collins), pp. 110–53. J. B. Lippincott, Philadelphia.

Allegra, C. J., Chabner, B. A., Tuazon, C. U. et al. (1987). Trimetrexate for the treatment of pneumocystis carinii pneumonia in patients with the acquired immunodeficiency syndrome. *N. Engl. J. Med.*, **317**, 978–85.

Aschele, C., Sobrero, A., Faderan, M. A. and Bertino, J. R. (1992). Novel mechanism(s) of resistance to 5-fluorouracil in human colon cancer (HCT-8) sublines following exposure to two different clinically relevant dose schedules. *Cancer Res.*, **52**, 1855–64.

Bertino, J. R. and Göker, E. (1993). Drug resistance in acute leukemia. *Leukemia & Lymphoma*, **11**, 37–41.

Carman, M. D., Schornagel, J. H., Rivest, R. S. et al. (1984). Resistance to methotrexate due to gene amplification in a patient with acute leukemia. *J. Clin. Oncol.*, **2**, 16–20.

Cheson, B. D. (1992). The purine analogs – a therapeutic beauty contest. *J. Clin. Oncol.*, **10**, 352–4.

Chu, E., Takimoto, C. H., Voeller, D. et al. (1993). Specific binding of human dihydrofolate reductase protein to dihydrofolate reductase messenger RNA in vitro. *Biochemistry*, **32**, 4756–60.

Creaven, P. J. and Rustum, Y. M. (1990). Principles of chemotherapy: drugs and biochemical determinants. In *Leukemia*, 5th edn (ed. E. S. Henderson and T. A. Lister), pp. 391–415. Saunders, Philadelphia.

Dixon, K. H., Lanpher, B. C., Chiu, J. et al. (1994). A novel cDNA restores reduced folate carrier activity and methotrexate sensitivity to transport deficient cells. *J. Biol. Chem.*, **269**, 17–20.

Ercikan, E., Banerjee, D., Waltham, M. et al. (1993). Translational regulation of the synthesis of dihydrofolate reductase. In *Chemistry and Biology of Pteridines and Folates*, vol. 338 (ed. J. E. Ayling, M. G. Nair and C. M. Baugh), pp. 537–40. Plenum Press, New York.

Fanin, R., Banerjee, D., Volkenandt, M. et al. (1993). Mutations leading to antifolate resistance in Chinese hamster ovary cells after exposure to the alkylating agent ethylmethane sulfonanate. *Mol. Pharm.*, **44**, 13–21.

Farber, S., Diamond, L. K., Mercer, R. D. et al. (1948). Temporary remissions in acute leukemia in children produced by folic acid antagonist, 4-aminopteroyl-glutamic acid (aminopterin). *N. Engl. J. Med.*, **238**, 787–93.

Flasshove, M., Strumberg, D., Ayscue, L. et al. (1994). Structural analysis of the deoxycytidine kinase gene in patients with acute myeloid leukemia and resistance to cytosine arabinoside. *Leukemia*, **8**, 780–5.

Göker, E., Lin, J. T., Trippett, T. M. (1993). Decreased polyglutamylation of methotrexate in acute lymphoblastic leukemia in adults as compared to children with this disease. *Leukemia*, **7**, 1000–4.

Göker, E., Waltham, M., Kheradpour, A. et al. (1995). Amplification of the dihydrofolate reductase gene is a mechanism of acquired resistance to methotrexate in patients with acute lymphoblastic leukemia and is correlated with p53 gene mutations. *Blood*, **86**, 677–84.

Göker, E., Kheradpour, A., Waltham, M. *et al.* (1995). Acute monocytic leukemia: a myeloid subset that may be sensitive to methotrexate. *Leukemia*, **9**, 174–6.

Goldman, I. D. and Matherly, L. H. (1986). The cellular pharmacology of methotrexate. In *Membrane Transport of Antineoplastic Agents* (International Encyclopedia of Pharmacology and Therapeutics; Section 118) (ed. I. D. Goldman), pp. 241–81. Pergamon Press, Oxford.

Gorlick, R., Goker, E., Trippett, T. *et al.* (1997a). Intrinsic and acquired resistance to methotrexate in acute leukemia. *N. Engl. J. Med.*, **335**, 1041–8.

Gorlick, R., Goker, E., Trippett, T. et al. (1997b). Defective transport is a common mechanism of acquired methotrexate resistance in acute lymphocytic leukemia and is associated with decreased reduced folate carrier expression. Blood, **89**, 1013–8.

Grem, J. L. (1990). Fluorinated pyrimidines. In *Cancer Chemotherapy: Principles and Practice* (ed. B. A. Chabner and J. M. Collins), pp. 180–24. J. B. Lippincott, Philadelphia.

Grogan, L., Sotos, G. E. and Allegra, C. J. (1993). Leucovorin modulation of fluorouracil. *Oncology*, 7, 63–72.

Harris, C. C. and Hollstein, M. (1993). Clinical implications of the p53 tumor suppressor gene. *N. Engl. J. Med.*, 329, 1318–27.

Heidelberger, C., Chaudhuari, N. K., Danenberg, P. *et al.* (1957). Fluorinated pyrimidines: a new class of tumor inhibitory compounds. *Nature*, 179, 663–6.

Henderson, E. S., Hoelzer, D. and Freeman, A. I. (1990). The treatment of acute lymphoblastic leukemia. In *Leukemia*, 5th edn (ed. E. S. Henderson and T. A. Lister), pp. 443–84. Saunders, Philadelphia.

Hiddemann, W. (1991). Cytosine arabinoside in the treatment of acute myeloid leukemia: the role and place of high dose regimens. *Ann. Hematol.*, 62, 119–28.

Kheradpour, A., Berman, E., Goker, E. et al. (1997). A phase II study of continuous infusion of trimetrexate in patients with refractory acute leukemia. *Cancer Invest.* (In Press).

Kufe, D. W., Major, P. P., Egan, M. and Beardsley, P. (1980). Incorporation of araC into L1210 DNA as a correlate of cytotoxicity. *J. Biol. Chem.*, 255, 8997–9000.

Lenz, H. J., Leichman, C., Danenberg, P. V. et al. (1993a). Thymidilate synthase gene expression predicts response of primary gastric cancer to 5-fluorouracil, leucovorin, cisplatin. *Proc. Am. Soc. Clin. Oncol.*, 12, 129 (abstr).

Lenz. H. J., Schnieders, B., Danenberg, K. et al. (1993b). A polymerase chain reaction (PCR) assay for folylpolyglutamate synthetase (FPGS) gene expression: marked variation in human leukemia blast samples. *Proc. Am. Soc. Can. Res.*, 34, 504(a).

Li, M. C., Hertz, R. and Spencer, D. B. (1956). Effect of methotrexate therapy upon choriocarcinoma and chorioadenoma. *Proc. Soc. Exp. Biol. Med.*, 93, 361–6.

Li, W. W., Fan, J. G., Zielenski, Z. *et al.* (1994). Absence of retinoblastoma protein mediates intrinsic resistance to antimetabolites in sarcoma cell lines. *Proc. Am. Assoc. Can. Res.*, 35, 418(a).

Lin, J. T. and Berlino, J. R. (1987). Trimetrexate: a second generation folate antagonist in clinical trial. *J. Clin. Oncol.*, 5, 2032–40.

Lin, J. T., Tong, W. P., Trippett, T. M. et al. (1991). Basis for natural resistance to methotrexate in human acute non-lymphoblastic leukemia. *Leukemia Res.*, 15, 1191–6.

Livingstone, L. R., White, A., Sprouse, J. et al. (1992). Altered cell cycle arrest and gene amplification potentiate accompany loss of wild type p53. *Cell*, 70, 923–35.

McCormack, J. J. and Johns, D. G. (1990). Purine and purine nucleoside antimetabolites. In *Cancer Chemotherapy: Principles and Practice* (ed. B. A. Chabner and J. M. Collins), pp. 234–52. J. B. Lippincott, Philadelphia.

Reichard, P., Skold, O., Klein, G. et al. (1962). Studies on resistance against 5-fluorouracil. I. Enzymes of the uracil pathway during the development of resistance. *Cancer Res.*, 22, 235–43.

Rosman, M., Lee, M. H., Creasey, W. A. and Sartorelli, A. C. (1974). Mechanisms of resistance to 6-thiopurines in human leukemia. *Cancer Res.*, 34, 1952–6.

Rutman, R. J., Cantarow, A. and Paschkis, K. E. (1954). Studies on 2-acetylaminofluorene carcinogenesis: III. The utilization of uracil-2-C[14] by pre-neoplastic rat liver. *Cancer Res.*, 14, 119–26.

Schimke, R. T. (1988). Gene amplification in cultured cells. *J. Biol. Chem.*, **263**, 5989–92.

Schweitzer, B. I., Dicker, A. P. and Bertino, J. R. (1990). Dihydrofolate reductase as a therapeutic target. *FASEB J.*, **4**, 2441–52.

Seifert, P., Baker, L. H., Reed, M. L. et al. (1975). Comparison of continuously infused 5-fluorouracil with bolus injection in treatment of patients with colorectal adenocarcinoma. *Cancer*, **36**, 123–8.

Seto, S., Carrera, C. J., Kubato, M. et al. (1985). Mechanism of deoxyadenosine and chlorodeoxyadenosine toxicity to nondividing human lymphocytes. *J. Clin. Invest.*, **75**, 377–83.

Shewach, D. S., Reynolds, K. K. and Hertel, L. (1992). Nucleotide specificity of human deoxycytidine kinase. *Mol. Pharm.*, **42**, 518–24.

Sirotnak, F. M. (1986). Correlates of folate analog transport, pharmacokinetics and selective antitumor action. In *Membrane Transport of Antineoplastic Agents* (International Encyclopedia of Pharmacology and Therapeutics; section 118) (ed. I. D. Goldman), pp. 241–81. Pergamon Press, Oxford.

Sobrero, A. F., Aschele, C., Guglielmi, A. P. et al. (1993). Synergism and lack of cross-resistance between short-term and continuous exposure to fluorouracil in human colon adenocarcinoma cells. *J. Natl. Cancer Inst.*, **85**, 1937–44.

Spiegelman, S., Nayaak, R., Sawyer, R. et al. (1980). Potentiation of the antitumor activity of 5-FU by thymidine and its correlation with the formation of (5-FU)RNA. *Cancer (Phil.)*, **45**, 1129–34.

Steuart, C. D. and Burke, P. J. (1971). Cytidine deaminase and the development of resistance to arabinosyl cytosine. *Nature New Biol.*, **223**, 109–10.

Trippett, T., Schlemmer, S., Elisseyeff, Y. et al. (1992). Defective transport as a mechanism of acquired resistance to methotrexate in patients with acute leukemia. *Blood*, **80**, 1158–62.

Whelan, J., Smith, T., Phear, G. et al. (1994). Resistance to cytosine arabinoside in acute leukemia: the significance of mutations in CTP synthetase. *Leukemia*, **8**, 264–5.

Wiley, J. S., Jones, S. P., Sawyer, W. H. et al. (1982). Cytosine arabinoside influx and nucleoside transport sites in acute leukemia. *J. Clin. Invest.*, **69**, 479–89.

Williams, F. M. R., Murray, R. C., Underhill, T. M. and Flintoff, W. F. (1994). Isolation of a hamster cDNA clone coding for a function involved in methotrexate uptake. *J. Biol. Chem.*, **269**, 5810–16.

Yin, Y., Tainsky, M. A., Bischoff, F. Z. et al. (1992). Wild-type p53 restores cell cycle control and inhibits gene amplification in cells with mutant p53 alleles. *Cell*, **70**, 937–48.

2

Resistance to antitumor alkylating agents and cisplatin

BEVERLY A. TEICHER and EMIL FREI III

Introduction

Therapeutic resistance to the antitumor alkylating agents, as to any other type of molecular therapy, can be envisioned at three levels: (1) at the cellular level where biochemical alterations in the tumor cells confer resistance, (2) at the level of the tumor mass where physiological abnormalities and properties of the tumor confer resistance and (3) at the level of tumor/host interaction where the tumor as a tissue recruits and involves normal cells in its growth and survival. Targets for the therapeutic modulation (potentiation) of the antitumor alkylating agents can be divided into similar classes. Modulators that act at the level of individual tumor cells include: (1) enzyme inhibitors such as inhibitors of topoisomerase I and II, inhibitors of glutathione-S-transferase and S-glutamylcysteinyl synthase, inhibitors of DNA repair and mitochondrial toxins and (2) depletors of cellular protectors such as glutathione depletors. Modulators that act at the level of properties related to the tumor mass include: (1) agents that reverse hypoxic protection and agents that are selectively active under hypoxic conditions and (2) direct inhibitors of extracellular matrix degrading enzymes. Finally, modulators that act by inhibiting the ability of the tumor to mobilize host normal cells include: (1) inhibitors of endothelial cell proliferation such as antiangiogenic and angiostatic agents and (2) inhibitors of intercellular signaling pathways such as cyclooxygenase and lipoxygenase inhibitors. This review will demonstrate the potential of each of these strategies of therapeutic modulation using antitumor alkylating agents as the cytotoxic therapy.

14

Cellular mechanisms of resistance and strategies for modulation

Non-protein and protein sulfhydryls

Increases in thiol content and glutathione-S-transferase activity have been shown to occur frequently in CDDP (*cis*-diamminedichloroplatinum(II))-resistant cell lines (Bakka et al., 1981; Endresen, Schjerven and Rugstad, 1984; Bedford et al., 1987; Teicher et al., 1987; Kelley et al., 1988; Andrews, Murphy and Howell, 1989; Sakiya et al., 1989; Wang et al., 1989; Teicher et al., 1991e,f). The depletion of cellular thiols by use of buthionine sulfoximine has been shown to sensitize cells to the cytotoxic actions of platinum-containing drugs (Bedford et al., 1987). Although only three of the four CDDP-resistant cell lines in our study demonstrated an increase in glutathione, there was an increase in both protein sulfhydryl and glutathione-S-transferase activity in each of the five CDDP-resistant lines (Table 2.1). Kelley et al. (1988) have shown that, in four of these same cell lines, there was a good correlation between non-protein sulfhydryl increases, metallothionein increases and resistance to CDDP, although the magnitudes of the changes in protein sulfhydryl do not correlate directly with the magnitudes of resistance to CDDP. It is interesting that these increases in protein sulfhydryl content and glutathione-S-transferase are a significant factor in cellular resistance to alkylating agents in general. These changes must then occur in specific isozymes or in specific subcellular compartments in order to account for the lack of cross-resistance to other alkylating drugs in cell lines showing similar increases in total glutathione-S-transferase activity.

Glutathione is a ubiquitous tripeptide that plays a central role in the protection of cells against a spectrum of toxic insults (Arrick and Nathan, 1984). Previous studies have demonstrated an association between elevated glutathione levels and resistance of neoplastic cells to alkylating agents such as melphalan and cyclophosphamide (McGown and Fox, 1986; Ahmad et al., 1987). More recently, glutathione conjugates of melphalan, nitrogen mustard, chlorambucil and cyclophosphamide have been demonstrated by high-pressure liquid chromatography, raising the suggestion that glutathione can detoxify all of these alkylating agents and prevent cross-link formation (Dulik, Fenselau and Hilton, 1986; Dulik, Colvin and Fenselau, 1990; Gamcsik, Hamill and Colvin, 1990; Yuan et al., 1990). Consistent with this suggestion, depletion of glutathione levels by treatment with L-buthione-*R*,*S*-sulfoximine, an inhibitor of the enzyme glutathione synthetase, has resulted in increased

Table 2.1. *Comparison of the characteristics of five parental human tumor cell lines and CDDP-resistant sublines*

Cell line	CDDP IC90 (μM)	Fold resistance	Generation time (h)	Sulfhydryl content (nmol/10/cells)		Glutathione-S-transferase activity[c] (nmol/min mg protein)
				non-protein[a]	protein[b]	
G3361	65		33	165 (50)[d]	287 (87)	52±4 (134±10)[e]
G3361/CDDP	600	9.2	32	148 (43)	388 (113)	282±59 (1087±230)
SL6	60		28	145 (55)	213 (80)	114±11 (240±23)
SL6/CDDP	250	4.2	29	155 (183)	409 (481)	153±17 (290±32)
SW2	15		64	96 (50)	95 (50)	3.8±4.4 (2.4±2.8)
SW2/CDDP	50	3.3	104	92 (86)	207 (193)	5.6±2.8 (5.1±2.5)
MCF-7	40		36	203 (35)	537 (94)	1.9±1.7 (4.3±3.8)
MCF-7/CDDP	250	6.3	78	262 (98)	636 (238)	6.6±3.2 (18.1±8.8)
SCC-25	15		48	250 (55)	230 (50)	231±25 (503±55)
SCC-25/CDDP	255	17	49	210 (54)	390 (100)	447±73 (1145±186)

[a] Measured by fluorescence emission at 420 nm of an OPT (ortho-phthaldialdehyde) derivative.
[b] Measured by the difference between total sulfhydryl content and non-protein sulfhydryl content using Ellman's method. Absorbance was measured at 412 nm.
[c] Activity determined by absorption at 340 nm of product formed by the reaction of glutathione with 1-chloro-2,4-dinitrobenzine. Mean ± S.E.M.
[d] Numbers in parentheses, nmol per mg protein.
[e] Numbers in parentheses, nmol per mg protein.

sensitivity to alkylating agents in vitro and in vivo (Green et al., 1984; Somfai-Relle et al., 1984; Andrews, Murphy and Howell, 1986; Kramer et al., 1987; Ozols et al., 1987; Skapek et al., 1988). In a recent study relating to cyclophosphamide resistance in medulloblastoma, Friedman et al. (1992a) showed that the Daoy (4-HCR) cell line contained 2-fold more glutathione than the parental cell line. Resistance of the Daoy (4-HCR) cell line to 4-hydroperoxycyclophosphamide was diminished approximately 2-fold in the presence of buthionine sulfoximine. These results indicate that the resistance of the Daoy (4-HCR) cell line to 4-hydroperoxycyclophosphamide results in part from the elevated expression of aldehyde dehydrogenase and in part from the elevated level of glutathione.

Ethacrynic acid, a clinically used diuretic agent, is also an inhibitor of glutathione-S-transferase. Ethacrynic acid has been shown to increase cell kill by chlorambucil or melphalan in Walker 256 and HT29 in vitro and human tumors xenografted into nude mice (Tew, Bomber and Hoffman, 1988; Clapper, Hoffman and Tew, 1990). Rhodes and Twentyman studied alterations in glutathione levels and glutathione-S-transferase activity in a series of in vitro derived multidrug resistant and CDDP resistant sublines of the human lung cancer lines NCI-H69 (small cell), COR-L23 (large cell) and MOR (adenocarcinoma) (Rhodes and Twentyman, 1992). They also investigated the effects of ethacrynic acid, a putative inhibitor of glutathione-S-transferases, on levels of glutathione and glutathione-S-transferase activity and on cellular sensitivity to melphalan and to CDDP. Neither glutathione content nor glutathione-S-transferase activity were significantly greater in the resistant sublines compared with their respective parental lines. Treating with ethacrynic acid reduced glutathione content in the CDDP resistant subline H69/CPR and increased it to over 140% of control in the MOR parental line. Exposure of parental line COR-L23/P to ethacrynic acid increased the glutathione content to over 300–500% of control. Variable effects of ethacrynic acid on glutathione-S-transferase activity were seen in these cell lines. Doses of 1 µg ml^{-1} and 3 µg ml^{-1} respectively of ethacrynic acid. Addition of ethacrynic acid to treatment of the cell lines with melphalan or with CDDP did not alter the dose-response curves to these agents (Rhodes and Twentyman, 1992).

Alaoui-Jamali et al. (1992) examined the relationship between intracellular levels of glutathione, glutathione-S-transferase activity and the kinetics of DNA cross-links induced by melphalan in a rat mammary carcinoma cell line and in a subline selected in vitro for primary resistance to melphalan (MLNr, 16-fold resistance) (Alaoui-Jamali et al., 1992). The melphalan resistant cells had a 2-fold increase in intracellular glutathione concentration and an approximately 5-fold increase in gluta-thione-S-transferase activity as compared with the parent cells. They were cross-resistant to a variety of drugs, including chlorambucil (6-fold) and nitrogen mustard (14-fold). Treatment of parent cells with 30 μM mel-phalan induced a significant accumulation of DNA–DNA cross-links for up to 8 h, which decreased over a 24 h period. In the cells, no significant cross-link formation was induced by melphalan at any time between 0 and 24 h. Formation of cross-links was observed immediately after treatment with nitrogen mustard in both cell lines and was followed by a subsequent decrease during a 24 h incubation in drug-free medium. The numbers of nitrogen mustard-induced cross-links were significantly lower in resistant cells than in parent cells. The 35% decrease in mel-phalan accumulation observed in resistant cells could not entirely explain the absence of cross-links, since thin-layer chromatographic analysis demonstrated that both cell lines accumulate a significant amount of melphalan and metabolize it to the same extent. Significant amounts of melphalan were also detected in nuclei isolated from parent and resistant cells that had been treated with [^{14}C]-melphalan. Intracellular depletion of glutathione by a nontoxic concentration of L-buthionine(S,R)-sulfoximine significantly sensitized the resistant cells to melphalan and increased cross-link formation. A nontoxic concentration (50 μM) of ethacrynic acid also sensitized the resistant cells to melphalan and increased cross-link formation (Alaoui-Jamali et al., 1992).

Nitrosoureas: O^6-alkylguanine–DNA alkyltransferase

Chloroethylnitrosoureas (CENUs), are moderately effective in the treat-ment of gliomas in adults (Levin, 1985). They produce cytotoxicity by alkyl substitution of DNA guanine residues, with subsequent formation of DNA interstrand cross-links (Kohn, 1977). The alkyl group can be removed from the O^6 position by a DNA repair protein, O^6-alkylguanine–DNA alkyltransferase (AGAT), with restoration of an intact guanine. Resistance to nitrosoureas and methylating agents such as procarbazine can be mediated by this protein, which is expressed in the majority of tumors studied to date, including those arising in the central nervous system (Wiestler, Kleihues and Pegg, 1984; Pegg, 1990). Depletion of AGAT with alkylguanines or methylating agents sensitizes cells to the cytotoxic action of CENU (Dolan, Corsico and Pegg, 1985;

Dolan, Morimoto and Pegg, 1985; Dolan, Young and Pegg, 1986; Yarosh, Hurst-Calderone and Babich, 1986; Gerson, Trey and Miller, 1988; Dolan, Larkin and English, 1989; Dolan, Moschel and Pegg, 1990; Dolan, Stine and Mitchell, 1990; Dolan, Mitchell and Mummert, 1991; Mitchell, Moschel and Dolan, 1992) and provides the opportunity for the use of combination therapy designed to restore sensitivity to tumor cells resistant to the CENU carmustine (BCNU; N,N-bis(2-chloroethyl)-N-nitrosourea).

Friedman et al. (1992b) recently reported studies evaluating therapy with BCNU plus O^6-benzylguanine in the treatment of human glioblastoma multiforme and medulloblastoma xenografts growing subcutaneously in athymic mice. Both D341 Med and D-456 MG xenografts were resistant to BCNU administered at 1.0 LD_{10}. D341 Med exhibited a growth delay of 0.5 day, and D-456 MG exhibited a growth delay of ×0.9 day (Table 2.2). No tumor regressions were observed in either group. Pretreatment with O^6-benzylguanine restored BCNU sensitivity in both D341 Med and D-456 MG, with growth delays of 12.2 days and 26.5 days, respectively, following therapy with BCNU at 0.38 LD_{10}. Furthermore, treatment with BCNU plus O^6-benzylguanine produced eight to ten (no complete) and ten of ten (five complete) regressions of D341 MED and D-456 MG, respectively.

Treatment with BCNU plus O^6-methylguanine did not produce growth delays or tumor regressions distinguishable from those produced by BCNU alone (Table 2.2). Administration of O^6-benzylguanine prior to administration of BCNU (at 0.38 LD_{10}) produced prolonged growth delays and tumor regressions in almost all animals bearing D341 Med or D-456 MG xenografts, whereas BCNU alone (at 0.38–1.0 LD_{10}) showed little activity. No additional toxicity was seen using BCNU plus O^6-benzylguanine compared with BCNU alone at these doses. Conversely, O^6-methylguanine did not alter the activity of BCNU against either xenograft, reflecting the more efficient alkyltransferase depletion characteristic of O^6-benzylguanine (Dolan et al., 1990a,b).

O^6-benzylguanine, which demonstrates greater affinity for the alkyltransferase protein compared with O^6-methylguanine, effectively enhances nitrosourea activity both in vitro and in vivo. Previous studies (Dolan et al., 1990; Mitchell et al., 1992) have demonstrated cessation of growth by no tumor regressions using combination therapy with O^6-benzylguanine plus a nitrosourea. The results of Friedman et al. (1992b) demonstrate substantial growth delays and are the first to demonstrate complete and partial tumor regressions in almost all the tumors

Table 2.2. *Tumor growth delay and regression resulting from treatment of D341 Med and D-456 MG xenografts growing subcutaneously in athymic BALB/c mice with BCNU alone or with BCNU plus O^6-benzylguanine, O^6-methylguanine or streptozocin*

Expt No. Treatment[a]	D341 Med		D-456 MG[b]		Toxicity, D341 Med and D-456 MG	
	T–C[c]	Regression[d]	T–C	Regressions	% mean weight loss nadir	Deaths from toxic effects
1 BCNU (1.0 LD_{10})	0.5	0 of 9	–0.9	0 of 9	3.6	0 of 18
2 BCNU (0.38 LD_{10})	1.0	0 of 10	1.5	1 of 10	1.9	0 of 20
O^6-benzylguanine	1.2	0 of 8	1.0	0 of 10	0	0 of 18
BCNU (0.38 LD_{10}) + O^6-benzylguanine	12.2	8 of 10**(0)[e]	26.5	10 of 10**(5)[e]	2.7	0 of 20
3 BCNU (0.38 LD_{10})	1.7	0 of 10	1.08	1 of 8	1.9	0 of 20
O^6-methylguanine	0.3	0 of 10			1.5	0 of 10
BCNU (0.38 LD_{10}) + O^6-methylguanine	1.2	0 of 10	3.9	0 of 8	2.5	0 of 18
4 BCNU (0.75 LD_{10})	2.2	0 of 10	3.7	1 of 8	1.0	1 of 18
Streptozocin	–1.7	0 of 10	2.0	0 of 8	0	0 of 18
BCNU (0.75 LD_{10}) + streptozocin	3.2	0 of 10	4.5	2 of 9	4.7	0 of 19

[a] BCNU was administered as a single intraperitoneal injection in 3% ethanol. In combination studies, BCNU was administered 1 hour after treatment with O^6-benzylguanine or O^6-methylguanine and 1 hour after the fourth daily injection of streptozocin. The BCNU doses were 1.0 LD_{10}, 100 mg/m²; 0.75 LD_{10}, 75 mg/m²; and 0.38 LD_{10}, 38 mg/m². The doses of O^6-benzylguanine and O^6-methylguanine were 240 mg/m² administered as a single intraperitoneal injection in 10% and 15% Cremophor, respectively. The doses of streptozocin was 600 mg/m² administered daily intraperitoneally in 0.9% saline for a total of four doses.

[b] $P>0.05$ except where noted by **, where $P<0.01$.

[c] T–C, growth delay in days defined as the difference between the median time for tumors in treated (T) and control (C) animals to reach five times the volume at initation of treatment.

[d] Regression was defined as a decrease in tumor volume over two successive measurements.

[e] No. of complete tumor regressions shown in parentheses.

treated with O^6-benzylguanine plus BCNU, in contrast to near absolute drug resistance in tumor treated with BCNU alone. Furthermore, no additional toxicity was seen using reduced doses of BCNU.

In a series of human tumor cell lines made resistant to BCNU by dose escalation, three out of five of the BCNU resistant sublines showed an increase in methyltransferase activity compared with the parental cell lines (Dr Leona Samson, personal communication).

Nuclear factors: topoisomerase I and II and ATP

Chromosomal DNA is maintained in a supercoiled state via attachment to the nuclear matrix (Paulson and Laemmli, 1977; Vogelstein, Pardol and Coffey, 1980). During active processes such as DNA replication, transcription, recombination and repair the DNA topoisomerases I and II are required for unwinding of the supercoiled structure (Mattern and Painter, 1979; DiNardo, Voelkel and Sternglanz, 1984; Wang, 1985; Wu et al., 1988). Topoisomerase I binds covalently to DNA forming a single-strand break in the DNA through a phosphodiester bond. The topoisomerase I allows passage of a single DNA strand, the strand break is then resealed using the energy preserved in the DNA phosphodiester bond (Champoux, 1978, 1981). Topoisomerase II cleaves both strands of DNA and becomes covalently bound to a 5'-phosphoryl end of the DNA (Wang, 1985). Topoisomerase II allows passage of a double helix of DNA before resealing the strand breaks (Wang, 1987; Liu, 1989; Gedick and Collins, 1990), a process that requires ATP hydrolysis (Osheroff, 1986). Experimental evidence thus far supports a direct role for topoisomerase I in transcription (Gilmour et al., 1986; Gilmour and Elgin, 1987; Stewart and Schutz, 1987; Giaver and Wang, 1988; Stewart, Herrera and Nordheim, 1990) and a direct role for topoisomerase II in DNA organization and replication (Berrios, Osheroff and Fisher, 1985; Earnshaw et al., 1986; Gasser and Laemmli, 1986; Nelson, Liu and Coffey, 1986; Yang et al., 1987; Heck, Hittelman and Earnshaw, 1988; Fernandes, Danks and Beck, 1990; Adachi, Luke and Laemmli, 1991). In the course of their activity both topoisomerases cause unwinding of the double helix, rendering the DNA less compact and perhaps more susceptible to bifunctional antitumor alkylating agents or metallating agents such as the antitumor platinum complexes (Eder et al., 1987, 1989, 1990).

Camptothecin and several of its analogs have been shown to be inhibitors of topoisomerase I (Mattern et al., 1987; Eng et al., 1988; Giovanella et al., 1989; Johnson et al., 1989; Hertzberg et al., 1990; Giovanella et al., 1991; Mattern et al., 1991). Topotecan, a water soluble analog of camptothecin, has shown a broad spectrum of activity in preclinical systems and has recently completed phase I clinical trial (Mattern et al., 1987; Johnson et al., 1989; Mattern et al., 1991; Rowinsky et al., 1992). Novobiocin, an inhibitor of topoisomerase II, has myriad effects that occur at pharmacologically relevant concentrations and likely involve multiple mechanisms (Edenberg, 1980; Mattern, Paone and Day III, 1982; Downes et al., 1985; Catten et al., 1986; Gottesfeld, 1986; Utsumi et al., 1990; Lee, Flannery and Siemann, 1992). Several clinical trials of novobiocin with antitumor alkylating agents have been carried out (Eder et al., 1991; Ellis et al., 1991).

Depletion of ATP can protect L1210 cells from the cytotoxic actions of topoisomerase II inhibitors such as VM-26 and m-AMSA but not from the cytotoxic actions of the topoisomerase I inhibitor camptothecin (Kupfer, Bodley and Liu, 1987). Lonidamine, a drug that affects the energy metabolism of cells, could be an important component of a combined modality regimen if repair of damage by cytotoxic treatment is an energy dependent process (Floridi, Paggi and D'Atri, 1981; Floridi, Paggi and Marcante, 1981; Floridi and Lehninger, 1983; DeMartino, Battelli and Paggi, 1984; Floridi, Bagnato and Bianchi, 1986; DeMartino, Malorni and Accinni, 1987; Szekely, Lobreau and Delaney, 1989). Lonidamine inhibited the repair of potentially lethal damage caused by X-rays, methyl methane sulfonate, bleomycin, and hyperthermia in Chinese hamster HA-1 cells. In murine tumor models lonidamine potentiated the effects of radiation and the effects of hyperthermia (Hahn, vanKersen and Silvestrini, 1984; Kim, Alfieri and Kim, 1984; Kim, Kim and Alfieri, 1984; Kim, Alfieri and Kim, 1986). Lonidamine has also been shown to enhance the cytotoxicity of several antitumor alkylating agents in vitro and in vivo as well as adriamycin in culture (Zupi, Greco and Laudino, 1986; Rosbe, Brann and Holden, 1989; Teicher et al., 1991a,b,c).

To discern the effects of these modulators on the tumor cell killing by antitumor alkylating agents in vivo, animals bearing the FSaIIC fibrosarcoma were treated with the modulators singly or in combination administered as five i.p. injections over 36 h (Schwartz et al., 1993). The antitumor alkylating agents were administered in single i.p. injections alone or along with the third dose of the modulators. Twenty-four hours after treatment with the antitumor alkylating agents the tumors were excised and tumor cell survival was determined CDDP produced

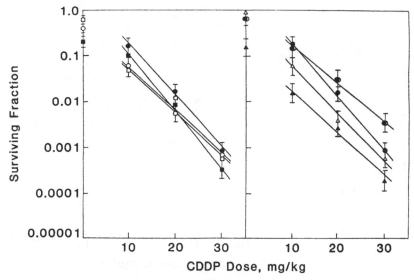

Figure 2.1. Survival of F SaIIC cells from F SaIIC tumors treated with various doses of CDDP alone (●) or along with the third dose of a five-dose regimen of novobiocin (50 mg/kg) (○), topotecan (50 mg/kg) (■), lonidamine (50 mg/kg) (□), novobiocin/topotecan (▲), novobiocin/lonidamine (△) or topotecan/lonidamine (◑). Points, mean of three independent experiments; bars, S.E.M.

log-linear killing of F SaIIC tumor cells with increasing dose of the drug (Figure 2.1). Singly, the modulators produced relatively modest increases in the killing of F SaIIC cells by CDDP. The combination of novobiocin/topotecan produced a surviving fraction of 0.15 ± 0.08, which was less than additive killing by the individual modulators as determined by product of the surviving fractions. Novobiocin modulation resulted in about a 10-fold increase in F SaIIC tumor cell killing with 10 mg/kg of CDDP, which decreased to about a 3-fold increase in the killing of F SaIIC tumor cells with the lower doses of CDDP but no significant increase in tumor cell killing with 30 mg/kg of CDDP. Topotecan/lonidamine did not alter the killing of F SaIIC tumor cells with lower doses of CDDP and was protective against tumor cell killing by high dose CDDP.

Melphalan also produced a log-linear increase in F SaIIC tumor cell killing with increasing dose of the drug (Figure 2.2) (Schwartz et al., 1993). Although novobiocin and lonidamine as single modulators did not significantly alter tumor cell killing by melphalan, topotecan was an effective modulator of melphalan, especially at higher doses of the

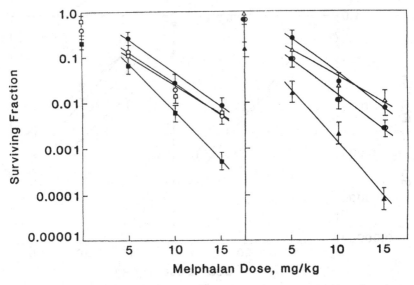

Figure 2.2. Survival of FSaIIC cells from FSaIIC tumors treated with various doses of melphalan alone (●) or along with the third dose of a five-dose regimen of novobiocin (50 mg/kg) (○), topotecan (50 mg/kg) (■), lonidamine (50 mg/kg) (□), novobiocin/topotecan (▲), novobiocin/lonidamine (△) or topotecan/lonidamine (◐). Points, mean of three independent experiments; bars, S.E.M.

drug. Novobiocin/topotecan modulation increased tumor cell killing by more than 1 log with the lower doses of melphalan and by 2 logs with the high dose of melphalan. Novobiocin/lonidamine did not alter FSaIIC tumor cell killing from that obtained with melphalan alone. Topotecan/lonidamine increased FSaIIC tumor cell killing by melphalan by about 3-fold over the dosage range of melphalan studied.

Cyclophosphamide over the dosage range from 100 mg/kg to 500 mg/kg produced log-linear increasing killing of FSaIIC tumor cells with increasing dose of the drug (Figure 2.3). The single modulators only modestly affected the tumor cell killing by cyclophosphamide. Novobiocin/topotecan administration increased FSaIIC tumor cell killing by about 1 log at the lower doses of cyclophosphamide, which increased to about 1.5 logs at the higher doses of cyclophosphamide. Novobiocin/lonidamine did not significantly alter the tumor cell killing from that produced by cyclophosphamide alone. Modulation by topotecan/lonidamine increased the tumor cell killing by cyclophosphamide by about 5-fold (Schwartz et al., 1993).

Like the other antitumor alkylating agents, BCNU kills FSaIIC tumor cells in a log-linear manner (Figure 2.4). The single modulators

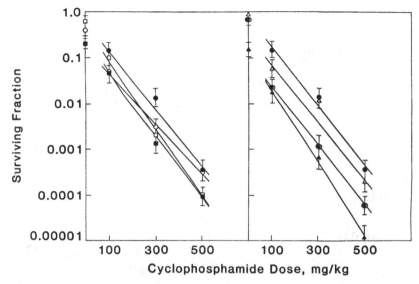

Figure 2.3. Survival of F SaIIC cells from F SaIIC tumors treated with various doses of cyclophosphamide alone (●) or along with the third dose of a five-dose regimen of novobiocin (50 mg/kg) (○), topotecan (50 mg/kg) (■), lonidamine (50 mg/kg) (□), novobiocin/topotecan (▲), novobiocin/lonidamine (△) or topotecan/lonidamine (◐). Points, mean of three independent experiments; bars, S.E.M.

did not significantly alter the tumor cell killing from that obtained with BCNU alone. Modulation by novobiocin/topotecan resulted in about 1 log increased tumor cell killing by BCNU at the lower dose of BCNU, which increased to about 2 logs increased tumor cell killing at the higher dose of the drug. Novobiocin/lonidamine modulation resulted in an enhancement in tumor cell killing by BCNU that increased from 3-fold to 10-fold over the dosage range of BCNU studied. Modulation by topotecan/lonidamine resulted in an enhancement in the killing of F SaIIC tumor cells that increased from 5-fold to 12-fold over the dosage range of BCNU studied (Schwartz *et al.*, 1993).

Tumor growth delay studies were conducted in the F SaIIC fibrosarcoma with the single modulators and modulator combinations along with antitumor alkylating agents administered in full, standard dosage regimens (Tables 2.3 and 2.4). The single modulators were variably effective in increasing the tumor growth delay produced by the various antitumor alkylating agents. Lonidamine was the most effective modulator of CDDP, increasing the tumor growth delay produced by CDDP about 1.2-fold. Treatment with the combination of topotecan/cyclophos-

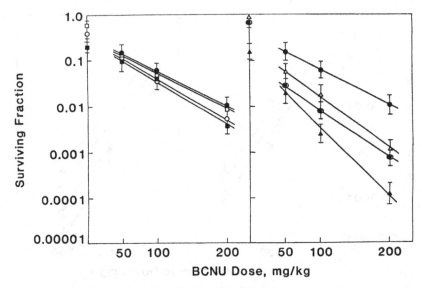

Figure 2.4. Survival of FSaIIC cells from FSaIIC tumors treated with various doses of BCNU alone (●) or along with the third dose of a five-dose regimen of novobiocin (50 mg/kg) (○), topotecan (50 mg/kg) (■), lonidamine (50 mg/kg) (□), novobiocin/topotecan (▲), novobiocin/lonidamine (△) or topotecan/lonidamine (◐). Points, mean of three independent experiments; bars, S.E.M.

phamide or topotecan/ifosfamide resulted in a tumor growth delay which was 2.3-fold and 1.6-fold greater than that produced by cyclophosphamide or ifosfamide alone, respectively. The most effective modulator of melphalan and thiotepa was novobiocin, which increased the tumor growth delay produced by 2.3-fold and 1.4-fold for melphalan and thiotepa, respectively. None of the single modulators significantly increased the tumor growth delay produced by BCNU (Schwartz et al., 1993).

Overall, the tumor growth delays resulting from treatment of animals bearing the FSaIIC fibrosarcoma with the antitumor alkylating agents and combined modulators were improved over those obtained with the antitumor alkylating agents and single modulators (Table 2.4). The most effective modulator combination was novobiocin/topotecan. Novobiocin/topotecan modulated CDDP such that the tumor growth delay produced by the combined treatment was 1.4-fold increased over that produced by treatment with CDDP. The tumor growth delay produced by cyclophosphamide with novobiocin/topotecan was 5.2-fold greater than that from treatment with cyclophosphamide alone. Melphalan was modulated by novobiocin/topotecan such that the tumor growth delay

Table 2.3. *Growth delay of the FSaIIC fibrosarcoma produced by various antitumor alkylating agents in combination with novobiocin, topotecan or lonidamine as modulators.*[a]

Alkylating agent treatment	Tumor growth delay (days)			
	Alone	+Novo	+Topo	+Lond
CDDP (10 mg/kg)	7.7±0.7	9.2±1.3	8.6±1.1	9.5±1.2
Cyclophosphamide (3 × 150 mg/kg)	9.3±1.2	14.4±1.8	21.3±2.3	17.4±2.4
Melphalan (10 mg/kg)	2.9±0.5	6.8±0.9	5.2±0.7	4.1±0.6
BCNU (3 × 15 mg/kg)	4.9±0.7	5.4±0.8	5.3±0.6	5.1±1.9
Thiotepa (5 × 5 mg/kg)	5.7±1.1	8.1±0.8	7.7±0.9	6.8±0.9
Ifosfamide (3 × 150 mg/kg)	6.2±1.0	9.0±0.7	10.1±1.3	8.3±1.1

[a] Tumor growth delay is the difference in the number of days for treatment tumors to reach 500 mm^3 compared to untreated control tumors. The data are presented as the means of 15 animals ± S.E.M.
The tumor growth delays produced by the modulators alone were:
(1) novobiocin, 1.2±0.5 days; (2) topotecan, 2.9±0.5 days and
(3) lonidamine, 2.0±0.4 days.

Table 2.4. *Growth delay of the FSaIIC fibrosarcoma produced by various antitumor alkylating agents and two modulator combinations*[a]

Alkylating agent treatment	Tumor growth delay (days)			
	Alone	+Novo/ Topo	+Novo/ Lond	+Topo/ Lond
CDDP (10 mg/kg)	7.7±0.7	11.0±1.2	10.6±1.1	7.9±0.8
Cyclophosphamide (3×150 mg/kg)	9.3±1.2	48.5±2.7^{b*}	19.3±2.4**	39.2±2.7*
Melphalan (10 mg/kg)	2.9±0.5	10.2±1.4**	8.4±0.9**	9.5±1.1**
BCNU (3×15 mg/kg)	4.9±0.7	8.4±0.7	5.9±0.6	6.0±0.6
Thiotepa (5×5 mg/kg)	5.7±1.1	16.5±1.8**	8.7±1.1	9.9±1.3
Ifosfamide (3×150 mg/kg)	6.2±1.0	11.7±1.5	10.9±1.2	11.2±1.3

[a] Tumor growth delay is the difference in the number of days for treated tumors to reach 500 mm^3 compared to untreated control tumors. The data are presented as the means of 15 animals ± S.E.M. The tumor growth delays produced by the modulators alone were: (1) novobiocin/topotecan, 4.0±0.6 days; (2) novobiocin/lonidamine, 2.9±0.5 days and (3) topotecan/lonidamine, 2.4±0.5 days.
[b] Significantly different from the corresponding drug along group:
* $P<0.001$; ** $P<0.01$.

produced by the combination was 3.5-fold greater than that produced by melphalan alone. The tumor growth delay produced by treatment with BCNU was increased 1.7-fold by the addition of novobiocin/topotecan to treatment with the drug. Thiotepa was modulated by novobiocin/topotecan such that the tumor growth delay produced by the combination was 2.9-fold greater than that produced by thiotepa alone. The tumor growth produced by treatment with ifosfamide was increased 1.9-fold by the addition of novobiocin/topotecan to treatment with the drug (Schwartz et al., 1993).

Antagonism between topoisomerase I and topoisomerase II inhibitors in cell culture has been described several times (Markovits et al., 1987; Zwelling et al., 1987; Utsumi et al., 1990; Lee et al., 1992). Although combinations of topoisomerase II inhibitors or topoisomerase I and topoisomerase II inhibitors may be cytotoxically antagonistic in vitro and in vivo, this effect does not inhibit the ability of these agents to be effective modulators of antitumor alkylating agent tumor cell killing.

Etoposide, a podophyllotoxin derivative, has been shown to cause both single-strand and double-strand DNA breaks and DNA protein cross-links in mammalian cells in a process that requires a nuclear protein. Etoposide does not bind directly to DNA, and evidence indicates that the protein-associated DNA breaks resulting from etoposide treatment are mediated through an interaction between the drug and topoisomerase II and perhaps oxygen (Long and Minocha, 1983; Issell, Muggia and Carter, 1984; Long, Musial and Brattain, 1984; Ross, 1985; Pommier et al., 1986; van Maanen et al., 1988). Flow cytometry in etoposide-treated cells shows a delay in S phase transit before arrest of cells in G2. Correlating with the S phase delay is a selective inhibition of thymidine incorporation into DNA as well as a concentration-dependent scission of DNA strands. Etoposide shows a selective cytotoxicity to normally oxygenated cells in vitro and, when combined with an oxygen-carrying perfluorochemical emulsion, the antitumor activity and therapeutic efficacy of etoposide are enhanced (Teicher, Holden and Rose, 1985b).

In an effort to improve the efficacy of the anti-tumor alkylating agents, we have examined the possibility of using etoposide as a modulator for several alkylating agents alone or in combination with a second modulator, lonidamine or pentoxifylline (Tanaka et al., 1991). Lonidamine, as described above, is a putative mitochondrial toxin that may interfere with cellular respiration and energy supplies (Floridi et al., 1981a,b; Floridi and Lehninger, 1983; DeMartino et al., 1984; Floridi et al., 1986; DeMartino et al., 1987). Pentoxifylline has significant hemorrheologic

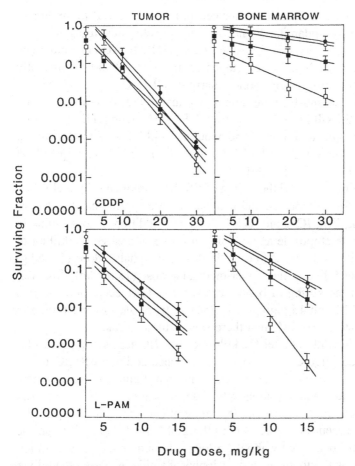

Figure 2.5. Survival of FSaIIC tumor cells and bone-marrow CFU-GM from animals treated in vivo with single doses of CDDP or L-PAM alone (•), preceded by a single dose of lonidamine (100 mg/kg) (○), preceded by a single dose of etoposide (20 mg/kg) (■), or with the combination of the two modulators (□). Points, means of three independent experiments; bars, S.E.M.

effects, increasing red blood cell deformability, inhibiting platelet aggregation and inhibiting fibrolytic activity, and thus may improve tumor blood flow (Ehrly, 1979; Aviado and Porter, 1984; Poggesi et al., 1985; Perego et al., 1986; Ward and Clissold, 1987).

Utilizing the FSaIIC murine fibrosarcoma tumor excision model following in vivo treatment, lonidamine did not significantly alter the killing of FSaIIC cells by CDDP (Figure 2.5). Etoposide produced additive FSaIIC tumor cell killing with CDDP at the lower CDDP dosage range but did not affect the tumor cell killing by CDDP at the higher dosage range. Lonidamine did not significantly alter the killing achieved with the combination of etoposide and CDDP. However, lonidamine added to the combination of etoposide and CDDP did significantly increase the killing of bone marrow CFU-GM (granulocyte–macrophage colony-forming units), so that there was about 5-fold increase in the killing of bone marrow CFU-GM with CDDP at 5 mg/kg and etoposide at 20 mg/kg and about a 10-fold increase in the killing of bone marrow CFU-GM with CDDP at 30 mg/kg and etoposide at 20 mg/kg (Tanaka et al., 1991).

Lonidamine increased the killing of FSaIIC tumor cells by melphalan by about 2-fold. Etoposide and melphalan were approximately additive in producing FSaIIC tumor cell killing. The addition of lonidamine to treatment with etoposide and melphalan further increased the killing of FSaIIC cells by about 2-fold at the lower melphalan dose (5 mg/kg) and by about 6-fold at the higher melphalan dose (15 mg/kg); however, it measured the killing of bone marrow CFU-GM even more, so that at doses of 10 and 15 mg/kg of melphalan there was greater killing of bone marrow CFU-GM than there was of tumor cells.

Lonidamine did not alter the killing of FSaIIC tumor cells by cyclophosphamide (Figure 2.6). Etoposide produced additive FSaIIC tumor cell killing with cyclophosphamide. Addition of lonidamine to treatment with etoposide and cyclophosphamide appeared to have a dose-modifying effect. At a dose of 300 mg/kg of cyclophosphamide, lonidamine co-treatment increased tumor killing of FSaIIC cells by etoposide and cyclophosphamide by about 1.5 logs. Although lonidamine addition to treatment with etoposide and cyclophosphamide increased the killing of bone marrow CFU-GM, the level of increase was only 3- to 4-fold.

Lonidamine increased FSaIIC tumor cell killing by BCNU by about 2-fold, but this difference was not significant. Etoposide produced a dose-modifying effect on BCNU that resulted in an increase in FSaIIC tumor cell killing ranging from about 3-fold at 25 mg/kg of BCNU to about 50-fold at 100 mg/kg of BCNU. The addition of lonidamine to treatment with etoposide and BCNU resulted in an additional dose-modifying effect. There was about a 3-fold increase in tumor cell killing at 25 mg/kg of BCNU, which increased to about 10-fold at 100 mg/kg of BCNU. The combination treatment had much less effect on the cytotoxicity of BCNU to bone marrow CFU-GM, which resulted in about a 5-fold increase in the killing of bone marrow CFU-GM.

Pentoxifylline increased the FSaIIC tumor cell killing by CDDP by

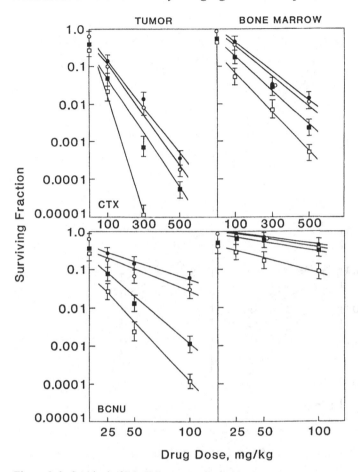

Figure 2.6. Survival of FSaIIC tumor cells and bone-marrow CFU-GM from animals treated in vivo with single doses of cyclophosphamide (CTX) or BCNU alone (●), preceded by a single dose of lonidamine (100 mg/kg) (○), preceded by a single dose of etoposide (20 mg/kg)(■), or with the combination of the two modulators (□). Points, means of three independent experiments; bars, S.E.M.

about 2-fold, but this increase was not significant (Figure 2.7). Pentoxifylline also did not alter the tumor cell killing of etoposide plus CDDP, which was additive at the low end of the CDDP dose range and less than additive in the higher range. In the bone marrow CFU-GM, there was a 3- to 50-fold increase in cytotoxicity with the addition of pentoxifylline to treatment with CDDP across the CDDP dosage range examined; however, etoposide did not further increase the cytotoxicity to bone marrow CFU-GM of the combination of pentoxifylline plus CDDP.

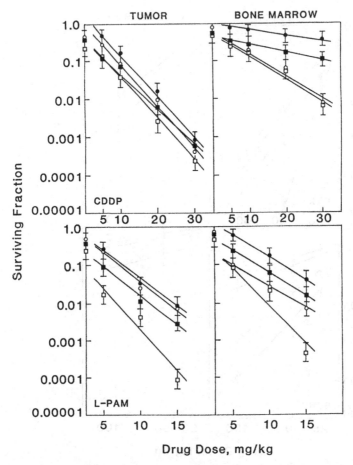

Figure 2.7. Survival of FSaIIC tumor cells and bone-marrow CFU-GM from animals treated in vivo with single doses of CDDP or L-PAM alone (●), preceded by a single dose of pentoxifylline (100 mg/kg) (○), preceded by a single dose of etoposide (20 mg/kg) (■), or with the combination of the two modulators (□). Points, means of three independent experiments; bars, S.E.M.

Etoposide alone increased the bone marrow toxicity of CDDP by 2- to 3-fold across the dose range examined, which was probably additive (Tanaka et al., 1991).

Pentoxifylline did not alter the killing of FSaIIC tumor cells by melphalan (L-PAM) but did significantly increase tumor cell killing by the combination of etoposide and melphalan in a dose-modifying manner. The increase in tumor cell killing by the combination etoposide/pentoxifylline/melphalan ranged from about 20- to 100-fold over the melphalan dosage range examined, as compared with melphalan alone, and by about 9- to 40-fold as compared with the combination of etoposide and melphalan, where the combination was 2- to 3-fold more cytotoxic than melphalan alone. There was about a 6-fold increase in the killing of bone marrow CFU-GM by the addition of pentoxifylline to treatment with melphalan. As with the tumor cells, pentoxifylline had a dose-modifying effect on treatment with the combination of etoposide and melphalan and at the highest dose tested; bone marrow CFU-GM killing was increased by about 2 logs. Etoposide alone increased killing of bone marrow by melphalan by 2- to 3-fold.

Pentoxifylline increased the killing of FSaIIC tumor cells by cyclophosphamide by 1.5- to 2-fold, but this difference was not significant (Figure 2.8). Pentoxifylline also did not increase tumor cell killing by the combination of etoposide and cyclophosphamide (100 mg/kg); however, there was about a 5-fold increase in tumor cell killing by the combination of etoposide and cyclophosphamide (500 mg/kg). Etoposide alone increased the tumor cell cytotoxicity of cyclophosphamide in about 0.5 to 1 log. Although pentoxifylline did not significantly increase the cytotoxicity of cyclophosphamide toward bone marrow CFU-GM, the addition of pentoxifylline to the combination of etoposide and cyclophosphamide increased the killing of bone marrow CFU-GM by 10- to 50-fold over the dosage range of cyclophosphamide examined compared with cyclophosphamide alone. Etoposide alone increased bone marrow killing by cyclophosphamide by 0.4 to 0.7 log.

Pentoxifylline had a dose-modifying effect on the killing of FSaIIC tumor cells by BCNU. Tumor cell killing was increased from 2- to 10-fold with the addition of pentoxifylline to the BCNU treatment. A similar dose-modifying effect was observed when pentoxifylline was added to treatment with the combination of etoposide and BCNU, so that overall there was a 15- to 1000-fold increase in tumor cell killing with pentoxifylline/etoposide/BCNU as compared with BCNU alone and about a 4- to 12-fold increase as compared with etoposide plus BCNU. Interestingly, there was little increase in the killing of bone marrow CFU-GM by the addition of pentoxifylline to treatment with BCNU and etoposide. Overall, there was about a 2- to 3-fold increase in the killing of bone marrow CFU-GM with the combination of pentoxifylline/etoposide/BCNU as compared with BCNU alone. Thus, of all the combinations tested, the greatest differential between tumor and marrow killing was seen with pentoxifylline/etoposide added to BCNU, especially at the highest BCNU dose tested.

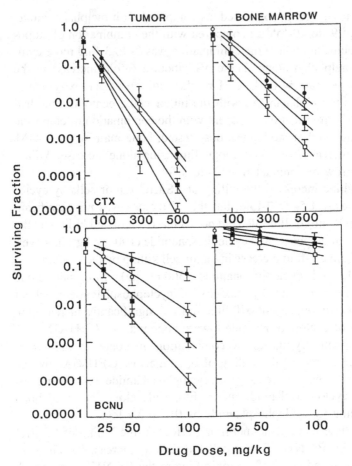

Figure 2.8. Survival of F S aIIC tumor cells and bone marrow C F U -G M from animals treated in vivo with single doses of cyclophosphamide (CTX) or BCNU alone (●), preceded by a single dose of pentoxifylline (100 mg/kg) (o), preceded by a single dose of etoposide (20 mg/kg) (■), or with the combination of the two modulators (□). Points, means of three independent experiments; bars, S.E.M.

The diffusion of Hoechst 33342 followed by fluorescent-activated cell sorting was used to assess the effect of these therapies on tumor subpopulations. The bright cells represent a subpopulation near to tumor vasculature and so presumably enriched in normally oxygenated cells, while the dim cells represent a subpopulation distant from the vasculature and so enriched the hypoxic cells. Cyclophosphamide was about 7-fold more cytotoxic toward bright cells than toward dim cells (Figure 2.9). Etoposide addition to treatment with cyclophosphamide did not alter the

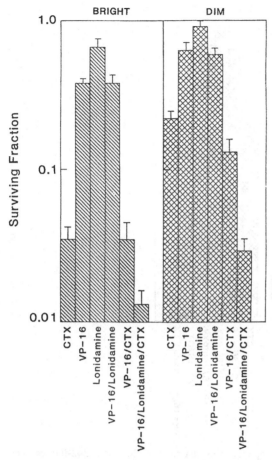

Figure 2.9. Survival of subpopulations based on Hoechst-33342-fluorescence intensity of FSaIIC cells from FSaIIC tumors treated with a single dose of cyclophosphamide (150 mg/kg) with or without lonidamine (100 mg/kg) and/or etoposide (VP-16) (20 mg/kg). Columns are means of three independent determinations, bars are S.E.M.

killing of the bright cells, but increased the killing of the dim cells by about 1.7-fold compared with the drug alone. The combination of lonidamine with etoposide and cyclophosphamide was more effective, producing increases in tumor cell killing of 2.7-fold in the bright cells and 7.6-fold in the dim cells compared with cyclophosphamide alone (Tanaka et al., 1991).

Pentoxifylline added to treatment with etoposide and cyclophosphamide resulted in a 1.7-fold increase in bright-tumor cell killing compared with cyclophosphamide alone or etoposide/cyclophosphamide

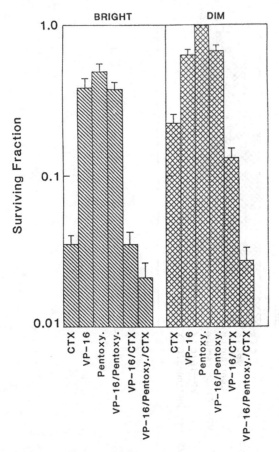

Figure 2.10. Survival of subpopulations based on Hoechst-33342-fluorescence intensity of FSaIIC cells from FSaIIC tumors treated with a single dose of cyclophosphamide (150 mg/kg) with or without pentoxifylline (100 mg/kg) and/or etoposide (VP-16) (20 mg/kg). Columns are means of three independent determinations, bars are S.E.M.

(Figure 2.10). However, in the dim cells, addition of pentoxifylline to treatment with etoposide and cyclophosphamide resulted in an 8.1-fold increase in tumor cell killing compared with cyclophosphamide alone and in a 4.8-fold increase in tumor cell killing compared with etoposide/ cyclophosphamide (Tanaka et al., 1991).

The combination of etoposide and CDDP is active in a variety of human tumors including small cell lung cancer, non-small cell lung cancer, lymphomas and testicular cancer (Sierocki et al., 1979; Natale and Wittes, 1982; Long and Minocha, 1983; Einhorn, 1986; Klastersky,

1986; Von Heyden, Scherpe and Nagel, 1987, Turrisi III, Glover and Mason, 1988). Positive results have also been reported for a regimen including concurrent, twice-daily radiotherapy plus etoposide and CDDP for limited small cell lung cancer (Turrisi III et al., 1988). Although etoposide inhibition of topoisomerase II could cause cellular DNA to become more susceptible to attack by CDDP or radiation, a more-than-additive interaction between CDDP and etoposide (Long and Minocha, 1983; Long et al., 1984; Ross, 1985) has been difficult to prove in the laboratory (Teicher et al., 1988; Tsai et al., 1989). In spheroids of V79 Chinese hamster cells, however, a degree of supra-additivity was observed between CDDP and etoposide (Durand and Goldie, 1987). Paradoxically, the scheduling of CDDP and etoposide radiation in several studies has temporally separated the CDDP and etoposide, markedly decreasing the possibilities of positive interaction (Sierocki et al., 1979; Natale and Wittes, 1982; Turrisi III et al., 1988). In addition, since etoposide was given on multiple days with concurrent chest irradiation in one study (Turrisi III et al., 1988), scheduling the combined modalities in a manner suitable to achieve synergy is clinically feasible.

The FSaIIC fibrosarcoma is responsive to treatment with CDDP and radiation. Three Gy daily × 5 produced a growth delay of about 6.3 days in this tumor (Herman and Teicher, 1988). For the combination treatments reported in this study, a dose of 5 mg/kg CDDP, which yielded about 4.4 days of tumor growth delay, was used (Table 2.5). Treatment with hyperthermia alone (43°C, 30 minutes) produced a minimal effect on the tumor, giving about 1.4 days of tumor growth delay. When treatment at 43°C was immediately preceded by CDDP or followed by radiation on day 1, tumor growth delays of about 5.9 days and about 8.4 days, respectively, resulted, which appeared to reflect additivity of the individual treatments. The sequence drug → hyperthermia → radiation (if radiation was given) was used in the present studies because our previous investigations in the FSaIIC tumor system showed this sequence to be most effective for CDDP in this trimodality regimen.

CDDP → hyperthermia → radiation produced a tumor growth delay of about 25.2 days (Hermann and Teicher, 1988). A single dose of etoposide (van Maanen et al., 1988) caused a tumor growth delay of about 3.4 days, which increased to about 5.3 days when drug administration was followed by hyperthermia treatment. Etoposide given just prior to radiation on day 1 of the five daily treatments with 300 cGy also improved a growth delay to approximately 10.6 days.

Table 2.5. *Growth delay of the FSaIIC fibrosarcoma produced by combinations of etoposide and cisplatin with hyperthermia and X-rays*

	Tumor growth delay (days)[a]			
Treatment group	No drug	Cisplatin (5 mg/kg)[b]	Etoposide (20 mg/kg)[b]	Etoposide (20 mg/kg) + cisplatin (5 mg/kg)
Drug	—	4.4±0.9	3.4±0.6	5.2±0.7
Drug → Heat[c]	1.4±0.7	5.9±1.1	5.3±0.7	7.8±1.2
Drug → X-rays[d]	6.3±1.5	11.7±1.8	10.6±1.7	12.2±2.0
Drug → Heat → X-rays	8.4±2.2	25.2±2.8	14.1±2.3	34.4±3.5

[a] Tumor growth delay is the difference in the number of days for treated tumors to reach 500 mm³ compared to untreated control tumors. The data are presented as the means of 14 animals ± S.E.M.
[b] Cisplatin (CDDP) and etoposide were injected in normal saline as a single dose i.p. on day 1 of the treatment.
[c] Heat was delivered as a single dose on day 1 of the treatment locally to the tumor-bearing limb by immersion in a water bath at 44°C, which allowed the tumors to reach 43°C.
[d] X-rays were delivered locally to the tumor-bearing limb at a dose of 3 Gy daily for 5 days. No anesthetic was used.

Etoposide was not as effective as CDDP in this trimodality regimen. When etoposide was followed by hyperthermia and then by radiation treatment on day 1 of the 5 day radiation schedule, a tumor growth delay of only about 14 days resulted.

Treatment with single doses of etoposide and CDDP in immediate succession i.p. resulted in a tumor growth delay of about 5.2 days. When this drug combination was followed by hyperthermia (43°C, 30 minutes), the tumor growth delay increased to about 7.8 days, which was 1.5-fold increase in tumor growth delay compared to the drugs alone. The addition of etoposide to CDDP and X-rays did not significantly alter the tumor growth delay produced with CDDP and X-rays alone. Treatment with either regimen resulted in tumor growth delays of about 12 days. On the other hand, a significant additional effect from etoposide was evident in tumor growth delay produced by the trimodality regimen. Treatment with etoposide/CDDP/hyperthermia/X-rays produced a tumor growth delay of about 34 days, which was an increase of about 9 days over the tumor growth delay resulting from treatment with CDDP/ hyperthermia and radiation (Pfeffer et al., 1991).

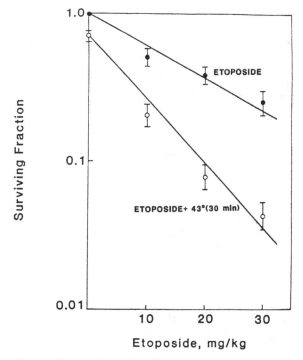

Figure 2.11. Survival of F S aIIC cells from F S aIIC tumors treated with various doses of etoposide with (○) hyperthermia (43°C, 30 minutes) delivered immediately after drug administration or without (●) hyperthermia. Points, means of three independent determinations ± S.E.M. (bars).

F S aIIC tumor cell kill by etoposide increased linearly with increasing dose of the drug over the dosage range from 10 mg/kg to 30 mg/kg as measured by tumor cell survival (Figure 2.11). Delivery of hyperthermia had a dose modifying effect (~2.0) on the tumor cell killing produced by etoposide as determined from the slopes of the tumor cell survival curves. In the therapeutic dosage range for single-dose etoposide, from 15 to 20 mg/kg, there was about a 5-fold increase in the tumor cell killing produced by the addition of hyperthermia to the drug treatment.

F S aIIC tumor cell kill by CDDP increased linearly with increasing dose of the drug as measured by tumor cell survival (Figure 2.12). As shown in Figure 2.11, hyperthermia (43°C, 30 minutes) killed only about 30% of the tumor population. However, treatment with CDDP followed by hyperthermia led to approximately a 2-log increase in cell kill compared to drug alone across the dosage range of CDDP (Herman et al., 1990; Pfeffer et al., 1991). The addition of etoposide to treatment with

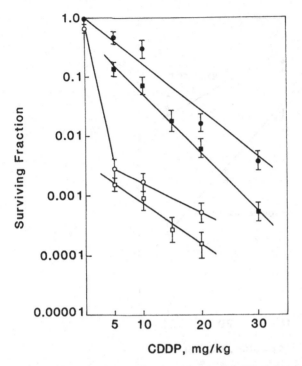

Figure 2.12. Survival of F S aIIC cells from F S aIIC tumors treated with various doses of CDDP with (o) hyperthermia (43°C, 30 minutes) delivered immediately after drug administration or without (•) hyperthermia, or various doses of cisplatin and etoposide (20 mg/kg) with (□) hyperthermia or without (■) hyperthermia. Points, means of three independent determinations ± S.E.M. (bars).

CDDP at 37°C increased tumor cell killing 3.7- to 6.5-fold over the dosage range of CDDP examined. Adding treatment with etoposide to CDDP and hyperthermia also increased tumor cell killing by about 2- to 3.4-fold over the CDDP dosage range examined.

Tumor mass targets for modulation

Hypoxic cells in solid tumors are presumed to be an obstacle to success-ful cancer treatment because these cells are relatively protected from the cytotoxic effects of radiotherapy and certain anticancer drugs (Ken-nedy et al., 1980, 1981; Teicher *et al.*, 1986c; Teicher and Rose, 1986). The importance of hypoxic cells in limiting the curability of human tumors remains a controversial issue, although some clinical (Duncan, 1973; Busse et al., 1977) and laboratory data (Fowler, Thomlinson and

Howes, 1970; Duncan, 1973; Teicher, Lazo and Sartorelli, 1981; Sartorelli, 1988) strongly suggest that hypoxic cells are a cause of in vivo treatment failure. With the greater availability of stable O_2-microelectrode systems suitable for use in the clinic, data supporting the notion that therapeutically significant hypoxia frequently exists in human tumors is well-established (Gatenby et al., 1988; Fleckenstein, 1990; Kallinowski et al., 1990; Vaupel, 1990; Vaupel et al., 1991; Vaupel, 1993).

Increasing tumor oxygenation

Solid tumors are aberrant tissues composed of stroma and malignant cells. Amongst the properties that distinguish normal tissues from solid tumors are physiological characteristics related to the disregulated proliferation of the neoplastic and normal cells that comprise the tumor mass. Although signals for vascular growth are present in solid tumors, the growth of blood vessels in tumors is irregular, and the vasculature is often poorly formed and inadequate, lacking vasoresponsive elements. Thus, solid tumors often exhibit highly heterogeneous oxygen tension distributions, pH, glucose delivery and utilization, etc. (Kennedy et al., 1980; Teicher et al., 1981; Sartorelli, 1988; Vaupel, Kallinowski and Okunieff, 1989; Dewhurst, 1993; Vaupel, 1993).

It has been well established that oxygen is rapidly metabolized by cells and, therefore, in tissues has a limited diffusion distance from vasculature (Gullino, 1975; Vaupel, Frinak and Bicher, 1981; Hasegawa et al., 1987; Song et al., 1987; Vaupel et al., 1987; Gatenby et al., 1988; Jain, 1988; Sevick and Jain, 1989). Regions of hypoxia have been demonstrated in many solid tumor model systems (Gullino, 1975; Vaupel et al., 1981; Hasegawa et al., 1987; Song et al., 1987; Vaupel et al., 1987; Jain, 1988; Sevick and Jain, 1989) and in human solid tumors (Vaupel et al., 1989) by several different methods. In cell culture and in some cases in vivo, significant differences in the effectiveness of many antineoplastic agents and treatment modalities have been demonstrated to be dependent on cellular oxygenation (Teicher et al., 1981; Keyes, Rockwell and Sartorelli, 1985; Teicher et al., 1985b, 1987a; Teicher, Holden and Jacobs, 1987b; Teicher, McIntosh-Lowe and Rose, 1988; Teicher et al., 1989). Solid tumors may also have regions of more acidic or more basic pH than are found in normal tissues (Gullino, 1975; Vaupel et al., 1981; Kallinowski and Vaupel, 1988). The actions of some chemotherapeutic agents and hyperthermia have been shown to

be affected by changes in both intra- and extracellular pH (Hahn and
Shiu, 1986; Herman, Teicher and Collins, 1988a; Herman et al., 1988b;
Herman et al., 1989).

Position in the cell cycle is also critical to the cytotoxic action of
some chemotherapeutic agents and is an important variable in the actions
of many others (Born, Hug and Trott, 1976; Momparler, 1980). Although
a difficult question to approach experimentally (Siemann and Keng,
1988), it is likely that the great proportion of cells that are distal from
the vasculature and in a hypoxic and acidotic environment are noncycling. Cells that are noncycling would be expected to be less sensitive
to many agents but may be more sensitive to nitrosoureas and bleomycin
(Barranco, Novak and Humphrey, 1973; Barranco and Novak, 1974;
Twentyman, 1976; Bhuyan, Fraser and Day, 1977).

The ability of drugs to penetrate through cell layers to reach cells
farther from the vasculature in concentrations adequate to be therapeutically effective is a variable dependent to a large degree on the lipophilicity
and metabolic stability of the drug molecule. Furthermore, the intracellular concentrations of the cytotoxic agents that can be achieved may
differ for oxygenated and hypoxic cells. Although molecular oxygen
diffuses only a short distance through tumor tissue because of its rapid
metabolic utilization, some dyes and some drugs can diffuse into the
tumor mass over much greater distances (Vaupel, 1977; Vaupel et al.,
1987; Jain, 1988; Teicher et al., 1990; Vaupel, 1993).

Hypoxia protects tumor cells from damage by cytotoxic therapies that
are directly and/or indirectly oxygen dependent. Hypoxia can lead to
therapeutic resistance through: (1) direct effects due to lack of O_2, which
some drugs and radiation require to be maximally cytotoxic, (2) indirect
effects via altered cellular metabolism, which decreases drug cytotoxicity
and (3) enhanced genetic instability, which can lead to more rapid development of drug resistant tumor cells.

Hemoglobin preparations

Bovine blood is a ready source of hemoglobin (Bunn, 1971; Cochen et
al., 1974; Breepel, Kreuzer and Hazevoet, 1981; Cunnington et al.,
1981). The molecular structure of bovine hemoglobin is similar to that
of human hemoglobin (Breepel et al., 1981) although it has a higher P_{50}
(26 ± 3 mmHg vs. 16 ± 3 mmHg; 3.5 ± 0.4 kPa vs. 2.1 ± 0.4 kPa)
than human hemoglobin (Breepel et al., 1981). The oxygen affinity of
bovine hemoglobin is regulated by chloride ions, whereas the oxygen

affinity of human hemoglobin is influenced by the presence of 2,3-diphosphoglycerate (Bunn, 1971; Laver et al., 1977). In addition, in contrast to human hemoglobin, bovine hemoglobin has low concentrations of organic phosphates (Rapoport and Guest, 1941), and has more pronounced Haldane (CO_2) and Bohr (pH) effects (Breepel et al., 1981). Ultrapurified bovine hemoglobin has been shown in preclinical studies to have low antigenicity among mammals (Cochen et al., 1974; Cunnington et al., 1981).

An ultrapurified polymerized bovine hemoglobin solution administered i.v. to C3H mice bearing the FSaIIC fibrosarcoma has been shown to increase both the tumor growth delay and tumor cell killing by radiation therapy and by a variety of chemotherapeutic agents with little increase in the toxicity of these agents to the bone marrow (Teicher et al., 1992b,c). Tumor oxygen tensions were measured using a computer control pO_2 microelectrode in two preclinical solid tumor models, the rat 9L gliosarcoma and the rat 13672 mammary carcinoma. Tumor oxygenation profiles were determined under four conditions: (1) normal air breathing, (2) carbogen breathing, (3) after intravenous administration of a solution of ultrapurified polymerized bovine hemoglobin with normal air breathing and (4) after intravenous administration of a solution of ultrapurified polymerized bovine hemoglobin with carbogen breathing. Both tumors had severely hypoxic regions under normal air breathing conditions. Although carbogen breathing increased the oxygenation of the better oxygenated portions of the tumor, it did not impact on the severely hypoxic tumor regions. Administration of the hemoglobin solution was effective in increasing the oxygenation throughout both tumors under normal air breathing conditions. The addition of carbogen breathing to administration of the hemoglobin solution eliminated severe hypoxia in the 9L gliosarcoma and markedly reduced the severely hypoxic regions of the 13672 mammary carcinoma (Teicher et al., 1992b,c).

Perfluorochemical emulsions/oxygen

The use of perfluorochemical emulsions and carbogen or oxygen breathing has been explored extensively in preclinical solid tumor models in conjunction with very positive results (Teicher and Rose, 1984a,b; Rockwell et al., 1986; Teicher and Rose, 1986; Lee, Levitt and Song, 1987; Martin et al., 1987; Moulder and Fish, 1987; Song et al., 1987; Moulder et al., 1988; Teicher, Herman and Rose, 1988; Teicher, Herman and Jones, 1989a; Lee, Levitt and Song, 1990). Some initial clinical trials of the perfluorochemical emulsion, Fluosol and oxygen breathing with radiation therapy have been carried out (Rose et al., 1986; Lustig et al., 1989; Evans et al., 1990; Lustig et al., 1990; Evans et al., 1993). Long-term follow-up of patients with high-grade brain tumors demonstrated a benefit from administration of Fluosol and oxygen breathing along with radiation therapy (Evans et al., 1993).

Effect of oxygenation on therapeutic response

Three times more radiation is required to kill fully anoxic cells than normally oxygenated cells. Radiosensitization, however, occurs at relatively low concentrations of oxygen: a concentration of 0.25% oxygen moves the dose-response curve halfway toward the fully aerated condition, with essentially identical dose-response curves obtained for cells in 2, 20 or 100% oxygen. Therefore, a small amount of oxygen delivered to hypoxic regions of a solid tumor would significantly increase the radiosensitivity of those tumor regions.

In two solid rat tumors there was a correlation in the oxygen-related and hypoxia-related parameters with a measure of therapeutic response. It appeared that the relative change in these parameters with the oxygen delivery treatments, rather than the absolute levels of these parameters, correlated best with endpoints related to response to various therapies. The two rat tumors, the 13672 mammary carcinoma and the 9L gliosarcoma, had similar levels of hypoxia and similar responses to the oxygen delivery agents. There appeared to be some correlation between the decrease in the % of pO_2 readings ≤ 5 mmHg achieved in these tumors and the level of enhancement in response to radiation produced by the oxygen delivery agent. The theoretical maximum for the radiation dose-modifying agents is 3.0 (Fowler et al., 1970; Duncan, 1973; Hall, 1978). As the % of pO_2 readings ≤ 5 mmHg decreased, the radiation response of the tumors increased. In the 9L gliosarcoma, administration of the hemoglobin solution along with carbogen breathing ablated hypoxia in this tumor and radiation sensitivity approached the theoretical maximum for a fully oxygenated tissue.

Several parameters related to the oxygen content of the murine F SaII fibrosarcoma are shown in Table 2.6. The oxygen profiles from which the data on Table 2.6 was derived were made up of at least 500 pO_2 readings. Shown are the median pO_2 (50th percentile), the 90th percentile pO_2, the modal pO_2 (highest reading under the given condition) and the

Table 2.6. *Oxygen-related parameters for the murine FSaII fibrosarcoma under several conditions*

| Measurement condition | pO_2 (mmHg) | | | |
	Median	90th Percentile	Maximum	Volume-weighted pO_2
Air	0.4	8.5	15	2.5
Carbogen	2.1	34.1	55	7.5
Perflubron/air	6.6	38	40	11
Perflubron/carbogen	12.8	76	116	21
Hemoglobin/air	1.0	19.1	22	3.7
Hemoglobin/carbogen	3.4	66.9	123	8.4
Pentoxifylline/air	0.4	5.9	18	2.4
Pentoxifylline/carbogen	1.1	22	56	11

volume-weighted pO_2 for the tumor under each condition (Gatenby et al., 1988). The median pO_2 of the FSaII tumor was 0.4 mmHg, the 90th percentile reading was 8.5 mmHg, the modal pO_2 was 15 mmHg and the volume weighted pO_2 of the tumor was 2.5 mmHg. Carbogen breathing increased the oxygen parameters of the FSaII tumor by about 4- to 5-fold and increased the volume-weighted pO_2 by about 3-fold. Administration of the perflubron emulsion along with air breathing increased the oxygen content of the FSaII tumor to a greater level than did carbogen breathing. The perflubron emulsion and air breathing increased the median pO_2 16.5-fold and the 90th percentile and modal pO_2s about 3- to 4.5-fold and increased the volume weighted pO_2 4.4-fold. The addition of carbogen breathing to administration of the perflubron emulsion further increased the oxygen content of the tumor such that there was a 32-fold increase in the median pO_2, an 8- to 9-fold increase in the 90th percentile reading and the modal pO_2s and an 8-fold increase in the volume weighted pO_2 compared with air breathing controls.

    Administration of the hemoglobin solution with maintenance of normal air breathing resulted in a 2- to 3-fold increase in the oxygen parameters of the tumor. The addition of carbogen breathing to the administration of the hemoglobin solution further increased the oxygen content of the tumor such that there was about an 8-fold increase in the oxygen parameters. As opposed to the rat tumors, administration of pentoxifylline did not alter the oxygen levels of the FSaII tumor (Lee

Table 2.7. *Hypoxia related parameters for the murine FSaII fibrosarcoma under several conditions*

Measurement condition	pO_2 (mmHg) 10th percentile	% of readings ≤ 5 mmHG	Decrease in % of readings ≤ 5 mmHg
Air	0.0	89	—
Carbogen	0.0	64	25
Perflubron/air	0.0	48	41
Perflubron/carbogen	0.0	44	45
Hemoglobin/air	0.0	74	15
Hemoglobin/carbogen	0.0	63	26
Pentoxifylline/air	0.0	88	1
Pentoxifylline/carbogen	0.0	70	19

et al., 1992; Teicher et al., 1993a). Carbogen breathing along with administration of pentoxifylline increased the oxygen content of the tumor to levels similar to those seen with carbogen alone.

Table 2.7 shows several parameters related to the hypoxic portions of the FSaII tumor under each of the conditions tested. The murine FSaII fibrosarcoma is very hypoxic, having 89% of the measured pO_2 values < 5 mmHg. Although carbogen breathing decreased the % of pO_2 readings < 5 mmHg to 64%, the 10th percentile pO_2 remained 0.0 mmHg to 48% of the measured values, a decrease of 41% compared with controls. Carbogen breathing, in addition to administration of the perflubron emulsion, produced a small further reduction in the hypoxia in the tumor so that the % of pO_2 readings < 5 mmHg was 44%.

Administration of the hemoglobin solution with maintenance of air breathing produced a 15% reduction in the % of pO_2 readings < 5 mmHg in the FSaII fibrosarcoma. The addition of carbogen breathing to administration of the hemoglobin solution further reduced the % of pO_2 readings < 5 mmHg in this tumor to 63%, a 26% reduction compared to air breathing controls. Administration of pentoxifylline to animals bearing the FSaII fibrosarcoma did not alter the hypoxia-related characteristics of this tumor. The addition of carbogen breathing to administration of pentoxifylline moderately decreased the % of pO_2 readings < 5 mmHg to 70%, a 19% reduction compared to controls.

As with radiation therapy (Figure 2.13), there appears to be a relationship between decrease in the % of pO_2 readings < 5 mmHg and sensi-

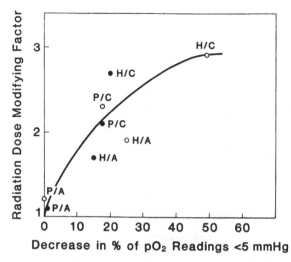

Figure 2.13. Relation between the dose-modifying factors obtained from single dose (10, 20 and 30 Gy) radiation tumor growth delay data and the decrease in the % of pO_2 readings ≤ 5 mmHg for the rat 13762 mammary carcinoma (●) and the rat 9L gliosarcoma (○), under various oxygenation conditions. P/A, perfluorochemical emulsion/air breathing; P/C, perfluorochemical emulsion/carbogen breathing; H/A, hemoglobin solution/air breathing; H/C, hemoglobin solution/carbogen breathing.

tivity to many chemotherapeutic agents. In the F S aII fibrosarcoma there is a 10-fold increase in tumor cell killing by 10 mg/kg of melphalan (L - P A M) as the % of pO_2 readings < 5 mmHg in the tumor decreased (Figure 2.14). Similarly there was a 40-fold increase in the killing of F S aII tumor cells by 300 mg/kg of cyclophosphamide (C T X) as the % of pO_2 readings < 5 mmHg in the tumor decreased. Both the hemoglobin solution and the perflubron emulsion/carbogen breathing were effective oxygen delivery agents in these settings. Interestingly, carbogen breathing was not effective in enhancing the effects of radiation therapy or chemotherapy in the three tumors studied here or several others. Some investigators have observed small increases in tumor response with carbogen breathing alone.

Hypoxia post therapy

Under normal air breathing conditions the rat 13672 mammary carcinoma has a broad range of oxygenation with a higher mean pO_2 (12.3 mmHg) than median pO_2 (5.8 mmHg), indicating a skewing of the oxygen distribution toward more hypoxic values. One day (24 h) after

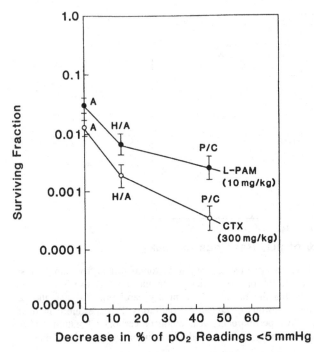

Figure 2.14. Survival of FSaII tumor cells from animals treated with a single dose of melphalan (L-PAM) (10 mg/kg, i.p.) (●) or a single dose of cyclophosphamide (CTX) (300 mg/kg, i.p.) at various levels of tumor hypoxia expressed as decrease in % of pO_2 readings ≤ 5 mmHg compared with controls. Values at 0 decrease are normal air breathing controls. H/A, hemoglobin solution/air breathing; P/C, the perfluorochemical emulsion Oxygent-CA/carbogen. Points, means of three experiments; bars, S.E.M.

administration of a single dose of cyclophosphamide (300 mg/kg, i.p.) the tumors were much more hypoxic. The mean pO_2 was 4.0 mmHg and the median pO_2 was essentially 0.0 mmHg. This level of hypoxia persisted at 48 h after cyclophosphamide administration such that the mean pO_2 in the tumors was 3.8 mmHg and the median pO_2 was 0.7 mmHg. Twenty-four hours after administration of CDDP (8 mg/kg, i.p.) there was also decreased oxygenation of the tumors compared with the de novo controls. One day after CDDP the mean pO_2 was 6.2 mmHg and the medial pO_2 was 2.1 mmHg. At 48 h post CDDP administration there was a further decrease in tumor oxygenation such that the mean pO_2 was 3.5 mmHg and the median pO_2 was 1.3 mmHg. Radiation therapy was administered locally to the tumor-bearing limb of the animals in a once-daily regimen of 3 Gy for 5 days. Twenty-four hours after the last fraction, the tumors were much more hypoxic than the de novo untreated controls. The level of oxygenation was similar to that observed one day after cyclophosphamide administration. The mean pO_2 was 3.7 mmHg and the median pO_2 was 0.0 mmHg. Two days after the last radiation fraction, the tumors remained quite hypoxic with a mean pO_2 of 3.8 mmHg and a median pO_2 of 1.6 mmHg.

Administration of perfluorochemical emulsions/carbogen breathing has increased the response of a wide variety of preclinical solid tumors to radiation and chemotherapy, presumably by increasing the oxygen level in the tumor (Teicher, Holden and Rose, 1985a; Teicher, Holden and Rose, 1986b; Teicher et al., 1987a,c; Teicher and Holden, 1987; Teicher et al., 1988a,b.c, 1989, 1990). Upon administration of the per-flubron emulsion (8 ml/kg, i.v.) and initiation of carbogen breathing the mean pO_2 in the de novo tumors increased to 46.4 mmHg and the median pO_2 increased to 18.7 mmHg. Although after treatment with cyclophosphamide the oxygen level in tumors was decreased, the oxygenation of the tumors was increased by administration of the perflubron emulsion and carbogen breathing. The mean pO_2 in tumors 24 h after cyclophosphamide in the presence of the perflubron emulsion/ carbogen breathing was 29.1 mmHg and the median pO_2 9.7 mmHg, while 48 h after cyclophosphamide in the presence of the perflubron emulsion/ carbogen breathing the mean pO_2 was 35.4 mmHg and the median pO_2 was 6.5 mmHg. These results tend to indicate that the increase in oxygen in the tumors occurred to a greater degree in the more oxygenated cells. At 24 h post administration of CDDP (8 mg/kg) in the presence of the perflubron emulsion/carbogen, the tumors achieved a mean pO_2 of 40.0 mmHg and median pO_2 of 25.4 mmHg while 48 h after the fifth radiation fraction the mean pO_2 in the tumors was 28.9 mmHg and the median pO_2 was 7.2 mmHg.

All three of the treatments administered in this study resulted in increased hypoxia in the tumors both 24 h and 48 h after treatment. It appears, therefore, that 'reoxygenation' was either not occurring or was occurring very slowly in this tumor. The factors contributing to the increased hypoxia are manifold. The dose of cyclophosphamide (300 mg/kg) and the dose of radiation (5×5 Gy) produced about a 2-log kill of the tumor cells while the dose of CDDP (8 mg/kg) produced about a 1-log kill of the tumor cells (unpublished results). In addition to decreased respiration, inflammatory processes including increased interstitial pressure (Jain, 1988; Sevick and Jain, 1989) are probably contributing to the increased hypoxia. Administration of the perflubron emulsion/carbogen breathing was able to increase the oxygenation of the tumors under all of the conditions studied.

These data indicate that hypoxia induced during treatment may be an important factor in treatment outcome and that an oxygen delivery agent such as the perflubron emulsion/carbogen breathing can increase tumor oxygenation during treatment.

Hypoxic cell selective cytotoxic agents as chemosensitizers

It has been well established that the nitroimidazole radiosensitizing agents can also act as selective cytotoxic drugs in hypoxic cells (Chaplin et al., 1986; Franko, 1986; Hill, 1986; Teicher et al., 1992). In addition, these compounds, which are said to mimic the effect of oxygen in cells, have been shown to enhance the cytotoxicity of several antitumor alkylating agents including melphalan, cyclophosphamide, BCNU and 1-(2-chloroethyl)-3-cyclohexyl-1-nitrosourea in vitro and in vivo. This phenomenon has been termed chemosensitization (Clement et al., 1980; Fowler, 1985; Teicher et al., 1991b, 1992b). The presence of hypoxic cells in solid tumors may account for the preferential effect, since chemo-sensitization in vitro occurs only when cells are exposed to misonidazole under hypoxic condition, i.e. conditions in which reduction of misonida-zole through formation of oxygen-mimicking free radicals can occur. Tumor cell survival assay in the FSaIIC murine fibrosarcoma demon-strated that when the modulator Fluosol-DA was administered just prior to an alkylating agent plus carbogen breathing for 6 h or the modulator etanidazole was administered just prior to an alkylating agent, the combi-nation treatment produced significantly more tumor cell killing across the dosage range of each alkylating agent tested compared with the alkylating agent alone (Teicher et al., 1991d). Each alkylating agent produced a dose-dependent log-linear tumor cell survival curve. There was an increase in tumor cell killing of 5–10-fold when either Fluosol-DA/carbogen or etanidazole was added to treatment with the alkylating agent. For CDDP and thiotepa, the modulators used in combi-nation increased tumor cell killing by only 2–3-fold over that obtained with a single modulator, but for the other alkylating agents, tumor cell killing was increased by 10–50-fold when the combination of modu-lators was used. Bone marrow CFU-GM survival assays showed that the combination of modulators with the alkylating agents resulted in only small increases in bone marrow toxicity of the alkylating agents except for thiotepa and melphalan, for which the toxicity to the bone marrow CFU-GM was increased by 5–10-fold compared with the alkylating agents alone. The Hoechst 33342 dye diffusion defined tumor cell subpopulation assay, also in the FSaIIC tumor, demonstrated that the combination of modulators increased the toxicity of CDDP, cyclophosphamide, melphalan and BCNU by 9–55-fold compared with alkylating agent alone in both the bright (euoxic-enriched) and dim (hypoxic-enriched) cells. For each alkylating agent except BCNU, the increase in tumor cell killing was greater in the dim cells than in the bright cells (Teicher et al., 1991d). Finally, tumor growth delay studies in both the FSaIIC tumor and EMT-6 murine mammary adenocarcinoma confirmed that the combination of modulators significantly increased the tumor growth delay caused by CDDP, carboplatin, cyclophosphamide, thiotepa, melphalan and BCNU (Table 2.8). The greatest increases (4–5-fold) were observed for carboplatin and melphalan in the FSaIIC tumor and CDDP and cyclophosphamide in the EMT-6 tumor.

To examine the ability of SR-4233, a new cytotoxic agent, to overcome the resistance of hypoxic tumor cells to antitumor alkylating agents, the cytotoxic effect of SR-4233 alone and in combination with varying doses of CDDP, cyclophosphamide, BCNU or melphalan on tumor cells and bone marrow cells isolated from C3H mice bearing the FSaIIC fibrosarcoma was examined (Holden et al., 1992). When SR-4233 alone was given, tumor cell killing was limited. When SR-4233 was administered just before single-dose treatment with CDDP, cyclophosphamide, BCNU or melphalan, however, marked dose enhancement leading to increased cytotoxic effects on tumor cells and on bone marrow cells was observed (Figure 2.15). Similar experiments with tumor cell subpopulations, selected by Hoechst 33342 dye diffusion, confirmed that while cytotoxicity to both bright (oxygenated) and dim (hypoxic) cells was increased by combining each alkylating agent with SR-4233, the enhancement of the effect was relatively greater in the subpopulation of dim cells. The delay in the growth of tumors in animals treated with the combination of SR-4233 and CDDP, cyclophosphamide or melphalan was 1.6-fold to 5.3-fold greater than that in animals treated with each alkylating agent alone (Holden et al., 1992).

Table 2.8. *Growth delay of the FSaIIC and EMT-6 tumors by alkylating agents with or without the combined modulation of etanidazole and Fluosol-DA/carbogen*

	Tumor growth delays (days)[b]			
Treatment group[a]	Drug alone	Fluosol-DA/ carbogen[c]	Etanidazole[d]	Etanidazole/ Fluosol-DA/ carbogen
FSaIIC fibrosarcoma		0.2±0.3	0.3±0.5	2.7±0.5
CDDP (10 mg/kg)	7.7±0.7	12.8±1.3	12.3±1.6	16.1±1.1
Carboplatin (50 mg/kg)	5.2±0.5	16.4±1.7	7.8±1.3	22.1±3.2
Cyclophosphamide (150 mg/kg)	4.2±0.5	13.9±1.5	5.3±0.7	15.1±1.2
Thiotepa (10 mg/kg)	3.0±0.4	6.2±1.2	4.2±0.4	8.9±1.3
BCNU (15 mg/kg)	2.5±0.4	5.5±0.9	4.3±0.7	9.4±1.3
L-PAM (10 mg/kg)	2.9±0.5	9.9±1.7	5.2±0.5	15.2±2.0
EMT-6 mammary carcinoma				3.8±1.1
CDDP (10 mg/kg)	7.5±0.8	32.7±3.2		
Carboplatin (50 mg/kg)	4.5±0.5	12.4±1.2		
Cyclophosphamide (150 mg/kg)	6.3±0.5	25.2±2.1		
Thiotepa (10 mg/kg)	3.0±0.4	10.7±1.5		
BCNU (15 mg/kg)	2.7±0.4	10.5±1.3		
L-PAM (10 mg/kg)	3.0±0.4	11.4±1.4		

[a] All drugs given i.p.
[b] Tumor growth delay is the difference in days for treatment tumors to reach 500 mm^3 compared with untreated control tumors. Mean of 14 animals ± S.E.M.
[c] Fluosol-DA dose was 0.3 ml; 12 ml/kg i.v. just prior to alkylating agents. Carbogen breathing began just after Fluosol-DA and continued for 6 h.
[d] Etanidazole dose was 1 g/m^2 i.p. just prior to alkylating agents.

Tumor/host: in vivo resistance and targets for modulation

The in vivo resistant EMT-6 mammary carcinoma lines

The group of drugs classified as the antitumor alkylating agents comprises small chemically reactive molecules that covalently attach to cellular components. The lethal lesion associated with exposure of cells to the antitumor alkylating agents is believed to be bifunctional binding of the drugs to DNA (Teicher et al., 1986a; Teicher and Frei III, 1988; Teicher et al., 1990). The EMT-6 mammary carcinoma sublines resistant to the antitumor alkylating agents cyclophosphamide (CTX), thiotepa, cisplatin (CDDP) and carboplatin were produced by repeated exposure

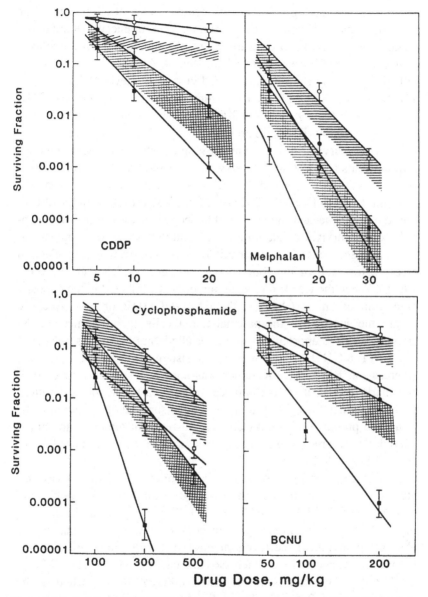

Figure 2.15. Survival of F SalIC tumor cells (•, ■) and bone marrow CFU-GM (○, □) from animals treated in vivo with single doses of one of four antitumor alkylating agents given either alone (•, ○), or combined with prior treatment with SR-4233 (50 mg/kg) (■, □). Shaded areas indicate the envelopes of additivity determined by isobologram analysis of the survival curves for each drug combination. Points, means of three independent determinations ± S.E.M. (bars).

of fresh tumor-bearing hosts to each drug (Teicher et al., 1990). After ten treatments, metastable resistant tumors were produced. Although the tumors were resistant to drug treatment, the tumor cells in monolayer culture were not (Teicher et al., 1990, 1993b). As determined the tumor cell survival assay from tumors treated in vivo at a level of 1 log (90%) of cell killing, the EMT-6/CDDP tumor is 4-fold resistant to CDDP and the EMT-6/CTX tumor is 3-fold resistant to cyclophosphamide as compared with the EMT-6/Parent tumor (Teicher et al., 1990).

When the survival of bone marrow granulocyte–macrophage colony-forming units (CFU-GM), an alkylating agent-sensitive normal tissue, was assessed in mice bearing the EMT-6 parental tumor or the in vivo resistant EMT-6/CDDP, EMT-6/CTX, EMT-6/Thio and EMT-6/Carbo tumors, the survival pattern of the bone marrow CFU-GM recapitulated the survival of the tumor cells, mimicking the development of resistance and reversion to sensitivity upon removal of the selection pressure for each of the four alkylating agents (Teicher et al., 1990, 1993b). When the EMT-6 parental tumor was implanted in the opposite hind limb of animals bearing the EMT-6/CDDP or EMT-6/CTX tumor, the survival of the parental tumor cells after treatment of the animals with the appropriate antitumor alkylating agent was enhanced. The EMT-6/CDDP tumor was cross-resistant to CTX and melphalan, whereas the EMT-6/CTX tumor was somewhat resistant to CDDP and markedly sensitive to etoposide. In each case, the survival pattern of the bone marrow CFU-GM reflected the survival of the tumor cells. Thus, the presence of an alkylating agent-resistant tumor in an animal altered the drug response of tissues distal to the resistant tumor (Teicher et al., 1990, 1993b).

When the expression of several early response genes and genes associated with malignant disease was assessed in the EMT-6/Parent tumor and the EMT-6/CTX and EMT-6/CDDP in vivo resistant lines growing as tumors or as monolayers in culture, it was found that in the absence of treatment the levels of mRNA for the genes c-*jun*, c-*fos*, c-*myc*, Ha-*ras* and *p53* were increased in the EMT-6/CTX and EMT-6/CDDP as compared with the EMT-6/Parent tumor, whereas the expression of *erb*-2 was similar in all three tumors (Teicher et al., 1990; Chatterjee et al., 1995). Although the cells from each of the three tumors showed increased expression of early response genes after exposure to CDDP or 4-hydroxyperoxycyclophosphamide in culture, in mRNA extracted from tumor tissue these changes were absent or very small. There was increased expression of both c-*jun* and *erb*-2 in the livers of tumor-bearing animals. The highest expression of both c-*jun* and *erb*-2 occurred in the livers of animals bearing the EMT-6/CDDP tumor. Treatment of the animals with CDDP or cyclophosphamide, in general, resulted in increased expression of both genes at 6 h post-treatment. The increased expression of these genes may impart metabolic changes in the tumors and/or hosts that contribute to the resistance of these tumors to specific antitumor alkylating agents (Chatterjee et al., 1995).

Several observations, including the fibrous nature of the resistant tumors, the increased metastatic potential of the resistant tumors and the altered pharmacokinetics of the drugs in the resistant tumor-bearing hosts, led to the hypothesis that transforming growth factor β might be integrally involved in in vivo antitumor alkylating agent resistance in the EMT-6 tumor lines.

Transforming growth factor β is a positive factor in breast cancer progression

TGF-β effects on increasing angiogenesis and stroma formation and decreasing immune function indicate that it may play a critical role in tumor progression. Some of the earliest in vivo work on the potential critical role of TGF-βs in breast cancer was carried out by Welch et al. (Welch, Fabra and Motowo, 1990), who treated rat 13762 mammary carcinoma cells with TGF-β1 in cell culture for 4 h then injected the cells i.v. into the appropriate host (female Fisher 344 rats) and counted the number of lung metastases 2 weeks later. Pretreatment of the 13762 cells with TGF-β1 (50 pg/ml) resulted in a 2- to 3-fold increase in the number of lung metastases on day 14. The 13762 cells treated with TGF-β1 had increased invasive capability, increased production of type IV collagenase and increased heparinase activity. Using a different approach, Arteaga et al. (1993) transfected a mouse TGF-β1 cDNA into human MCF-7 breast carcinoma cells. The transfected cells were tumorigenic in nude mice in the absence of estrogen while the parental MCF-7 cells were not unless the animals were given injections of TGF-β1 (1 μg/day, i.p., 3 weeks). These investigators also found that administration of the 2G7IgG2b antibody, which neutralizes TGF-β1, -β2 and -β3 to nude mice prevented the growth and metastases of the estrogen-independent human MDA-231 breast carcinoma in these animals. Implantation of MDA-231 cells in nude mice decreased the murine spleen natural killer cell activity. Administration of the 2G7 TGF-β neutralizing antibody restored the natural killer cell activity in these animals and decreased tumor formation suggesting that suppression of the host immune surveillance may be a functional component in the ability of TGF-β to support tumor progression (Arteaga et al., 1993). Both the TGF-β protein and TGF-β mRNA have been detected in human breast cancer tissue and their expression correlated with the invasive nature of the disease (MacCallum et al., 1994; Walker, Dearing and Gallacher, 1994). In a cell culture study, Herman and Katzenellenbogen (1994) found that MCF-7 cells deprived of steroid hormones transiently for about 8 weeks increased production of the TGF-β proteins 3- to 10-fold and then decreased expression of these proteins once again.

Transforming growth factor β is a positive factor in the progression of solid tumors

Most cells can produce as well as respond to TGF-β, thus TGF-β levels are significant in controlling many physiological processes that involve interactions between cells of different types, thereby influencing the metabolic balance among tissues and/or organs (Roberts and Sporn, 1988, 1990; Ueki et al., 1992). To model the potential effects of TGF-β1 production, Ueki et al. (1993) transfected the human TGF-β1 cDNA into CHO(Chinese hamster ovary) cells. After subcutaneous implantation in nude mice the transfected cells were highly tumorigenic, producing vascularized tumors and lung metastases, while the parental CHO cells were weakly tumorigenic and non-metastatic. Hsu et al. (1994) found that U9 human colon carcinoma cells that show autocrine-positive growth regulation by TGF-β1 were more tumorigenic in vivo than a similar human colon carcinoma line HD3 that demonstrated autocrine-negative regulation by TGF-β1. In a study of clinical prostate carcinoma biopsies, Muir et al. (1994) found that TGF-β was up-regulated in the extracellular space in tumors by hormonal manipulation in vivo and that this up-regulation of TGF-β persisted after tumor relapse in many cases. Using clinical materials and Northern blot analysis, Merz, Arnold and Studer (1994) found a progressive increase in the expression of TGF-β1 in normal prostate, benign prostatic hyperplasia and prostate carcinoma. In a detailed study, Gold et al. (1994) investigated the potential role of the TGF-β2 in the normal proliferative endometrium as well as in the transition to complex hyperplasia and then to endometrial carcinoma. Their results suggested a greater paracrine than autocrine mechanism for TGF-β in the pathological state and an association between overexpression of TGF-β and progression toward malignancy. Exposure to TGF-β in cell culture has been shown to increase the production of both 72 kDa and 92 kDa metalloproteinases in human cervical carcinoma cells (Agarwal et al., 1994). In melanoma and glioma cell lines loss of growth inhibition upon exposure to TGF-β has been associated with tumor progression to a more invasive phenotype (Fujiwara et al., 1994; Jennings et al., 1994; Merzak et al., 1994; Rodeck et al., 1994).

Resistance reversal with TGF-β neutralizing antibody

In vivo it is likely, especially after multiple exposures to antitumor alkylating agents, that the cells that comprise the resistant tumor lines are highly heterogeneous. One of the goals in developing these drug resistant tumor lines in vivo was to allow the expression of community characteristics rather than single clonal properties. Several studies have demonstrated that even very small subpopulations of cells producing a growth factor within a tumor can significantly alter the properties of that tumor without becoming a dominant population (Picard, Rolland and Poupon, 1986; Nicolson, Dulski and Trosko, 1988; Pritchett, Wang and Jones, 1989; Camps et al., 1990; Miller and Heppner, 1990; Ohmura et al., 1990. Chen et al., 1991; Korczak, Kerbel and Dennis, 1991; Mukaida et al., 1991; Miller et al., 1993; Jouanneau et al., 1994).

The number of lung metastases formed after subcutaneously implanting the EMT-6/Parent or each of the four antitumor alkylating agent EMT-6 tumor lines was determined over a time course of primary tumor growth (Figure 2.16). The antitumor alkylating agent resistant tumor lines were much more aggressively metastatic than the EMT-6/Parent tumor. The differential in the number of lung metastases between the parent and resistant tumors increased over time. The number of lung metastases formed by the EMT-6/CDDP and EMT-6/Carbo tumors was about 2-fold greater than the EMT-6/Parent tumor by day 16 while the number of lung metastases formed by the EMT-6/CTX tumor was about 2.5-fold greater and by the EMT-6/thiotepa tumor was about 3-fold greater than by the EMT-6/Parent tumor.

The EMT-6 in vivo alkylating agent resistant tumors are markedly less responsive to the drugs to which resistance was developed than is the EMT-6/Parent tumor when growth as solid tumors subcutaneously in the hind legs of female Balb/C mice (Teicher et al., 1990, 1993b; Chatterjee et al., 1995). When animals bearing the EMT-6/Parent tumor

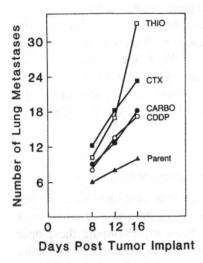

Figure 2.16 Numbers of lung metastases firmed over time from subcutaneously implanted EMT-6/Parent, EMT-6/CTX, EMT-6CDDP, EMT-6/Carbo or EMT-6/Thio tumors. Tumor cells (2×10^6) were implanted on day 0 in a hind limb.

or the EMT-6/CTX tumor were treated with a single dose of cyclophosphamide, the tumor cell killing shown in Figure 2.17 was obtained. Cyclophosphamide at a dose of 300 mg/kg killed 2 logs of EMT-6/Parent tumor cells and less than 1 log of EMT-6/CTX tumor cells. Cyclophosphamide at a dose of 500 mg/kg killed 3.5 logs of EMT-6/Parent tumor cells but only 1.5 logs of EMT-6/CTX tumor cells. To assess the possibility that TGF-β might have a role in in vivo alkylating agent resistance, animals bearing the EMT-6/Parent or EMT-6/CTX tumor were treated with anti-TGF-β 2G7, anti-TGF-β 4A11 or anti-TGF-β 2G7 and anti-TGF-β 4A11 daily by intraperitoneal injection on days 4−8 or daily on days 0−8 post tumor cell implantation. No significant difference was observed in tumor growth rate by administration of these antibody treatments. There was no significant effect of the administration of anti-TGF-β 2G7 or anti-TGF-β 4A11 on days 4−8 on tumor cell killing by cyclophosphamide (300 mg/kg) in animals bearing either the EMT-6/Parent or EMT-6/CTX tumor; however, treatment with anti-TGF-β 2G7 and anti-TGF-β 4A11 on days 4−8 post tumor cell implantation resulted in increased tumor cell killing on both EMT-6/Parent and EMT-6/CTX tumors by cyclophosphamide (300 mg/kg) ($P < 0.1$). When treatment with antibodies to TGF-β was extended to the full period of tumor growth, days 0−8, a significant increase in the tumor cell killing

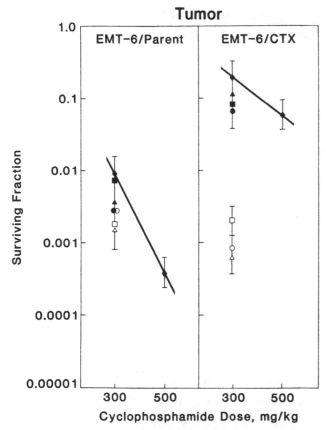

Figure 2.17. Survival of EMT-6/Parent tumor cells and EMT-6/CTX tumor cells from tumors treated in vivo with cyclophosphamide alone (♦), anti-TGF-β 2G7 (1 mg/kg, i.p.) days 4–8 then cyclophosphamide (■), anti-TGF-β 4A11 (1 mg/kg, i.p.) days 4–8 then cyclophosphamide (▲), anti-TGF-β 2G7 (1 mg/kg, i.p.) anti-TGF-β 4A11 (1 mg/kg, i.p.) days 4–8 then cyclophosphamide (●), anti-TGF-β 2G7 (1 mg/kg, i.p.) days 0–8 then cyclophosphamide (□), anti-TGF-β 2G7 (1 mg/kg, i.p.) anti-TGF-β 4A11 (1 mg/kg, i.p.) days 0–8 then cyclophosphamide (○). Points are the means of three independent experiments; bars are the S.E.M.

of the EMT-6/Parent tumor by cyclophosphamide (300 mg/kg) was observed with each of the three antibody regimens ($P < 0.1$). A much greater effect on cyclophosphamide tumor cell killing was observed when animals bearing the EMT-6/CTX tumor were treated with any of the anti-TGF-β regimens on days 0–8. The effect of anti-TGF-β treatment on the EMT-6/CTX tumor cell killing was not only highly significant ($P < 0.001$) but also resulted in the restoration of drug sensitivity to the level of the parent tumor in the EMT-6/CTX tumor cells.

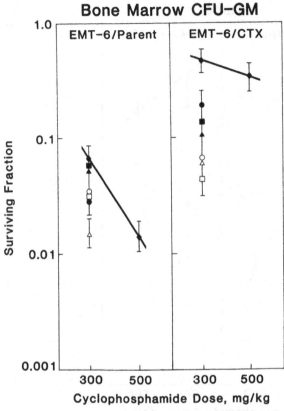

Figure 2.18. Survival of bone marrow CFU-GM from the same animals shown in Figure 2.17. Bone marrow was taken from the femurs of the animals at the time of tumor excision. Points are the means of three independent experiments; bars are the S.E.M.

The survival of bone marrow CFU-GM in bone marrow taken from the same animals described above was assessed (Figure 2.18). The bone marrow CFU-GM from animals bearing the EMT-6/Parent tumor was much more sensitive to treatment with cyclophosphamide than the bone marrow CFU-GM from the animals bearing the EMT-6/CTX tumor, such that 1 log and 2 logs greater killing of bone marrow CFU-GM occurred in animals bearing the EMT-6/Parent tumor than in animals bearing the EMT-6/CTX tumor after treatment with 300 mg/kg or 500 mg/kg of cyclophosphamide, respectively. Upon treatment of the tumor-bearing animals with antibodies to TGF-β on days 4–8 there was a significant increase in the killing of bone marrow CFU-GM by cyclophosphamide (300 mg/kg) in animals bearing the EMT-6/CTX tumors. When the anti-TGF-β regimens were extended to days 0–8 there was a significant ($P < 0.1$) increase in the killing of bone marrow CFU-GM from animals bearing the EMT-6/CTX tumor ($P < 0.001$) by cyclophosphamide. The increase in the killing of bone marrow CFU-GM in the EMT-6/CTX tumor bearing animals was sufficient to restore the sensitivity of the bone marrow CFU-GM in these animals to the level of the bone marrow CFU-GM in animals bearing the EMT-6/Parent tumor.

A similar study was carried out with animals bearing the EMT-6/Parent tumor and animals bearing the EMT-6/CDDP tumor treated with CDDP (Figure 2.19). Treatment of animals bearing the EMT-6/Parent tumor or the EMT-6/CDDP tumor with a dose of CDDP of 20 mg/kg resulted in 1 log less killing of the EMT-6/CDDP tumor cells than of the EMT-6/Parent tumor cells. Treatment of animals bearing the EMT-6/Parent tumor or the EMT-6/CDDP tumor with 50 mg/kg of CDDP produced 4 logs less killing of the EMT-6/CDDP tumor cells than of the EMT-6/Parent tumor cells. The anti-TGF-β treatment regimens were the same as those described above. Administration of the antibodies to TGF-β on days 4–8 did not alter the response of the EMT-6/Parent tumor to treatment with CDDP (20 mg/kg) but significantly increased the killing of the EMT-6/CDDP tumor cells by CDDP (20 mg/kg) ($P < 0.1$). Administration of the antibodies to TGF-β on days 0–8 increased the tumor cell killing of the EMT-6/Parent tumor cells by CDDP but increased the tumor cell killing of the EMT-6/CDDP tumor cells by CDDP to a much greater degree ($P < 0.001$). The increase in the tumor cell killing in the EMT-6/CDDP tumor by treatment with anti-TGF-β on days 0–8 in addition to CDDP (20 mg/kg) was sufficient to produce cell killing of the EMT-6/CDDP tumor cells that was equivalent to that of the EMT-6/Parent tumor.

The bone marrow was taken from the femurs of the same animals shown in Figure 2.19 and the survival of bone marrow CFU-GM was determined (Figure 2.20). Bone marrow CFU-GM are, in general, not very sensitive to CDDP; however, the bone marrow CFU-GM in the animals bearing the EMT-6/CDDP tumors was less sensitive to CDDP than the bone marrow CFU-GM in animals bearing the EMT-6/Parent tumor. Treatment of the EMT-6/Parent and EMT-6/CDDP tumor bearing animals with any of the three anti-TGF-β regimens on days 4–8 resulted in increased killing of bone marrow CFU-GM by CDDP (20 mg/kg) in animals bearing either tumor. Administration of the antibodies to TGF-β on days 0–8 produced increased bone marrow

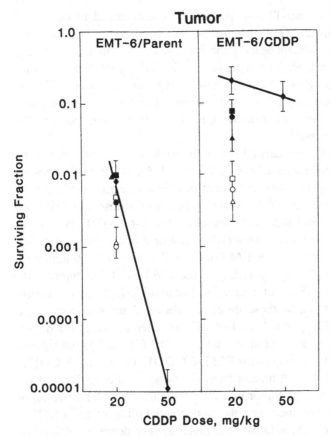

Figure 2.19. Survival of EMT-6/Parent tumor cells and EMT-6/CDDP tumor cells from tumors treated in vivo with CDDP alone (♦), anti-TGF-β 2G7 (1 mg/kg, i.p.) days 4–8 then CDDP (■), anti-TGF-β 4A11 (1 mg/kg, i.p.) days 4–8 then CDDP (▲), anti-TGF-β 2G7 (1 mg/kg, i.p.) anti-TGF-β 4A11 (1 mg/kg, i.p.) days 4–8 then CDDP (●), anti-TGF-β 2G7 (1 mg/kg, i.p.) days 0–8 then CDDP (□), anti-TGF-β 4A11 (1 mg/kg, i.p.) days 0–8 then CDDP (△), anti-TGF-β 2G7 (1 mg/kg, i.p.) anti-TGF-β 4A11 (1 mg/kg, i.p.) days 0–8 then CDDP (○). Points are the means of three independent experiments; bars are the S.E.M.

CFU-GM killing by CDDP (20 mg/kg) in animals bearing either the EMT-6/Parent or the EMT-6/CDDP tumors ($P < 0.01$) such that over-all the killing of bone marrow CFU-GM in animals bearing these tumors was equivalent.

To explore the systemic effects produced by the presence of the EMT-6/Parent, EMT-6/CTX or EMT-6/CDDP tumors in the presence or absence of treatment with antibodies to TGF-β, tumor bearing animals were either untreated or injected intraperitoneally with anti-

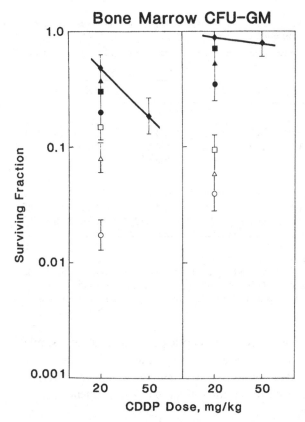

Figure 2.20. Survival of bone marrow CFU-GM from the same animals shown in Figure 2.19. Bone marrow was taken from the femurs of the animals at the time of tumor excision. Points are the means of three independent experiments; bars are the S.E.M.

TGF-β 2G7 and anti-TGF-β 4A11 on days 0–8 and several metabolic characteristics of the tumors and hosts were determined.

Glutathione levels were highest in the EMT-6/CTX tumors and lowest in the EMT-6/CDDP tumors with or without anti-TGF-β treatment (Table 2.9). Glutathione-S-transferase activity was highest in the EMT-6/CTX tumor and similar in the EMT-6/Parent and EMT-6/CDDP tumors. Glutathione reductase levels were similar in all of the tumor homogenates. Glutathione peroxidase activity as measured by the hydrogen peroxide assay was increased in the EMT-6/CTX and EMT-6/CDDP tumors compared with the EMT-6/Parent tumor and was decreased in the EMT-6/CTX and EMT-6/CDDP tumors after treatment of the animals with the anti-TGF-β regimen. Glutathione

Table 2.9. *Enzymatic characteristics of EMT-6 tumors from animals either treated or untreated with TGF-β antibodies*

| Tumor | GSH | GST | GSH red. | GSH peroxidase | | P-450 |
				H$_2$O$_2$	CuOOH	
Untreated						
EMT-6/Parent	30.0±2.7	194±9	188±6	163±3	285±11	14.1±3.0
EMT-6/CTX	38.8±3.1	291±11	172±4	224±9	271±11	9.2±2.1
EMT-6/CDDP	27.2±1.8	207±8	198±12	306±13	268±8	11.8±2.7
Anti-TGF-β treated						
EMT-6/Parent	28.7±3.8	149±11	186±7	164±11	286±13	22.0±3.6
EMT-6/CTX	41.4±4.1	180±9	204±12	154±9	255±11	17.4±3.2
EMT-6/CDDP	18.6±3.1	99±7	191±9	178±13	235±10	16.1±2.7

Glutathione (GSH) is expressed as nmol/mg protein.
Glutathione-S-transferase activity (GST), glutathione reductase activity (GSH red.), glutathione peroxidase activity (GSH peroxidase), and cytochrome *P*-450 reductase activity (*P*-450 red.) are expressed as substrate conversion, nmol/min mg protein.

peroxidase activity as measured by the cupric peroxide assay was similar in the three tumors in the presence and absence of anti-TGF-β treatment. Cytochrome *P*-450 reductase activity was similar in the three tumors and was increased in each of the three tumors after treatment with the anti-TGF-β regimen.

Livers were collected from the same animals described above. Glutathione levels were similar in the liver homogenates from non-tumor bearing animals and from animals bearing the EMT-6/Parent, EMT-6/CTX and EMT-6/CDDP tumors (Table 2.10). Treatment with the anti-TGF-β regimen decreased hepatic glutathione levels to about 60% of normal in both the non-tumor bearing and the tumor bearing animals. Glutathione-S-transferase activity in the livers of tumor bearing animals was decreased compared to the non-tumor bearing control animals. Treatment of the animals with the anti-TGF-β regimen decreased the glutathione-S-transferase activity in both the tumor-bearing and non-tumor bearing animals. Glutathione reductase activity was highest in the livers of the non-tumor bearing animals and similar in the livers of the tumor-bearing animals. After treatment with the anti-TGF-β regimen, glutathione reductase activity was decreased to similar levels in the livers of both tumor-bearing and non-tumor bearing animals. Glutathione peroxidase activity as measured by hydrogen peroxide assay was highest

Table 2.10. *Enzymatic characteristics of livers from EMT-6 tumor-bearing animals either treated or untreated with TGF-β antibodies*

Tumor	GSH	GST	GSH red.	GSH peroxidase H_2O_2	CuOOH	*P*-450
Untreated						
Non-tumor-bearing control	84±11	1183±129	129±12	1652±200	2435±289	134±9
EMT-6/Parent	75±10	734±88	99±13	645±127	1657±125	109±16
EMT-6/CTX	68±12	856±95	80±9	1289±190	1818±180	98±12
EMT-6/CDDP	74±17	836±114	105±13	1337±153	1787±180	112±11
Anti-TGF-β treated						
Non-tumor-bearing control	52±10	749±59	65±12	647±76	948±120	182±16
EMT-6/Parent	73±11	692±65	71±13	625±68	1001±131	160±12
EMT-6/CTX	41±8	681±70	67±8	726±77	1139±125	179±18
EMT-6/CDDP	45±9	648±67	66±8	537±59	875±93	152±21

Glutathione (GSH) is expressed as nmol/mg protein.
Glutathione-S-transferase activity (GST), glutathione reductase activity (GSH red.), glutathione peroxidase activity (GSH peroxidase), and cytochrome *P*-450 reductase activity (*P*-450 red.) are expressed as substrate conversion, nmol/min mg protein.

in the livers of non-tumor-bearing animals, lowest in the livers of animals bearing the EMT-6/Parent tumor and intermediate in the livers of animals bearing the EMT-6/CTX and EMT-6/CDDP tumors. Treatment with the anti-TGF-β regimen resulted in decreased glutathione peroxidase activity in both the non-tumor bearing and the tumor bearing animals. Glutathione peroxidase activity as determined by the cupric peroxide was highest in the non-tumor bearing animals and similar in the livers of animals bearing each of the three tumors. After treatment with the anti-TGF-β regimen, this enzyme activity was decreased in both tumor bearing and non-tumor bearing animals. There is a trend towards lower cytochrome *P*-450 reductase activity in the livers of the tumor bearing compared with non-tumor bearing animals. Interestingly, upon treatment with the anti-TGF-β regimen there was increased cytochrome *P*-450 reductase activity in livers of both non-tumor bearing and tumor bearing animals.

Integration with other studies

Transforming growth factor β is a widely occurring cytokine (Border and Noble, 1994). TGF-β1, the most intensely studied of the three TGF-β isoforms, is secreted as an inactive latent high molecular weight protein that in the extracellular matrix is cleaved to form active TGF-β. TGF-β1 along with other cytokines such as basic fibroblast growth factor, platelet-derived growth factor, tumor necrosis factor and inter-leukin-1 are involved in tissue remodeling, that is wound healing, after injury. Excessive or sustained production of TGF-β1 is a key factor in tissue fibrosis (Roberts et al., 1990; Beck et al., 1993; Roberts and Sporn, 1993; Sporn and Roberts, 1993). In breast cancer patients, high plasma concentrations of TGF-β1 measured after induction chemo-therapy but prior to high dose combination alkylating agent therapy with autologous bone marrow transplantation have been shown to correlate strongly with risk of hepatic venoclusive disease and idiopathic inter-stitial pneumonitis (Anscher et al., 1993). In another clinical study it was found that persistently elevated plasma TGF-β levels were a strong predictor for developing symptomatic pneumonitis after thoracic radio-therapy (Anscher et al., 1994). Muir et al. (1994) found that high levels of TGF-β expression in prostate carcinoma biopsies from patients corre-lated with failure of the tumors to respond to hormonal withdrawal. In a cell culture study using human MCF-7 breast carcinoma it was found that marked alterations in the levels of TGF-β (and TGF-α) may play a role in the molecular events that are involved in the progression of these cells from estrogen-responsive to estrogen-autonomous growth (Herman and Katzenellenbogen, 1994). Welch et al. (1990) tested the ability of TGF-β to alter the metastatic potential of a rat mammary carcinoma cell line. Lung colonies were measured 2 weeks after inocu-lation in syngeneic F344 rats, and a bell-shaped dose-response curve with 2- to 3-fold increase in number of surface lung metastases was seen. Maximal enhancement occurred at the 50 pg/ml dose level. The effect was specific because addition of neutralizing anti-TGF-β antibody blocked the stimulatory activity at all levels of TGF-β1 pretreatment, but when antibody was given alone, neutralizing anti-TGF-β antibody had no effect on untreated cells. Increased metastatic potential appears to be due to an increased propensity of cells to extravasate, as tested in the membrane invasion culture system. TGF-β1 treatment of the cells did not alter their growth rate or morphology in the presence of serum; however, growth was inhibited in serum-free medium. Likewise, adhesion to human umbilical vein endothelial cell monolayers or to immobilized reconstituted basement membrane or fibronectin matrices was unchanged. These results suggest that TGF-β1 may modulate metastatic potential of mammary tumor cells by controlling their ability to break down and penetrate basement-membrane barriers (Welch et al., 1990). TGF-β1 was found to strongly stimulate the ability of human glioma cells to migrate and invade in cell culture (Merzak et al., 1994). In the clinic, expression of TGF-β1 correlates with decreased survival presumably due to its invasion-promoting action (Merzak et al., 1994). The EMT-6 in vivo alkylating agent resistant tumor lines were developed by treatment of a tumor-bearing animal with the specific alkylating agent followed by transfer of the tumor cells to a fresh host. Therefore, the changes observed in the host metabolic characteristics amongst the tumors must be due to factors carried by the tumor cells, since the host was not exposed to the drugs. The resistant tumors are: (1) more fibrous with collagen bundles visible on electron micrographs of the tumors, (2) more aggressively metastatic than the parent tumor and (3) much less responsive to the drugs to which resistance was developed than the parent tumor and also somewhat cross-resistant to other cytotoxic therapies (Teicher et al., 1993b). Treatment with antibodies to TGF-β reversed the resistance of these tumors, if the tumors were grown in the presence of antibody treatment. A concentration range from 1 to 1000 pg/ml addition of TGF-β1 to the media of EMT-6/ Parent, EMT-6/CTX or EMT-6/CDDP cells did not alter the growth (proliferation) of the cells grown under adherent or non-adherent conditions in culture (data not shown).

TGF-β seems to have an important role in hepatic pathophysiology. It has been reported to be a potent inhibitor of hepatocyte proliferation in vitro (Nakamura et al., 1985; Carr et al., 1986; Braun et al., 1988). Moreover, hepatic TGF-β mRNA levels increased after partial hepatectomy in the nonparenchymal liver cells (Braun et al., 1988); thus, TGF-β may function in vivo as the effector of an inhibitory paracrine mechanism to prevent uncontrolled hepatocyte growth during liver regeneration. TGF-β dramatically decreased accumulation (> 95% inhibition) of the negative acute-phase protein albumin in both normal human hepatocyte and human hepatoma HepG2 cell line culture media (Busso et al., 1990). Several other proteins are also modulated by TGF-β in primary human hepatocytes and HepG2 cells; amongst these is plasminogen activator inhibitor type-1 PAI-1, a positive acute phase protein. In hepatoma cells, it has been recently reported that in addition to albumin, TGF-β decreases apolipoprotein A-1, another negatively regulated protein during acute phase reaction (Morrone, Cortese and Sorrentino, 1989). The fact that TGF-β is able to act on negative (albumin and apolipoprotein A-1) as well as on positive (PAI-1) acute phase proteins, suggests that this cytokine may be an important mediator of the acute phase response.

Kayanoki et al. (1994) investigated the effect of TGF-β1 on expression of antioxidative enzymes, manganese superoxide dismutase, copper, zinc superoxide dismutase, and catalase in cultured hepatocytes of rat. TGF-β1 suppressed expression of all these antioxidative enzymes in time- and cell density-dependent manners. Furthermore, expression of two major classes of the rat glutathione-S-transferase subunits 1 and 2 was also reduced by TGF-β1, although expression of glutathione peroxidase was not affected. Flow cytometric analysis indicated that production of peroxides was increased in hepatocytes treated with TGF-β1. Treatment of animals bearing the EMT-6/Parent, EMT-6/CTX and EMT-6/CDDP tumors with antibodies to TGF-β selectively decreased by 30–50% the activity of glutathione-S-transferase and glutathione peroxidase (H_2O_2) in homogenates of the resistant tumors (Table 2.9). The effects on normal liver function were profound with a 40–60% reduction in the activity of the three sulfhydryl related enzymes measured. The presence of a tumor in the animals decreased the activity of all the hepatic enzymes measured compared with the enzyme activities in the normal animals. However, the hepatic activities of glutathione-S-transferase and glutathione peroxidase were higher (closer to normal) in the liver homogenates from animals bearing the resistant tumors than in animals bearing the EMT-6/Parent tumor. Treatment of animals bearing the resistant tumors with the anti-TGF-β regimen decreased the activity of glutathione-S-transferase, glutathione reductase and glutathione peroxidase in the livers of these animals 30–50%. After treatment with the antibodies to TGF-β, the enzymatic activity in the livers of both tumor-bearing and non-tumor-bearing animals were similar. On the other hand, the activity of cytochrome P-450 reductase, a flavoprotein that transfers an electron to cytochrome P-450, required along with molecular oxygen to hydroxylate a substrate, is increased in both the livers and tumors of anti-TGF-β treated animals. Cytochrome P-450 reductase activity is intimately paired with cytochrome P-450 activity. Cytochrome P-450 is necessary for the conversion of the prodrug cyclophosphamide to 4-hydroxycyclophosphamide, which is further converted to phosphoramide mustard and other active alkylating species. Overall, therefore, anti-TGF-β treatment decreased the activity of drug-inactivating enzymes and increased the activity of a drug-activating enzyme in the livers of tumor-bearing animals.

Although it cannot be concluded from these studies that increased expression TGF-β is a direct cause of in vivo alkylating agent resistance, it can be concluded that treatment with TGF-β neutralizing antibodies restored drug sensitivity in the alkylating agent resistant tumors and that treatment with these antibodies alters both tumor and host metabolic states.

Host targets for modulation: inhibitors of processes involved in growth and invasion

In order to enlarge and invade, locally or distally tumor must continue to cause the breakdown and restructuring of the extracellular matrix including both basement membrane and interstitial matrices (Terranova, Hujanen and Martin, 1986; Tryggvason, Hoyhtya and Salo, 1987; Folkman, 1990; Vlodavsky et al., 1990; Weidner et al., 1991). It has been recognized for many years that the formation of a blood supply (angiogenesis) is critical for growth of both normal and malignant tissues (Willis, 1953; Rubin and Casarett, 1966; Folkman, 1987; Folkman et al., 1989). For over 20 years cancer researchers have been searching for agents that could inhibit the processes of malignant cell invasion and growth in normal tissues. One focus of that search has used the inhibition of the formation of blood vessels; usually in the normal tissue model system of the chick choroallantoic membrane (CAM) to discover potential therapeutic agents, which have been termed 'angiostatic' or 'antiangiogenic' (Folkman, 1987; Folkman and Klagsbrun, 1987; Folkman et al., 1989a; Folkman, 1990). Evidence has been accumulating that indicates that the actions of some of the agents discovered through the angiogenesis assay occur at the level of extracellular matrix enzymes (Ingber, Madri and Folkman, 1986; Folkman and Ingber, 1987; Tryggvason et al., 1987; Ingber and Folkman, 1988; Vlodavsky et al., 1990).

The angiostatic activity of several steroids was discovered some years ago. The method by which these steroids inhibit vessel growth and/or produce regression of growing vessels is only now being elucidated (Ingber et al., 1986; Folkman and Ingber, 1987; Folkman and Klagsbrun, 1987; Ingber and Folkman, 1988). Angiostatic steroids appear to induce basement membrane dissolution as part of their antiangiogenic action (Ingber et al.,

1986; Folkman and Ingber, 1987; Ingber and Folkman, 1988). In fact, in the CAM assay angiostatic steroids had a direct effect on extracellular matrix turnover resulting in a decrease in collagen accumulation when administered in combination with heparin. The steroids had a modest effect on collagen accumulation and heparin had no effect on collagen accumulation when administered alone (Ingber et al., 1986). Therefore, a direct effect on extracellular matrix metabolism resulted in inhibition of new capillary growth. Of the naturally occurring angiostatic steroids, tetrahydrocortisol was identified as the most potent (Folkman and Ingber, 1987).

In 1983, Folkman et al. reported that heparin or a heparin fragment administered in combination with cortisone presented angiogenesis in the CAM assay and inhibited the growth of several solid murine tumors. Inhibition of angiogenesis or tumor response has been reported in other model systems after treatment with cortisone or cortisone acetate; however, in most studies heparin did not increase the effect obtained with the steroid (Penhaligon and Camplejohn, 1985; Lee et al., 1987b). More recently, Folkman et al. (1989b) reported that β-cyclodextrin tetradeca-sulfate in combination with hydrocortisone inhibited capillary formation in the CAM assay and prevented neovascularization induced by endotoxin in the rabbit cornea (Folkman et al., 1989b).

Several enzymes are involved in the degradation of the extracellular matrix during malignant tumor growth and invasion. Serine proteases and metalloproteases are the most prominent of the enzymes (Terranova et al., 1986; Tryggvason et al., 1987; Alexander and Werb, 1989; Vlo-davsky et al., 1990; Liotta, Steeg and Stetler-Stevenson, 1991). Type IV collagen is the main component of the tight structure of the basement membrane (Terranova et al., 1986; Tryggvason et al., 1987; Vlodavsky et al., 1990). At least two specific type IV collagenases have been isolated and characterized (Salo and Oikarinen, 1985; Templeton and Stetler-Stevenson, 1991; Pyke et al., 1992). Activity of type IV collagenase has been associated with the metastatic phenotype. Relatively high concentrations of cortisol have been shown to inhibit type IV collagenase activity in human skin fibroblast cultures (Salo and Oikarinen, 1985). The interstitial collagen types (I, II and III) are remarkably resistant to the attack of proteinases but they can be degraded by highly specific metalloproteinases called interstitial collagenases, which have been isolated from a variety of mammalian cells and tissues including rabbit synovial fibroblasts, rheumatoid synovium, rabbit VX2-carcinoma, human skin and pig synovium (Harris Jr, Welgus and Krane, 1984; Harris Jr, 1985; Tryggvason et al., 1987). It has been recognized for some time that the tetracyclines can inhibit tissue collagenase activity and tetracycline administration has been used in the treatment of periodontal disease (Golub et al., 1983), gingival collagenolytic activity in diabetes (Golub et al., 1983, 1987) and to inhibit joint deterioration in patients with rheumatoid arthritis (Greenwald et al., 1987). This inhibitory activity has been associated with both type IV collagenase and interstitial collagenase (Golub et al., 1991). Tamargo et al. (1991) has reported that minocycline, a semisynthetic tetracycline with a relatively long circulating half-life, inhibited neovascularization in the rabbit cornea implanted with the VX2 carcinoma.

The Lewis lung carcinoma was chosen for primary tumor growth delay studies and tumor lung metastases studies (Sotomayor et al., 1992; Teicher, Alvarez Sotomayor and Huang, 1992a). Tetrahydrocortisol and β-cyclodextrin tetradecasulfate were administered in a 1:1 molar ratio by continuous infusion over 14 days and minocycline was administered i.p. over 14 days from day 4 to day 18 post tumor implant (Table 2.11). The combination of tetrahydrocortisol/β-cyclodextrin tetradecasulfate diminished the tumor growth delay produced by CDDP and melphalan and produced modest increases in the tumor growth delay produced by cyclophosphamide and radiation. Minocycline co-treatment increased the tumor growth delay produced by CDDP, melphalan, radiation, bleomycin and especially cyclophosphamide where 4 out of 12 animals receiving minocycline (14 × 5 mg/kg, days 4–18) and cyclophosphamide (3 × 150 mg/kg, days 7, 9, 11) were long-term survivors. The three modulators in combination produced further increase in tumor growth delay with all of the cytotoxic therapies and 5 out of 12 of the animals treated with the three modulator combinations and cyclophosphamide were long-term survivors. Although neither tetrahydrocortisol/β-cyclodextrin tetradecasulfate, minocycline nor the three modulator combination impacted the number of lung metastases, there was a decreased number of large lung metastases (Table 2.12). Treatment with the cytotoxic therapies alone reduced the number of lung metastases. Addition of the modulators to treatment with the cytotoxic therapies resulted in further reduction in the number of lung metastases. These results indicate that agents that inhibit the breakdown of the extracellular matrix can be useful additions to the treatment of solid tumors (Sotomayor et al., 1992; Teicher et al., 1992).

Table 2.11. Growth delay of the Lewis lung tumor produced by various anticancer treatments alone or in combination with β-cyclodextrin tetradecasulfate/tetrahydrocortisol, minocycline or the combination of modulators

Treatment group	Dose[a]	Tumor growth delay (days)[b]			
		Alone	+14(S0$_4$)βCD/THC	+Minocycline	+14(S0$_4$)βCD/THC/Mino
+14(S0$_4$)βCD/THC	1000 mg/kg		0.6+0.3		
	125 mg/kg over 14 days				
Minocycline	14×5 mg/kg			0.6+0.3	
+14(S0$_4$)βCD/THC	– as above				
CDDP	1×10 mg/kg	4.5±0.3	2.2±0.3	5.0±0.3	26.2±2.5
Melphalan	1×10 mg/kg	2.7±0.3	1.1±0.3	4.3±0.3	10.5±0.9
Cyclophosphamide	1×150 mg/kg	7.2±0.4	16.2±1.2	24.7±2.7	27.6±2.8
	3×150 mg/kg	21.5±1.7	36.8±3.4	45.2±2.9*	48.8±3.3**
Radiation	1×20 Gy	6.2±0.5	8.3±0.5	11.9±1.4	13.8±1.3
	5×3 Gy	4.4±0.3	7.1±0.7	7.8±0.6	12.6±1.2
Adriamycin	5×1.75mg/kg	7.0±0.6	—	9.8±0.8	11.7±1.2
Bleomycin	4×10 mg/kg	8.5±0.6	—	12.0±1.2	12.9±1.3

[a] β-Cyclodextrin tetradecasulfate (1000 mg/kg) and tetrahydrocortisol (125 mg/kg) were administered in a 1:1 molar ratio by continuous infusion over 14 days in an Alzet osmotic pump from days 4–18 post-tumor implant. Minocycline (5 mg/kg) was administered i.p. on days 4–18 post-tumor implant. CDDP (10 mg/kg), melphalan (10 mg/kg) and cyclophosphamide (150 mg/kg) were administered i.p. on day 7 post-tumor implant. Cyclophosphamide (150 mg/kg) was also administered on days 7, 9 and 11 post-tumor implant. Radiation was delivered locally to the tumor-bearing limb as 20 Gy on day 7 or 3 Gy daily on days 7–11. Adriamycin (1.75 mg/kg) was administered i.p. daily on days 7–11. Bleomycin (10 mg/kg) was administered i.p. on days 6, 10, 13 and 16.
[b] Tumor growth delay is the difference in days for treated tumors to reach 500 mm³ compared with untreated control tumors. Untreated control tumors reach 500 mm³ in about 14 days. Mean of 15 animals ± S.E.M.
* Four animals out of 12 were long-term survivors (>120 days).
** Five animals out of 12 were long-term survivors (>120 days).

Table 2.12. *Numbers of lung metastases on day 20 from subcutaneous Lewis lung tumors after various anticancer treatments or in combination with β-cyclodextrin tetradecasulfate/tetrahydrocortisol, minocycline or the combination of modulators*

Treatment group	Dose[b]	Mean number of lung metastases (Number and % of vascularized metastases)[a]			
		Alone	+14(SO₄)βCD/THC	+Minocycline	+14(SO₄)βCD/THC/Mino
Untreated controls					
+(S0₄)βCD/THC	100 mg/kg	15 (10; 66%)			
	125 mg/kg over 14 days	14.5 (10; 69%)			
Minocycline	14×5 mg/kg	12 (5; 43%)			
+14(S0₄)βCD/THC/Mino	as above	13 (6; 46%)			
CDDP	1×10 mg/kg	12	15 (10; 67%)	10.5 (5; 48%)	6 (2.5; 39%)
Melphalan	1×10 mg/kg	8	8 (4; 48%)	6 (3; 50%)	5 (2.5; 47%)
Cyclophosphamide	1×150 mg/kg	6.5	6 (2; 32%)	3 (1; 33%)	4 (0; 44%)
	3×150 mg/kg	3.5	3 (0.5; 16%)	0.5 (0; 18%)	0.5 (0; 20%)
Radiation	1×20 Gy	8	7 (3; 40%)	8 (1; 25%)	7 (3; 46%)
	5×3 Gy	7	7 (2.5; 35%)	6.5 (2; 30%)	7 (3; 47%)
Adriamycin	5×1.75 mg/kg	8	—	7.5 (5; 63%)	5 (3; 57%)
Bleomycin	4×10 mg/kg	7	—	7 (4.5; 64%)	4 (2; 45%)

[a] The number of external lung metastases on day 20 post-tumor implant were counted manually and scored as 2 mm³ in diameter. The data is shown as the means from 6–12 pairs of lungs. Parantheses indicated the number of large (vascularized) metastases and percentage of the total number of metastases that were large.
[b] The schedules of drug administration were as shown in Table 2.11.

Modulation by inhibition of intercellular signaling

Non-small cell lung cancer is traditionally regarded as a chemotherapy refractory disease (Selawry and Hansen, 1982). Numerous combinations of cytotoxic agents have been tried both preclinically and clinically against non-small-cell lung cancer. In cell culture human non-small-cell lung cancer lines tend to be among the more drug-resistant cell lines developed from other human solid tumor types (Teicher et al., 1991e; Frei III et al., 1993).

Growth in vivo requires that tumor cells restructure the surrounding extracellular matrix, initiate proliferation of critical normal cells such as endothelial cells and perhaps alter host defense systems (Marnett, 1992). Products of arachidonic acid metabolism are involved in intercellular signaling (Samuelsson et al., 1987; Oates et al., 1988; Smith, 1989; Fukushima, 1992). In a study of 55 human solid tumor cell lines, 15 of the 19 non-small cell lung carcinoma cell lines secreted prostaglandins E_2 and $F_2\alpha$ into the cell culture media at relatively high levels while only six of the remaining 36 cell lines produced any detectable prostaglandin E_2 (Hubbard et al., 1988a,b; 1989, 1991). The lung cancer cell lines that secreted the prostaglandin were bronchioalveolar cell (2 out of 2) adenocarcinoma (9 out of 10) and large cell undifferentiated carcinoma (3 out of 3). Two squamous cell carcinoma of the lung cell lines did not produce detectable prostaglandin E_2 and $F_2\alpha$. In a study comparing profiles of endogenous prostaglandin E_2 production in matched unstimulated normal lung and lung carcinoma tissue, prostaglandin E_2 levels were higher in all primary lung tumor histological cell types (squamous cell, $n = 20$; adenocarcinoma, $n = 7$; small cell, $n = 4$; mixed cell $n = 2$; bronchioalveolar cell, $n = 2$; bronchial carcinoid, $n = 1$) with the exception of large cell undifferentiated carcinomas ($n = 3$) (McLemore et al., 1988).

It has been recognized for some time that the murine Lewis lung carcinoma secretes prostaglandin E_2 and that administration of the prostaglandin synthesis inhibitor beginning at the time of tumor cell implantation could slow the growth and metastasis of the tumor (Young and Knies, 1984; Chiabrando et al., 1985; Young, Newby and Meunier, 1985; Young and Hoover, 1986; Young and Newby, 1986; Young, Wheeler and Newby, 1986; Young, Newby and Wepsic, 1987; Young, Young and Wepsic, 1987; Young, Young and Kim, 1988; Ellis et al., 1990a,b; Young et al., 1990). The secretion of prostaglandin E_2 by both the Lewis lung tumor cells and host macrophages correlated with the suppression of host natural killer cell and T-lymphocyte cytotoxic activity in mice bearing the tumor (Young and Hoover, 1986; Young and Newby, 1986; Young et al., 1986; Maca, 1988; Young et al., 1990). The role of prostaglandin secretion in the metastatic potential of Lewis lung tumor cells remains under investigation and may be correlated with the level of lamin in receptor expression by these cells (Aliño, Unda and Pérez-Yarza, 1990; Ellis et al., 1990a,b).

Arachidonic acid is metabolized through three pathways (Oates et al., 1988; Smith, 1989). The first, which leads to the prostanoids (thromboxanes and prostaglandins) is initiated by the cyclooxygenase (PGG/H synthase) enzymes. The second, which leads to the leukotrienes, is initiated by the lipoxygenase enzymes and the third, which leads to the epoxyeicosatrienoic acids, is initiated by cytochrome P-450 epoxygenases. Most of the work examining the relationships between eicosanoids and malignant disease has focused on the prostanoids (Honn, Busse and Sloane, 1983; Watson and Chuah, 1985; Laekeman et al., 1986; Aitokallio-Tallberg, Viinikka and Ylikorkala, 1988; Castelli et al., 1989; Aitokallio-Tallberg et al., 1991; Baron and Greenberg, 1991). The enzyme cyclooxygenase is found in most tissues and intracellularly is found in greatest abundance in the endoplasmic reticulum (Smith, 1989; Buckley et al., 1991; Hla and Maciag, 1991). Cyclooxygenase metabolizes arachinoid acid to prostaglandin endoperoxide H_2, which goes on to thromboxane A_2, prostacyclin and various prostaglandins. These molecules are positive and negative effectors of various metabolic processes operating through specific plasma membrane receptors coupled to G proteins, which activate intracellular message transduction (Honn et al., 1983; Oates et al., 1988; Smith, 1989). Specifically, prostaglandins ($PGF_2\alpha$) have been implicated in the control of the production of collagenase IV, thromboxane A_2, and prostacyclin, which are positive and negative regulators of platelet aggregation in vasodilation as well as endothelial and perhaps malignant cell proliferation (Honn et al., 1983; Oates et al., 1988; Smith, 1989; Buckley et al., 1991; Hla and Maciag, 1991). The level of cyclooxygenase protein has been shown to be influenced in various cell and organ systems by steroids, growth factors, cytokines and tumor promoters, suggesting that regulation of the level of this enzyme is an important part of regulating prostanoid formation.

The Lewis lung carcinoma has been used as a model of both primary and metastatic disease to assess the ability of cyclooxygenase inhibitors (mefenamic acid, diflunisal, sulindac and indomethacin), the collagenase inhibitor minocycline and the lipoxygenase inhibitor phenidone to act as modulators of cytotoxic cancer therapies (Teicher et al., 1993c, 1994). Although none of the single modulators administered i.p. daily on days 4–18 altered tumor growth or the number of metastases on day 20, modulator combinations consisting of minocycline/a cyclooxygenase inhibitor and especially of phenidone/a cyclooxygenase inhibitor resulted in modest tumor growth delay and a decreased number of lung metastases on day 20 (Tables 2.13 and 2.14). The most effective modulators of CDDP were phenidone/sulindac and phenidone/indomethacin, which led to 2.4–2.5-fold increases in the tumor growth delay produced by CDDP. The most effective modulations of cyclophosphamide, resulting from administration of minocycline, minocycline/sulindac or phenidone/sulindac, led to 2.0–2.1-fold increases in tumor growth delay by cyclophosphamide. The most effective modulators of melphalan produced 4.5–4.7-fold increases in tumor growth delay by the drug and were minocycline/sulindac, minocycline/mefenamic acid and phenidone/sulindac. The most effective modulation of BCNU was obtained with minocycline/sulindac and minocycline/diflunisal leading to 2.8–3.1-fold increases in tumor growth delay by BCNU. Finally, the most effective modulation of radiation was obtained with minocycline/sulindac and phenidone/sulindac and resulted in 2.8–3.3-fold increases in tumor growth delay by radiation (Teicher *et al.*, 1993c, 1994). The modulator combination that, along with the cytotoxic therapies, was most effective against metastatic disease was phenidone/mefenamic acid. There was no clear relationship between effective modulation of the cancer therapies and degree of reduction in serum levels of prostaglandin E_2 and leukotriene B4 by the agents in Lewis lung tumor bearing mice (Teicher et al., 1993c, 1994).

Interleukin 1 is a distal mediator of immune and inflammatory responses. This pleiotropic cytokine is produced by many other cells including fibroblasts (Bouchelouche, Reimert and Bendtzen, 1988; Mauviel et al., 1988), keratinocytes (Nawroth et al., 1986; Kupper, 1988; Kupper et al., 1988; Blanton et al., 1989), squamous tumor cells (Nowak et al., 1990; Partridge et al., 1991), glial cells (Rothwell, 1991) and endothelial cells (Miossec, Cavender and Ziff, 1986; Cozzolino et al., 1990). These cells can also be targets for IL-1 stimulated activities (Howells, Chantry and Feldman, 1988; Gadient, Cron and Otten, 1990). Although IL-2 was cytostatic in some melanoma (Morinaga et al., 1990), ovarian carcinoma (Kilian et al., 1991), osteogenic sarcoma (Dedhar, 1989) and MCF-7 breast cancer (Sgagias, Kasid and Danforth, 1991)

Table 2.13. *Growth delay of the Lewis lung carcinoma and numbers of lung metastases on day 20 post subcutaneous tumor implantation produced by treatment with minocycline and a cyclooxygenase inhibitor along with cytotoxic cancer therapies*

Treatment	Tumor growth delay (days)	Lung metastases No.	(% large)
Minocycline/sulindac	3.1±0.4	16	(38)
Minocycline/diflunisal	1.4±0.4	16	(63)
Minocycline/indomethacin	3.0±0.3	16	(56)
Minocycline/mefenamic acid	0.9±0.5	13	(63)
CDDP (10 mg/kg)	4.5±0.3	13	(58)
Mino/sulin/CDDP	8.6±0.8	14	(36)
Mino/diflun/CDDP	7.6±0.7	15	(40)
Mino/indo/CDDP	5.9±0.6	14	(43)
Mino/mefen/CDDP	6.7±0.6	8	(30)
Cyclophosphamide (3×150 mg/kg)	21.5±1.7	12	(40)
Mino/sulin/CTX	43.7±3.6	13	(23)
Mino/diflun/CTX	32.3±3.3	12.5	(32)
Mino/indo/CTX	36.6±2.9	13.5	(33)
Mino/mefen/CTX	27.9±2.8	6.5	(44)
Melphalan (10 mg/kg)	2.7±0.3	13	(48)
Mino/sulin/PAM	12.1±1.3	7.5	(35)
Mino/diflun/PAM	10.2±1.2	6.5	(38)
Mino/indo/PAM	6.3±0.5	12	(41)
Mino/mefen/PAM	12.6±1.2	8	(43)
BCNU (3×15 mg/kg)	3.6±0.4	15.5	(53)
Mino/sulin/BCNU	9.9±0.9	16	(31)
Mino/diflun/BCNU	11.2±1.4	15.5	(35)
Mino/indo/BCNU	9.1±0.9	10	(30)
Mino/mefen/BCNU	7.6±0.7	10	(30)
X-Rays (5×3 Gy)	4.4±0.3	15	(40)
Mino/sulin/5×3 Gy	12.5±1.2	13	(38)
Mino/diflun/5×3 Gy	9.2±1.1	12.5	(40)
Mino/indo/5×3 Gy	8.8±0.9	13	(38)
Mino/mefen/5×3 Gy	11.1±0.9	13	(38)

cell lines, little or no effect was seen on the clonal growth of primary human tumor explant cultures (Hanauske et al., 1992). In vivo, IL-1α can have growth-inhibitory activity in highly immunogenic tumors, but little clonogenic cell kill or tumor growth inhibition is seen in non-immunogenic or weakly immunogenic solid tumors (Constantinidis et al., 1989; Braunschweiger et al., 1990). Marked pathophysiological perturbations including reduced tumor perfusion, reduced high-energy phos-

Table 2.14. *Growth delay of the Lewis lung carcinoma and numbers of lung metastases on day 20 post subcutaneous tumor implantation produced by treatment with phenidone and a cyclooxygenase inhibitor along with cytotoxic cancer therapies*

Treatment	Tumor growth delay (days)	Lung metastases No.	(% large)
Phenidone/sulindac	3.1±0.3	12	(40)
Phenidone/diflunisal	2.2±0.3	12	(48)
Phenidone/indomethacin	3.0±0.4	12	(45)
Phenidone/mefenamic acid	0.9±0.3	10	(45)
CDDP (10 mg/kg)	4.5±0.3	13	(58)
Phen/sulin/CDDP	10.9±1.1	9	(48)
Phen/diflun/CDDP	8.5±0.4	11	(36)
Phen/indo/CDDP	11.2±0.8	8	(45)
Phen/mefen/CDDP	9.3±0.7	5	(50)
Cyclophosphamide (3×150 mg/kg)	21.5±1.7	12	(40)
Phen/sulin/CTX	45.4±2.9	2.5	(32)
Phen/diflun/CTX	43.2±2.8	2.5	(52)
Phen/indo/CTX	40.9±3.0	3.3	(61)
Phen/mefen/CTX	40.7±2.8	2.5	(46)
Melphalan (10 mg/kg)	2.7±0.3	13	(48)
Phen/sulin/PAM	12.6±0.9	9	(48)
Phen/diflun/PAM	7.9±0.4	11	(36)
Phen/indo/PAM	11.2±0.7	10	(40)
Phen/mefen/PAM	3.9±0.4	4	(25)
BCNU (3×15 mg/kg)	3.6±0.4	15.5	(53)
Phen/sulin/BCNU	6.3±0.5	11	(36)
Phen/diflun/BCNU	5.3±0.3	15	(39)
Phen/indo/BCNU	6.7±0.5	15	(40)
Phen/mefen/BCNU	6.3±0.5	11	(40)
X-Rays (5×3 Gy)	4.4±0.3	15	(40)
Phen/sulin/5×3 Gy	14.5±1.3	11	(36)
Phen/diflun/5×3 Gy	7.3±0.7	14	(36)
Phen/indo/5×3 Gy	6.9±0.8	12	(40)
Phen/mefen/5×3 Gy	7.4±0.9	11	(36)

phate reserves, microvascular injuries and acute hemorrhagic necrosis were, however, observed within 4 h after administration of the cytokine to mice bearing nonimmunogenic tumors (Braunschweiger et al., 1988; Constantinidis et al., 1989; Braunschweiger et al., 1990, 1993). Braunschweiger et al. (1993) studied the antitumor activity of CDDP and human recombinant interleukin-1α in RIF-1 and SCC VII solid tumor models and in a CDDP resistant subline of RIF-1 designated RIF-

$R1_{CDDP}$. In RIF-1 tumors, clonogenic cell survival after CDDP plus IL-1α combinations was highly schedule and IL-1α dose dependent. More than additive clonogenic cell kill was seen when CDDP was given 6 h before, but not 8 h before or at least 24 h after IL-1α. Time-course studies indicated that maximal clonogenic cell killing was achieved within 4–6 h after the CDDP plus IL-1α combination, with little or no recovery for up to 4 h. In vivo dose-response studies indicated that CDDP plus IL-1α combinations induced more clonogenic cell kill than CDDP alone in all three tumor models and analysis by the median effect principle indicated highly synergistic antitumor activity. IL-1α had no effect on the cytotoxicity of CDDP in SCC VII cells in vitro and neither in vitro hypoxia nor in vivo schema, induced by clamping tumor blood supply, significantly affected CDDP clonogenic cell killing. Increased clonogenic cell killing was seen, however, after removal of the clamp, implicating repercussion events, such as oxyradical stress, as a potential mechanism for increased CDDP cytotoxicity in SCC VII solid tumors.

References

Adachi, Y., Luke, M. and Laemmli, U. K. (1991). Chromosome assembly *in vitro*: toposiomerase II is required for condensation. *Cell*, **64**, 137–48.

Agarwal, C., Hembree, J. R., Rorke, E. A. and Eckert, R. L. (1994). Transforming growth factor β1 regulation of metalloproteinase production in cultured human cervical epithelial cells. *Cancer Res.*, **54**, 943–9.

Ahmad, S., Okine, L., Le, B. et al. (1987). Elevation of glutathione in phenylalanine mustard-resistant murine L1210 leukemia cells. *J. Biol. Chem.*, **262**, 15048–53.

Aitokallio-Tallberg, A. M., Viinikka, L. U. and Ylikorkala, R. O. (1988). Increased synthesis of prostacyclin and thromboxane in human ovarian malignancy. *Cancer Res.*, **48**, 2396–8.

Aitokallio-Tallberg, A. M., Jung, J. K., Kim, S. J. et al. (1991). Urinary excretion of degradation products of prostacyclin and thromboxane is increased in patients with gestational choriocarcioma. *Cancer Res.*, **51**, 4146–8.

Alaoui-Jamali, M. A., Panasci, L., Centurioni, G. M. et al. (1992). Nitrogen mustard–DNA interaction in melphalan-resistant mammary carcinoma cells with elevated intracellular glutathione and glutathione-S-transferase activity. *Cancer Chemother. Pharmacol.*, **30**, 341–7.

Alexander, C. M. and Werb, Z. (1989). Proteinases and extracellular matrix remodelling. *Curr. Opin. Cell Biol.*, **1**, 974–82.

Aliño, S.-F., Unda, F.-J., Perez-Yarza, G. and Cañavate, M.-L. (1989). Are laminin binding sites on tumor cell surface involved in the indomethacin-induced sensitivity to natural cytotoxic cells? *Biology of the Cell*, **66**, 255–61.

Aliño, S. F., Unda, F. J. and Pérez-Yarza, G. (1990). Laminin surface binding sites and metastatic potential of 3LL tumor cells, increased by indomethacin. *Biochem. Biophys. Res. Comm.*, **167**(2), 731–8.

Andrews, P. A., Murphy, M. P. and Howell, S. B. (1986). Differential sensitization of human ovarian-carcinoma and mouse L1210 cells to cisplatin and melphalan by glutathione depletion. *Mol. Pharmacol.*, **30**, 643–50.

Andrews, P. A., Murphy, M. P. and Howell, S. B. (1989). Characterization of cisplatin-resistant COLO 316 human ovarian carcinoma cells. *Eur. J. Cancer Clin. Oncol.*, **25**, 619–25.

Anscher, M. S., Peters, W. P., Reisenbichler, H. et al. (1993). Transforming growth factor β as a predictor of liver and lung fibrosis after autologous bone marrow transplantation for advanced breast cancer. *N. Engl. J. Med.*, **328**, 1592–8.

Anscher, M. S., Murase, T., Prescott, D. M. et al. (1994). Changes in plasma TGFβ levels during pulmonary radiotherapy as a predictor of the risk of developing radiation pneumonitis. *Int. J. Rad. Oncol. Biol. Phys.*, **30**(3), 671–6.

Arrick, B. A. and Nathan, C. F. (1984). Glutathione metabolism as a determinant of therapeutic efficacy: a review. *Cancer Res.*, **44**, 4224–32.

Arteaga, C. L., Dugger, T. C., Winnier, A. R. and Forbes, J. T. (1993a). Evidence for a positive role of transforming growth factor-β in human breast cancer cell tumorigenesis. *J. Cell. Biochem.*, **17G**, 187–93.

Arteaga, C. L., Hurd, S. D., Winnier, A. R. et al. (1993b). Anti-transforming growth factor (TGF)-β antibodies inhibit breast cancer cell tumorigenicity and increase mouse spleen natural killer cell activity. *J. Clin. Invest.*, **92**, 2569–76.

Aviado, D. M. and Porter, J. M. (1984). Pentoxifylline: a new drug for treatment of intermittent claudication. *Pharmacotherapy*, **6**, 297–307.

Bakka, A., Endressen, L., Johnsen, A. B. S. et al. (1981). Resistance against cis-dichlorodiammineplatinum in cultured cells with a high content of metallothionein. *Toxicol. Appl. Pharmacol.*, **61**, 215–26.

Baron, J. A. and Greenberg, E. R. (1991). Could aspirin really prevent colon cancer? *N. Engl. J. Med.*, **325**, 1644–6.

Barranco, S. C. and Novak, J. K. (1974). Survival responses of dividing and nondividing mammalian cells after treatment with hydroxyurea, arabinosylcytosine, or Adriamycin. *Cancer Res.*, **34**, 1616–8.

Barranco, S. C., Novak, J. K. and Humphrey, R. M. (1973). Response of mammalian cells following treatment with bleomycin and 1,3-bis(2-chloroethyl)-1-nitrosourea during plateau phase. *Cancer Res.*, **33**, 691–4.

Beck, L. S., DeGuzman, L., Lee, W. P. et al. (1993). One systemic administration of transforming growth factor-β1 reverses age- or glucocorticoid-impaired wound healing. *J. Clin. Invest.*, **92**, 2841–9.

Bedford, P., Walker, M. C., Sharma, H. L. et al. (1987). Factors influencing the sensitivity of two human bladder carcinoma cell lines to cis-diamminedichloroplatinum(II). *Chem. Biol. Interact.*, **61**, 1–15.

Berrios, M., Osheroff, N. and Fisher, P. A. (1985). *In situ* localization of DNA topoisomerase II, a major polypeptide component of the *Drosophila* nuclear matrix fraction. *Proc. Natl. Acad. Sci. USA*, **82**, 4142–6.

Bhuyan, B. K., Fraser, T. J. and Day, K. J. (1977). Cell proliferation kinetics and drug sensitivity of exponential and stationary populations of cultured L1210 cells. *Cancer Res.*, **37**, 1057–63.

Blanton, R. A., Kupper, T. S. McDougall, J. K. and Dower, S. (1989). Regulation of interleukin 1 and its receptor in human keratinocytes. *Proc. Natl. Acad. Sciences USA*, **86**, 127312–77.

Border, W. A. and Noble, N. A. (1994). Transforming growth factor β in tissue fibrosis. *N. Engl. J. Med.*, **331**, 1286–92.

Born, R., Hug, O. and Trott, K. R. (1976). The effect of prolonged hypoxia on growth and viability of Chinese hamster ovary cells. *Int. J. Rad. Oncol. Biol. Phys.*, **1**, 687–97.

Bouchelouche, P. N., Reimert, C. and Bendtzen, K. (1988). Effects of natural and recombinant interleukin-α and -β on cytosolic free calcium in human and murine fibroblasts. *Leukemia (Balt.)*, **2**, 691–6.

Braun, L., Mead, J. E., Panzica, M. et al. (1988). Transforming growth factor β mRNA increases during liver regeneration: a possible paracrine mechanism of growth regulation. *Proc. Natl. Acad. Sci. USA*, **85**(5), 1539–43.

Braunscheweiger, P., Johnson, C. S., Kumar, N. et al. (1988). Antitumor effects of recombinant human interleukin 1α in RIF-1 and PancO$_2$ solid tumors. *Cancer Res.*, **48**, 6011–6.

Braunschweiger, P. G., Kumar, N., Constantinidis, I. et al. (1990). Potentiation of interleukin 1α mediated antitumor effects by ketoconazole. *Cancer Res.*, **50**, 4709–17.

Braunschweiger, P. G., Basrur, V. S., Santos, O. et al. (1993). Synergistic antitumor activity of cisplatin and interleukin 1 in sensitive and resistant solid tumor. *Cancer Res.*, **53**, 1091–7.

Breepel, P. M., Kreuzer, F. and Hazevoet, M. (1981). Interactions of organic phosphates with bovine hemoglobin: I. Oxylabile and phosphate-labile proton binding. *Pflugers Archives*, 389, 219–25.

Buckley, B. J., Barchowsky, A., Dolor, R. J. and Whorton, A. R. (1991). Regulation of arachidonic acid release in vascular endothelium Ca^2-dependent and -independent pathways. *Bioch. J.*, **280**, 281–7.

Bunn, H. F. (1971). Differences in the interaction of 2,3-diphosphoglycerate with certain mammalian hemoglobins. *Science*, 172, 1049–50.

Busse, P. M., Bose, S. K., Jones, R. W. and Tolmach, L. J. (1977). The action of caffeine on X-irradiated HeLa cells: II. Synergistic lethality. *Radiation Res.*, **71**, 666.

Busso, N., Chesne, C., Delers, F. et al. (1990). Transforming growth-factor-β (TGF-β) inhibits albumin synthesis in normal human hepatocytes and in hepatoma HepG2 cells. *Biochem. Biophy. Res. Comm.*, **171**(2), 647–54.

Camps, J. L., Chang, S. M., Hsu, T. C. et al. (1990). Fibroblast-mediated acceleration of human epithelial tumor growth in vivo. *Proc. Natl. Acad. Sci. USA*, **87**(1), 75–9.

Carr, B. I., Hayashi, I., Branum, E. L. and Moses, H. L. (1986). Inhibition of DNA synthesis in rat hepatocytes by platelet-derived type β transforming growth factor. *Cancer Res.*, **46**(5), 2330–4.

Castelli, M. G., Chiabrando, C., Fanelli, R. et al. (1989). Prostaglandin and thromboxane synthesis by human intracranial tumors. *Cancer Res.*, **49**, 1505–8.

Catten, M., Bresnahan, D., Thompson, S. and Chalkly, R. (1986). Novobiocin precipitates histones at concentrations normally used to inhibit eukaryotic type II topoisomerase. *Nucl. Acids Res.*, **14**, 3671–86.

Champoux, J. J. (1978). Mechanism of the reaction catalyzed by the DNA untwisting enzyme: attachment of the enzyme to the 3'-terminus of the nicked DNA. *J. Mol. Biol.*, **118**, 441–6.

Champoux, J. J. (1981). DNA is linked to the rat liver DNA nicking–closing enzyme by a phosphodiester bond to tyrosine. *J. Biol. Chem.*, **256**, 4805–9.

Chaplin, D. J., Durand, R. E., Stratford, I. J. and Jenkins, T. C. (1986). The radiosensitizing and toxic effects of RSU-1069 on hypoxic cells in a murine tumor. *Int. J. Rad. Oncol. Biol. Phys.*, **12**, 1091–5.

Chatterjee, D., Liu, J. T., Northey, D. and Teicher, B. A. (1995). Molecular characterization of the *in vivo* alkylating agent resistant murine EMT-6 mammary carcinoma tumors. *Cancer Chemother. Pharmacol.*, 35(5), 423–31.

Chen, S. C., Chou, C. K., Wong, F. H. et al. (1991). Overexpression of epidermal growth factor and insulin-like growth factor-I receptors and autocrine stimulation in human esophageal carcinoma cells. *Cancer Res.*, 51(7), 1898–903.

Chiabrando, C., Brogggini, M., Castagnoli, M. N. et al. (1985). Prostaglandin and thromboxane synthesis by Lewis lung carcinoma during growth. *Cancer Res.*, 45, 3605–8.

Clapper, M. L., Hoffman, S. J. and Tew, K. D. (1990). Sensitisation of human colon tumour xenografts to L-phenylalanine mustard using ethacrynic acid. *J. Cell. Pharmacol.*, 1, 71–6.

Clement, J. J., Gorman, M. S., Wodinsky, I. et al. (1980). Enhancement of antitumor activity of alkylating agents by the radiation sensitizer misonidazole. *Cancer Res.*, 40, 4165–72.

Cochen, A., Das Gupta, T. K., DeWoskin, R. and Moss, G. S. (1974). Immunologic properties of stroma vs. stroma-free hemoglobin solution. *J. Surg. Oncol.*, 4, 19–28.

Constantinidis, I., Braunschweiger, P. G., Wehrle, J. P. et al. (1989). ^{31}P-nuclear magnetic resonance studies of the effect of recombinant human interleukin 1α on the bionergetics of RIF-1 tumors. *Cancer Res.*, 49, 6379–82.

Cozzolino, F., Torcia, M., Aldinucci, D. et al. (1990). Interleukin 1 is an autocrine regulator of human endothelial cell growth. *Proc. Natl. Acad. Sci. USA*, 87, 6487–91.

Cunnington, P. G., Jenkins, S. N., Tam, S. C. and Wong, J. T. (1981). Oxygen-binding and immunological properties of complexes between dextran and animal hemoglobins. *Bioch. J.*, 193, 261–6.

Dedhar, S. (1989). Regulation of expression of the cell adhesion receptors, integrins, by recombinant human interleukin-1B in human ostersarcoma cells: inhibition of cell proliferation and stimulation of alkaline phosphatase activity. *J. Cell. Physiol.*, 138, 291–9.

DeMartino, C., Battelli, T. and Paggi, M. G. (1984). Effects of lonidamine on murine and human tumor cells *in vitro*. *Oncology*, 41, 15–29.

DeMartino, C., Malorni, W. and Accinni, L. (1987). Cell membrane changes induced by lonidamine in human erythrocytes and T lymphocytes, and Ehrlich ascites tumor cells. *Exp. Mol. Pathol.*, 46, 15–30.

Dewhirst, M. W. (1993). Angiogenesis and blood flow. In *Drug Resistance in Oncology* (ed. B. A. Teicher), pp. 3–24. Marcel Dekker, New York.

DiNardo, S., Voelkel, K. and Sternglanz, R. (1984). DNA toposiomerase II mutant of Saccaromyces cervisiae: toposiomerase II is required for segregation of daughter molecules at the termination of DNA replication. *Proc. Natl. Acad. Sci. USA*, 81, 2616–20.

Dolan, M. E., Corsico, C. D. and Pegg, A. E. (1985). Exposure of HeLa cells to O^6-alkylguanines increases sensitivity to the cytotoxic effects of alkylating agents. *Bioch. Biophy. Res. Comm.*, 132, 178–85.

Dolan, M. E., Morimoto, K. and Pegg, A. E. (1985). Reduction of O^6-alkylguanine–DNA alkyltransferase activity in HeLa cells treated with O^6-alkylguanines. *Cancer Res.*, 45, 6413–7.

Dolan, M. E., Young, G. S. and Pegg, A. E. (1986). Effect of O^6-alkylguanine pretreatment on the sensitivity of human colon tumor cells to the cytotoxic effects of chloroethylating agents. *Cancer Res.*, 46, 4500–4.

Dolan, M. E., Larkin, G. L. and English, H. F. (1989). Depletion of O^6-alkylguanine–DNA alkyltransferase activity in mammalian tissues and human tumor xenografts in nude mice by treatment with O^6-methylguanine. *Cancer Chemother. Pharmacol.*, **25**, 103–8.

Dolan, M. E., Moschel, R. C. and Pegg, A. E. (1990a). Depletion of mammalian O^6-alkylguanine-DNA alkyltransferase activity by O^6-benzylguanine provides a means to evaluate the role of this protein in protection against carcinogenic and therapeutic alkylating agents. *Proc. Natl. Acad. Sci. USA*, **87**, 5368–72.

Dolan, M. E., Stine, L. and Mitchell, R. B. (1990b). Modulation of mammalian O^6-alkylguanine-DNA alkyltransferase in vivo by O^6-benzylguanine and its effect on the sensitivity of a human glioma tumor to 1-(2-chloroethyl)-3-(4-methylcyclohexyl)-1-nitrosourea. *Cancer Comm.*, **2**, 371–7.

Dolan, M. E., Mitchell, R. B. and Mummert, C. (1991). Effect of O^6-benzylguanine analogues on sensitivity of human tumor cells to the cytotoxic effects of alkylating agents. *Cancer Res.*, **51**, 3367–72.

Downes, C. S., Ord, M. J., Mulligan, A. M. et al. (1985). Novobiocin inhibition of DNA excision repair may occur through effects on mitochondrial structure and ATP metabolism, not on repair topoisomerases. *Carcinogenesis*, **6**, 1343–52.

Dulik, D. M., Fenselau, C. and Hilton, J. (1986). Characterization of melphalan-glutathione adducts whose formation is catalyzed by glutathione transferases. *Biochem. Pharmacol.*, **35**, 3405–9.

Dulik, D. M., Colvin, O. M. and Fenselau, C. (1990). Characterization of glutathione conjugates of chlorambucil by fast atom bombardment and thermospray liquid chromatography mass spectrometry. *Biomed. Envir. Mass Spectrometry*, **19**, 248–52.

Duncan, W. (1973). Exploitation of the oxygen enhancement ratio in clinical practice. *Br. Med. Bull.*, **29**, 33.

Durand, R. E. and Goldie, J. H. (1987). Interaction of etoposide and cisplatin in an *in vitro* tumor model. *Cancer Treat. Rep.*, **71**, 673–9.

Earnshaw, W. C., Halligan, B., Cooke, C. A. et al. (1986). Topoisomerase II is a structural component of mitotic chromosome scaffolds. *J. Cell. Biol.*, **100**, 1706–15.

Edenberg, H. J. (1980). Novobiocin inhibition of simian virus 40 DNA replication. *Nature*, **286**, 529–31.

Eder, J. P., Teicher, B. A., Holden, S. A. et al. (1987). Novobiocin enhances alkylating agent cytotoxicity and DNA interstrand crosslinks in a murine model. *J. Clin. Invest.*, **79**, 1524–8.

Eder, J. P., Teicher, B. A., Holden, S. A. and Cathcart, K. N. S. (1989). Effect of novobiocin on the antitumor activity and tumor cell and bone marrow survivals of three alkylating agents. *Cancer Res.*, **49**, 595–8.

Eder, J. P., Teicher, B. A., Holden, S. A. et al. (1990). Ability of four topoisomerase II inhibitors to enhance the cytotoxicity of CDDP in Chinese hamster ovary cells and in an epipodophyllotoxin resistant subline. *Cancer Chemother. Pharmacol.*, **26**, 423–8.

Eder, J. P., Wheeler, C. A., Teicher, B. A. and Schnipper, L. E. (1991). A phase I clinical trial of novobiocin, a modulator of alkylating agent cytotoxicity. *Cancer Res.*, **51**, 510–3.

Ehrly, A. M. (1979). The effect of pentoxifylline on the deformability of erythrocytes and on the muscular oxygen pressure in patients with chronic arterial disease. *J. Med.*, **10**, 331.

Einhorn, L. (1986). Initial therapy with cisplatin plus VP-16 in small-cell lung cancer. *Sem. Oncol.*, **13**(3), 5–9.

Ellis, G. K., Crowley, J., Livingston, R. B. et al. (1991). Cisplatin and novobiocin in the treatment of non-small cell lung cancer. *Cancer*, **67**, 2969–73.

Ellis, L. M., Copeland, E. M., Bland, K. and Sitren, H. S. (1990a). Inhibition of tumor growth and metastasis by chronic intravenous infusion of prostaglandin E_1. *Ann. Surg.*, **212**, 45–50.

Ellis, L. M., Copeland, E. M., Bland, K. I. and Sitren, H. S. (1990b). Differential role of prostaglandin E_1 on tumor metastasis. *J. Surg. Oncol.*, **48**, 333–6.

Endresen, L., Schjerven, L. and Rugstad, H. E. (1984). Tumors from a cell strain with a high content of metallothionein show enhanced resistance against *cis*-dichlorodiammineplatinum. *Acta Pharmacol. Toxicol.*, **55**, 183–91.

Eng, W.-K., Faucette, L., Johnson, R. K. and Sternglanz, R. (1988). Evidence that DNA topoisomerase I is necessary for the cytotoxic effects of camptothecin. *Mol. Pharmacol.*, **34**, 755–60.

Evans, R. G., Kimmler, B. F., Morantz, R. A. et al. (1990). A phase I/II study of the use of Fluosol as an adjuvant to radiation therapy in the treatment of primary high-grade brain tumors. *Int. J. Rad. Oncol. Biol. Phys.*, **19**(2), 415–20.

Evans, R. G., Kimler, B. F., Morantz, R. A. and Batnitzky, S. (1993). Lack of complications in long-term survivors after treatment with Fluosol® and oxygen as an adjuvant to radiation therapy for high-grade brain tumors. *Int. J. Rad. Oncol. Biol. Phys.*, **26**, 649–52.

Fernandes, D. J., Danks, M. K. and Beck, W. T. (1990). Decreased nuclear matrix DNA topoisomerase II in human leukemia cells resistant to VM-26 and m-AMSA. *Biochemistry*, **29**, 4235–41.

Fleckenstein, W. (1990). *Distribution of Oxygen Pressure in the Periphery and Centre of Malignant Head and Neck Tumours*. Blackwell Ueberreuter Wissenchaft, Berlin.

Floridi, A. and Lehninger, A. L. (1983). Action of the antitumor and antispermatogenic agent lonidamine on electron transport in Ehrlich ascites tumor mitochondria. *Arch. Biochem. Biophys.*, **226**, 73–83.

Floridi, A., Paggi, M. G. and D'Atri, S. (1981a). Effect of lonidamine on the energy metabolism of Ehrlich ascites tumor cells. *Cancer Res.*, **41**, 4661–6.

Floridi, A., Paggi, M. G. and Marcante, M. L. (1981b). Lonidamine a selective inhibitor of aerobic glycolysis of murine tumor cells. *J. Natl. Cancer Inst.*, **66**, 497–9.

Floridi, A., Bagnato, A. and Bianchi, C. (1986). Kinetics of inhibition of mitochondrial respiration by antineoplastic agent lonidamine. *J. Exp. Clin. Cancer Res.*, **5**, 273–80.

Folkman, J. (1987). What is the role of angiogenesis in metastasis from cutaneous melanoma? *Eur. J. Cancer Clin. Oncol.*, **23**, 361–3.

Folkman, J. (1990). What is the evidence that tumors are angiogenesis dependent? *J. Natl. Cancer Inst.*, **82**, 4–6.

Folkman, J. and Ingber, D. E. (1987). Angiostatic steroids: method of discovery and mechanism of action. *Ann. Surg.*, **206**, 374–83.

Folkman, J. and Klagsbrun, M. (1987). Angiogenic factors. *Science*, **235**, 442–7.

Folkman, J., Langer, R., Lingardt, R. et al. (1983). Angiogenesis inhibition and tumour regression caused by heparin or a heparin fragment in the presence of cortisone. *Science*, **221**, 719–25.

Folkman, J., Watson, K., Ingber, D. and Hanahan, D. (1989a). Induction of, angiogenesis during the transition from hyperplasis to neoplasia. *Nature*, **339**, 58–61.

Folkman, J., Weisz, P. B., Joullie, M. M. et al. (1989b). Control of angiogenesis with synthetic heparin substitutes. *Science*, **243**, 1490–3.

Fowler, J. F. (1985). Chemical modifiers of radiosensitivity – theory and reality: a review. *Int. J. Rad. Oncol. Biol. Phys.*, **11**(4), 665–74.

Fowler, J. R., Thomlinson, R. H. and Howes, A. E. (1970). Time–dose relationships in radiotherapy. *Eur. J. Cancer*, **6**, 207.

Franko, A. J. (1986). Misonidazole and other hypoxia markers. Metabolism and applications. *Int. J. Rad. Oncol. Biol. Phys.*, **12**, 1195–202.

Frei III, E., Holden, S. A., Gonin, R. et al. (1993). Antitumor alkylating agents: *in vitro* cross-resistance and collateral sensitivity studies. *Cancer Chemother. Pharmacol.*, **33**, 113–22.

Friedman, H. S., Colvin, O. M., Kaufmann, S. H. et al. (1992a). Cyclophosphamide resistance in medulloblastoma. *Cancer Res.*, **52**, 5373–8.

Friedman, H. S., Dolan, M. E., Moschel, R. C. et al. (1992b). Enhancement of nitrosourea activity in medulloblastoma and glioblastoma multiforme. *J. Natl. Cancer Inst.*, **84**, 1926–31.

Fujiwara, T., Mukhopadhyay, T., Cai, D. W. et al. (1994). Retroviral-mediated transduction of *p53* gene increases TGF-β expression in a human glioblastoma cell line. *Int. J. Cancer*, **56**, 834–9.

Fukushima, M. (1992). Biological activities and mechanisms of action of PGJ2 and related compounds: an update. *Prostaglandins Leukotrienes and Essential Fatty Acids*, **47**, 1–12.

Gadient, R. A., Cron, K. C. and Otten, U. (1990). Interleukin-1β and tumor necrosis factor-α synergistically stimulate nerve growth factor (NGF) release from cultured rat astrocytes. *Neurosci. Letters*, **117**, 335–40.

Gamcsik, M. P., Hamill, T. G. and Colvin, M. (1990). NMR studies of the conjugation of mechlorethamine with glutathione. *J. Med. Chem.*, **33**, 1009–14.

Gasser, S. M. and Laemmli, U. K. (1986). The organization of chromatin loops: characterization of a scaffold attchment site. *EMBO J.*, **5**, 511–8.

Gatenby, R. A., Kessler, H. B., Rosenblum, J. S. et al. (1988). Oxygen distribution in squamous cell carcinoma metastases and its relationship to outcome of therapy. *Int. J. Rad. Oncol. Biol. Phys.*, **14**, 831–8.

Gedick, C. M. and Collins, A. R. (1990). Comparison of effects of fostriecin, novobiocin, and camptothecin, inhibitors of DNA topoisomerases, on DNA replication and repair in human cells. *Nucl. Acids. Res.*, **18**, 1007.

Gerson, S. L., Trey, J. E. and Miller, K. (1988). Potentiation of nitrosourea cytotoxicity in human leukemic cells by inactivation of O⁶-alkylguanine-DNA alkyltransferase. *Cancer Res.*, **48**, 1521–7.

Giaver, G. N. and Wang, J. C. (1988). Supercoiling of intracellular DNA can occur in eukaryotic cells. *Cell*, **55**, 849–56.

Gilmour, D. S. and Elgin, S. C. R. (1987). Localization of specific topoisomerase I interactions within the transcribed region of active heat shock genes by using the inhibitor camptothecin. *Mol. Cell. Biol.*, **7**, 141–8.

Gilmour, D. S., Pflugfelder, G., Wang, J. C. and Lis, J. T. (1986). Topoisomerase I interacts with transcribed regions in Drosophila cells. *Cell*, **44**, 401–7.

Giovanella, B. C., Stehlin, J. S., Wall, M. E. et al. (1989). DNA topoisomerase I-targeted chemotherapy of human colon cancer in xenografts. *Science*, **246**, 1046–8.

Giovanella, B. C., Hinz, H. R., Kozielski, A. J. et al. (1991). Complete growth inhibition of human cancer xenografts in nude mice by treatment with 20-(S)-camptothecin. *Cancer Res.*, **51**, 3052–5.

Gold, L. I., Saxena, B., Mittal, K. R. et al. (1994). Increased expression of transforming growth factor β isoforms and basic fibroblast growth factor in complex hyperplasia and adenocarcinoma of the endometrium: evidence for paracrine and autocrine action. *Cancer Res.*, **54**, 2347–58.

Golub, L. M., Lee, H. M., Nemiroff, L. A. et al. (1983). Minocycline reduces gingival collagenolytic activity during diabetes. Preliminary observations and a proposed new mechanism of action. *J. Periodontal Res.*, **18**, 516–26.

Golub, L. M., McNamara, T. F., D'Angelo, G. et al. (1987). A non-antibacterial chemically-modified tetracycline inhibits mammalian collagenase activity. *J. Dental Res.*, **66**, 1310–4.

Golub, L. M., Ramamurthy, N. S., McNamara, T. F. et al. (1991). Tetracyclines inhibit connective tissue breakdown: new therapeutic implications for an old family of drugs. *Crit. Rev. Oral. Biol. Med.*, **2**, 297–321.

Gottesfeld, J. (1986). Novobiocin inhibits RNA polymerase III transcription *in vitro* by a mechanism distinct from DNA topoisomerase II. *Nucl. Acids Res.*, **14**, 2075–88.

Green, J. A., Vistica, D. T., Young, R. C. et al. (1984). Potentiation of melphalan cytotoxicity in human ovarian cancer cell lines by glutathione depletion. *Cancer Res.*, **44**, 5427–31.

Greenwald, R. A., Golub, L. M., Lavietes, B. et al. (1987). Tetracyclines inhibit human synovial collagenase in vivo and in vitro. *J. Rheumatol.*, **14**, 28–32.

Gullino, P. M. (1975). *In vivo* utilization of oxygen and glucose by neoplastic tissue. *Adv. Exp. Med. Biol.*, **75**, 521–36.

Hahn, G. M. and Shiu, E. C. (1986). Adaptation to low pH modifies thermal and thermochemical responses of mammalian cells. *Int. J. Hyperthermia*, **2**, 379–87.

Hahn, G. M., vanKersen, I. and Silvestrini, B. (1984). Inhibition of the recovery from potentially lethal damage of lonidamine. *Br. J. Cancer*, **50**, 657–60.

Hall, E. J. (1978). *Radiobiology for the Radiobiologist*. Philadelphia, Harper & Row.

Hanauske, A. R., Degen, D., Marshall, M. H. et al. (1992). Effect of recombinant interleukin-1α on clonogenic growth of primary human tumors *in vitro*. *J. Immunother.*, **11**, 155–8.

Harris Jr, E. D. (1985). *Textbook of Rheumatology*. W. B. Saunders, Philadelphia.

Harris Jr, E. D., Welgus, H. B. and Krane, S. M. (1984). Collagen. *Relat. Res.*, **4**, 493–512.

Hasegawa, T., Rhee, J. G., Levitt, S. H. and Song, C. W. (1987). Increase in tumor pO_2 by perfluorochemicals and carbogen. *Int. J. Rad. Oncol. Biol. Phys.*, **13**, 569–74.

Heck, M. M. S., Hittelman, W. N. and Earnshaw, W. C. (1988). Differential expression of topoisomerases I and II during the eukaryotic cell cycle. *Proc. Natl. Acad. Sci. USA*, **85**, 1086–90.

Herman, M. E. and Katzenellenbogen, B. S. (1994). Alterations in transforming growth factor-α and -β production and cell responsiveness during the progression of MCF-7 human breast cancer cells to estrogen-autonomous growth. *Cancer Res.*, **54**, 5867–74.

Herman, T. S. and Teicher, B. A. (1988). Sequencing of trimodality therapy [*cis*-diamminedichloroplatinum(II)/hyperthermia/radiation] as determined by tumor growth delay and tumor cell survival in the FSaIIC fibrosarcoma. *Cancer Res.*, **48**, 2693–7.

Herman, T. S., Teicher, B. A. and Collins, L. S. (1988a). Effect of hypoxia and acidosis on the cytotoxicity of four platinum complexes at normal and hyperthermic temperatures. *Cancer Res.*, **48**, 2342–7.

Herman, T. S., Teicher, B. A., Jochelson, M. et al. (1988b). Rationale for use of local hyperthermia with radiation therapy and selected anticancer drugs in locally advanced human malignancies. *Int. J. Hyperthermia*, **4**, 143–58.

Herman, T. S., Teicher, B. A., Holden, S. A. and Collins, L. C. (1989). Interaction of hyperthermia and radiation: hypoxia and acidosis *in vitro*, tumor subpopulations *in vivo*. *Cancer Res.*, **49**, 3338–43.

Herman, T. S., Teicher, B. A., Holden, S. A. et al. (1990). Addition of 2-nitroimidazole radiosensitizers to trimodality therapy (*cis*-diamminedichloroplatinum II/hyperthermia/radiation) in the murine FSaIIC fibrosarcoma. *Cancer Res.*, **50**, 2734–40.

Hertzberg, R. P., Busby, R. W., Caranfa, M. J. et al. (1990). Irreversible trapping of the DNA-topoisomerase I covalent complex. *J. Biol. Chem.*, **265**, 19287–95.

Hill, R. P. (1986). Sensitizers and radiation dose fractionation: results and interpretations. *Int. J. Rad. Oncol. Biol. Phys.*, **12**, 1049–54.

Hla, T. and Maciag, T. (1991). Cyclooxygenase gene expression is down-regulated by heparin-binding (acidic fibroblast) growth factor-1 in human endothelial cells. *J. Biol. Chem.*, **266**(35), 24059–63.

Holden, S. A., Teicher, B. A., Ha, C. et al. (1992). Enhancement by perfusion emulsion (Oxygent®) and carbogen breathing of the tumor growth delay of the FSaIIC fibrosarcoma after treatment with antitumor alkylating agents. *Biomat. Artif. Cells Immob. Biotechnol.*, **20**, 895–8.

Honn, K. V., Busse, W. D. and Sloane, B. F. (1983). Commentary. Prostacyclin and thromboxanes: Implications for their role in tumor cell metastasis. *Biochem. Pharmacol.*, **32**, 1–11.

Howells, G. L., Chantry, D. and Feldman, M. (1988). Interleukin 1 (IL-1) and tumor necrosis factor synergise in the induction of IL-1 synthesis by human vascular endothelial cells. *Immunol. Letters*, **19**, 169–74.

Hsu, S., Huang, F., Hafez, M. et al. (1994). Colon carcinoma cells switch their response to transforming growth factor β1 with tumor progression. *Cell Growth Differ.*, **5**, 267–75.

Hubbard, W. C., Alley, M. C., McLemore, T. L. and Boyd, M. R. (1988a). Evidence for thromboxane biosynthesis in established cell lines derived from human lung adenocarcinomas. *Cancer Res.*, **48**, 2674–7.

Hubbard, W. C., Alley, M. C., McLemore, T. L. and Boyd, M. R. (1988b). Profiles of prostaglandin biosynthesis in sixteen established cell lines derived from human lung, colon, prostate, and ovarian tumors. *Cancer Res.*, **48**, 4770–5.

Hubbard, W. C., Alley, M. C., Gray, G. N. et al. (1989). Evidence for prostanoid biosynthesis as a biochemical feature of certain subclasses of non-small cell carcinomas of the lung as determined in established cell lines derived from human lung tumors. *Cancer Res.*, **49**, 826–32.

Hubbard, W. C., Alley, M. C., McLemore, T. L. and Boyd, M. R. (1991). Fatty acid cyclooxygenase metabolism of arachidonic acid in human tumor cells. In *Eicosanoids and other bioactive lipids in cancer and radiation injury*, ed. K. V. Honn, L. J. Marnett, S. Nigam and T. Walden Jr. pp. 27–32. Norwell, MA: Kluwer Academic Publishers.

Ingber, D. and Folkman, J. (1988). Inhibition of angiogenesis through modulation of collagen metabolism. *Lab. Invest.*, **59**, 44–51.

88 *B. A. Teicher & E. Frei III*

Ingber, D. E., Madri, J. A. and Folkman, J. (1986). A possible mechanism for inhibition of angiogenesis by angiostatic steroids: induction of capillary basement membrane dissolution. *Endocrinology*, **119**, 1768–75.

Issell, B. F., Muggia, F. M. and Carter, S. F. (1984). *Etoposide (VP-16): Current Status and New Developments*. Academic, New York.

Jain, R. K. (1988). Determinants of tumor blood flow: a review. *Cancer Res.*, **48**, 2641–58.

Jennings, M. T., Kaariainen, I. T., Gold, L. et al. (1994). TGFβ1 and TGFβ2 are potential growth regulators for medulloblastomas, primitive neuroectodermal tumors, and ependymomas: evidence in support of an autocrine hypothesis. *Human Pathol.*, **25**, 464–75.

Johnson, R. K., McCabe, F. L., Faucette, L. F. et al. (1989). SK&F 104864, a water-soluble analog of camptothecin with broad-spectrum activity in preclinical tumor models. *Proc. Am. Assoc. Cancer Res.*, **30**, 623.

Jouanneau, J., Moens, G., Bourgeois, Y. et al. (1994). A minority of carcinoma cells producing acidic fibroblast growth factor induces a community effect for tumor progression. *Proc. Natl. Acad. Sci. USA*, **91**, 286–90.

Kallinowski, F. and Vaupel, P. (1988). pH distributions in spontaneous and isotransplanted rat tumours. *Br. J. Cancer*, **58**, 134–321.

Kallinowski, F., Zander, R., Höckel, M. and Vaupel, P. (1990). Tumor tissue oxygenation as evaluated by computerized-pO_2-histography. *Int. J. Rad. Oncol. Biol. Phys.*, **19**, 953–61.

Kayanoki, Y., Fujii, J., Suzuki, K. et al. (1994). Suppression of antioxidative enzyme expression by transforming growth factor-β1 in rat hepatocytes. *J. Biol. Chem.*, **269**(22), 15488–92.

Kelley, S. L., Basu, A., Teicher, B. A. et al. (1988). Overexpression of metallothionein confers resistance to anticancer drugs. *Science*, **241**, 1813–5.

Kennedy, K. A., Teicher, B. A., Rockwell, S. A. and Sartorelli, A. C. (1980). The hypoxic tumor cell: a target for selective cancer chemotherapy. *Bioch. Pharmacol.*, **29**, 1–8.

Kennedy, K. A., Teicher, B. A., Rockwell, S. A. and Sartorelli, A. C. (1981). *Chemotherapeutic Approaches to Cell Populations in Tumors*. Academic Press, New York.

Keyes, S. R., Rockwell, S. and Sartorelli, A. C. (1985). Porfiromycin as a bioreductive alkylating agent with selective toxicity to hypoxic EMT6 tumor cells in vivo and in vitro. *Cancer Res.*, **45**, 3642–5.

Kilian, P. L., Kaffka, K. L., Biondi, D. A. et al. (1991). Antiproliferative effect of interleukin-1 on human ovarian carcinoma cell line (NIH:OVCAR-3). *Cancer Res.*, **51**, 1823–8.

Kim, J. H., Alfieri, A. and Kim, S. H. (1984a). Radiosensitization of Meth-A fibrosarcoma in mice by lonidamine. *Oncology*, **41**, 36–8.

Kim, J. H., Kim, S. H. and Alfieri, A. (1984b). Lonidamine: A hyperthermic sensitizer of HeLa cells in culture and of the Meth-A tumor *in vivo*. *Oncology*, **41**, 30–5.

Kim, J. H., Alfieri, A. A. and Kim, S. H. (1986). Potentiation of radiation effects of two murine tumors by lonidamine. *Cancer Res.*, **46**, 1120–3.

Klastersky, J. (1986). Therapy with cisplatin and etoposide for non-small cell lung cancer. *Sem. Oncol.*, **13**(3), 104–14.

Kohn, K. W. (1977). Interstrand cross-linking of DNA by 1,3-bis(2-chloroethyl)-1-nitrosourea and other 1-(2-haloethyl)-1-nitrosoureas. *Cancer Res.*, **37**, 1450–4.

Korczak, B., Kerbel, R. S. and Dennis, J. W. (1991). Autocrine and paracrine regulation of tissue inhibitor of metalloproteinases, transin, and urokinase gene expression in metastatic and nonmetastatic mammary carcinoma cells. *Cell Growth Differ.*, **2**(7), 335–41.

Kramer, R. A., Greene, K., Ahmad, S. and Vistica, D. T. (1987). Chemosensitization of L-phenylalanine mustard by the thiol-modulating agent buthionine sulfoximine. *Cancer Res.*, **47**, 1593–7.

Kupfer, G., Bodley, A. L. and Liu, L. F. (1987). Involvement of intracellular ATP in cytotoxicity of topoisomerase II-targetting antitumor drugs. *NCI Monograph*, **4**, 37–40.

Kupper, T. S. (1988). Interleukin 1 and other human keratinocyte cytokines: molecular and functional characterization. *Adv. Dermatol.*, **3**, 293–308.

Kupper, T. S., Lee, F., Birchall, N. et al., (1988). Interleukin 1 binds to specific receptors on human keratinocytes and induces granulocyte macrophage colony-stimulating factor mRNA and protein. A potential autocrine role for interleukin 1 in epidermis. *J. Clin. Invest.*, **82**, 1787–92.

Laekeman, G. M., Vergote, I. B., Keersmaekers, G. M. et al. (1986). Prostacyclin and thromboxane in benign and malignant breast tumours. *Br. J. Cancer*, **54**, 431–7.

Laver, M. D., Jackson, E., Scherperel, M. et al. (1977). Hemoglobin-O$_2$ affinity regulation; DPF, monovalent ions, and hemoglobin concentration. *J. Appl. Physiol.*, **43**, 632–42.

Lee, F. Y. F., Flannery, D. J. and Siemann, D. W. (1992). Modulation of the cell cycle-dependent cytotoxicity of adriamycin and 4-hydroperoxycyclophosphamide by novobiocin, an inhibitor of mammalian topoisomerase II. *Cancer Res.*, **52**, 3515–20.

Lee, I., Levitt, S. H. and Song, C. W. (1987a). Effects of Fluosol-DA 20% and carbogen on the radioresponse of SCK tumors and skin of A/J mice. *Rad. Res.*, **112**, 173–82.

Lee, I., Levitt, S. H. and Song, C. W. (1990). Radiosensitization of murine tumors by Fluosol-DA 20%. *Rad. Res.*, **122**, 275–9.

Lee, I., Kim, J. H., Levitt, S. H. and Song, C. W. (1992). Increases in tumor response by pentoxifylline alone or in combination with nicotinamide. *Int. J. Rad. Oncol. Biol. Phys.*, **22**, 425–9.

Lee, K.-E., Erturk, E., Mayer, R. and Cockett, A. T. K. (1987b). Efficacy of antitumor chemotherapy in C3H mice enhanced by the antiangiogenesis steroid, cortisone acetate. *Cancer Res.*, **47**, 5021–4.

Levin, V. A. (1985). Chemotherapy of primary brain tumors. *Neurol. Clin.*, **3**, 855–66.

Liotta, L. A., Steeg, P. S. and Stetler-Stevenson, W. G. (1991). Cancer metastasis and angiogenesis: an imbalance of positive and negative regulation. *Cell*, **64**, 327–36.

Liu, L. F. (1989). DNA topoisomerase poisons as anti-tumor drugs. *Ann. Rev. Biochem.*, **58**, 351–75.

Long, B. H. and Minocha, A. (1983). Inhibition of topoisomerase II by VP-16-213 (etoposide), VM-26 (teniposide) and structured congeners as an explanation for *in vivo* DNA breakage and cytotoxicity. *Proc. Am. Assoc. Cancer Res.*, **24**, 1271.

Long, B. H., Musial, S. T. and Brattain, M. G. (1984). Comparison of cytotoxicity and DNA breakage activity of congeners of epipodophyllotoxin including VP-16-213 and VM-26: a quantitative structure-activity relationship. *Biochemistry*, **23**, 1183–8.

90   *B. A. Teicher & E. Frei III*

Lustig, R., McIntosh-Lowe, N. L., Rose, C. et al. (1989). Phase I/II study of
    Fluosol-DA and 100% oxygen breathing as an adjuvant to radiation in the
    treatment of advanced squamous cell tumors of the head and neck. *Int. J. Rad.
    Oncol. Biol. Phys.*, **16**, 1587–94.
Lustig, R., Lowe, N., Prosnitz, L. et al. (1990). Fluosol and oxygen breathing as an
    adjuvant to radiation therapy in the treatment of locally advanced non-small
    cell carcinoma of the lung: results of a phase I/II study. *Int. J. Rad. Oncol.
    Biol. Phys.*, **19**(1), 97–102.
Maca, R. D. (1988). Inhibition of the growth of Lewis lung carcinoma by
    indomethacin in conventional, nude, and beige mice. *J. Biol. Response
    Modifiers*, **7**, 568–80.
MacCallum, J., Bartlett, J. M. S., Thompson, A. M. et al. (1994). Expression of
    transforming growth factor beta mRNA isoforms in human breast cancer. *Br.
    J. Cancer*, **69**, 1006–9.
Markovits, J., Pommier, Y., Kerrigan, D. et al. (1987). Topoisomerase II-mediated
    DNA breaks and cytotoxicity in relation to cell proliferation and the cell cycle
    in NIH 3T3 fibroblasts and L1210 leukemia cells. *Cancer Res.*, **47**, 2050–5.
Marnett, L. J. (1992). Aspirin and the potential role of prostaglandins in colon
    cancer. *Cancer Res.*, **52**, 5575–89.
Martin, D. F., Porter, E. A., Fischer, J. J. and Rockwell, S. (1987). Effect of a
    perfluorochemical emulsion on the radiation response of BA-1112
    rhabdomyosarcomas. *Rad. Res.*, **112**, 45–53.
Mattern, M. R. and Painter, R. B. (1979). Dependence of mammalian DNA
    replication on DNA supercoiling. *Biochim. Biophys. Acta*, **563**, 306–12.
Mattern, M. R., Paone, R. F. and Day III, R. S. (1982). Eukaryotic DNA repair is
    blocked at different steps by inhibitors of DNA topoisomerases and of DNA
    polymerases α and β. *Biochim. Biophys. Acta*, **697**, 6–13.
Mattern, M. R., Mong, S.-M., Bartus, H. F. et al. (1987). Relationship between the
    intracellular effects of camptothecin and the inhibition of DNA topoisomerase
    I in cultured L1210 cells. *Cancer Res.*, **47**, 1793–8.
Mattern, M. R., Hofmann, G. A., McCabve, F. L. and Johnson, R. K. (1991).
    Synergistic cell killing by ionizing radiation and topoisomerase I inhibitor
    topotecan (SK&F 104864). *Cancer Res.*, **51**, 5813–6.
Mauviel, A., Termine, N., Charron, D. et al. (1988). Interleukin-1α and β induce
    interleukin-1β gene expression in human dermal fibroblasts. *Biochem. Biophys.
    Res. Comm.*, **156**, 1209–14.
McGown, A. T. and Fox, B. W. (1986). A proposed mechanism of resistance to
    cyclophosphamide and phosphoramide mustard in a Yoshida cell line *in vitro*.
    Cancer Chemother. Pharmacol., **17**, 223–6.
McLemore, T. L., Hubbard, W. C., Litterst, C. L. et al. (1988). Profiles of
    prostaglandin biosynthesis in normal lung and tumor tissue from lung cancer
    patients. *Cancer Res.*, **48**, 3140–7.
Merz, V. W., Arnold, A. M. and Studer, U. E. (1994). Differential expression of
    transforming growth factor-β1 and β3 as well as *C-FOS* mRNA in normal
    human prostate, benign prostatic hyperplasia and prostatic cancer. *World J.
    Urol.*, **12**, 96–8.
Merzak, A., McCrea, S., Koocheckpour, S. and Pilkington, G. J. (1994). Control of
    human glioma cell growth, migration and invasion *in vitro* by transforming
    growth factor β1. *Br. J. Cancer*, **70**, 199–203.
Miller, B. E., Miller, F. R., Machemer, T. and Heppner, G. H. (1993). Melphalan
    sensitivity as a function of progressive metastatic growth in two
    subpopulations of a mouse mammary tumour. *Br. J. Cancer*, **68**(1), 18–25.

Miller, F. R. and Heppner, G. H. (1990). Cellular interactions in metastasis. *Cancer and Metastasis Reviews*, 9(1), 21–34.

Miossec, P., Cavender, D. and Ziff, M. (1986). Production of interleukin 1 by human endothelial cells. *J. Immunol.*, 136, 2486–91.

Mitchell, R. B., Moschel, R. C. and Dolan, M. E. (1992). Effect of O^6-benzylguanine on the sensitivity of human tumor xenografts to 1,3-bis(2-chloroethyl)-1-nitrosourea and on DNA interstrand cross-link formation. *Cancer Res.*, 52(5), 1171–5.

Momparler, R. L. (1980). *In vitro* systems for evaluation of combination chemotherapy. *Pharmacol. Ther. Part A Chemother. Toxicol. Metab. Inhib.*, 8, 21–35.

Morinaga, Y., Hayashi, H., Takeuchi, A. and Onozaki, K. (1990). Antiproliferative effect of Interleukin 1 (IL-1) on tumor cells: G0–G1 arrest of a human melanoma cell line by IL-1. *Biochem. Biophys. Res. Commun.*, 173, 186–92.

Morrone, G., Cortese, R. and Sorrentino, V. (1989). Post-transcriptional control of negative acute phase genes by transforming growth factor beta. *EMBO J.*, 8(12), 3767–71.

Moulder, J. E. and Fish, B. L. (1987). *Tumor sensitization by the intermittent use of perfluorochemical emulsions and carbogen breathing with fractionated radiotherapy.* Taylor and Francis, Inc., London.

Moulder, J. E., Dutreix, J., Rockwell, S. and Siemann, D. W. (1988). Applicability of animal tumor data to cancer therapy in humans. *Int. J. Rad. Oncol. Biol. Phys.*, 14, 913–27.

Muir, G. H., Butta, A., Shearer, R. J. et al. (1994). Induction of transforming growth factor beta in hormonally treated human prostate cancer. *Br. J. Cancer*, 69, 130–4.

Mukaida, H., Hirabayashi, N., Hirai, T. et al. (1991). Significance of freshly cultured fibroblasts from different tissues in promoting cancer cell growth. *Int. J. Cancer*, 48(3), 423–7.

Nakamura, T., Tomita, Y., Hirai, R. et al. (1985). Inhibitory effect of transforming growth factor-β on DNA synthesis of adult rat hepatocytes in primary culture. *Biochem. Biophys. Res. Comm.*, 133(3), 1042–50.

Natale, R. B. and Wittes, R. E. (1982). Combination *cis*-platinum and etoposide in small-cell lung cancer. *Cancer Treat. Rev.*, 9(A), 91–4.

Nawroth, P. P., Bank, I., Handley, D. et al. (1986). Tumor necrosis factor/cachectin interacts with endothelial cell receptors to induce release of interleukin 1. *J. Exp. Med.*, 163, 1363–75.

Nelson, W. G., Liu, L. F. and Coffey, D. S. (1986). Newly replicated DNA is associated with DNA topoisomerase II in cultured rat prostatic adenocarcinoma cells. *Nature*, 322, 187–9.

Nicolson, G. L., Dulski, K. M. and Trosko, J. E. (1988). Loss of intercellular junctional communication correlates with metastatic potential in mammary adenocarcinoma cells. *Proc. Natl. Acad. Sci. USA*, 85(2), 473–6.

Nowak, R. A., Morrison, N. E., Goad, D. L. et al. (1990). Squamous cell carcinomas often produce more than a single bone resorption-stimulating factor: role of interleukin-1α. *Endocrinology*, 127, 3061–9.

Oates, J. A., Fitzgerald, G. A., Branch, R. A. et al. (1988). Medical Progress: clinical implications of prostaglandin and thromboxane A_2 formation. *N. Engl. J. Med.*, 319(11), 689–98.

Ohmura, E., Okada, M., Onoda, N. et al. (1990). Insulin-like growth factor I and transforming growth factor alpha as autocrine growth factors in human pancreatic cancer cell growth. *Cancer Res.*, 50(1), 103–7.

Osheroff, N. (1986). Eukaryotic topoisomerase II. Characterization of enzyme turnover. *J. Biol. Chem.*, **261**, 9944–50.

Ozols, R. F., Louie, K. G., Plowman, J. et al. (1987). Enhanced melphalan cytotoxicity in human ovarian cancer in vitro and in tumor-bearing nude mice by buthionine sulfoximine depletion of glutathione. *Biochem. Pharmacol.*, **36**, 147–53.

Partridge, M., Chantry, D., Turner, M. and Feldmann, M. (1991). Production of interleukin-1 and interleukin-6 by human keratinocytes and squamous cell carcinoma cells. *J. Invest. Dermatol.*, **96**, 771–6.

Paulson, J. R. and Laemmli, U. K. (1977). The structure of histone-depleted metaphase chromosomes. *Cell*, **12**, 817–28.

Pegg, A. E. (1990). Mammalian O^6-alkylguanine-DNA alkyltransferase: regulation and importance in response to alkylating carcinogenic and therapeutic agents. *Cancer Res.*, **50**, 6119–29.

Penhaligon, M. and Camplejohn, R. S. (1985). Combination heparin plus cortisone treatment of two transplanted tumors in C3H/He mice. *J. Natl. Cancer Inst.*, **74**, 869–73.

Perego, M. S., Sergio, G., Artale, F. et al. (1986). Haemorheological improvement by pentoxifylline in patients with peripheral arterial occlusive disease. *Curr. Med. Res. Opin.*, **10**, 135.

Pfeffer, M. R., Teicher, B. A., Holden, S. A. et al. (1991). The interaction of cisplatin plus etoposide with radiation ± hyperthermia. *Int. J. Rad. Oncol. Biol. Phys.*, **19**, 1439–47.

Picard, O., Rolland, Y. and Poupon, M. F. (1986). Fibroplast-dependent tumorigenicity of cells in nude mice: implication for implantation of metastases. *Cancer Res.*, **46**(7), 3290–4.

Poggesi, L., Scarti, L., Boddi, M. et al. (1985). Pentoxifylline treatment in patients with occlusive peripheral vascular disease. *Angiology*, **36**, 268.

Pommier, Y., Schwartz, R. E., Zwelling, L. A. et al. (1986). Reduced formation of protein-associated DNA strand breaks in Chinese hamster cells resistant to topoisomerase II inhibitors. *Cancer Res.*, **46**, 611–6.

Pritchett, T. R., Wang, J. K. M. and Jones, P. A. (1989). Mesenchymal–epithelial interactions between normal and transformed human bladder cells. *Cancer Res.*, **49**(10), 2750–4.

Pyke, C., Ralfkiaer, E., Huhtala, P. et al. (1992). Localization of messenger RNA for Mr 72,000 and 92,000 type IV collagenases in human skin cancers by *in situ* hybridization. *Cancer Res.*, **52**, 1336–41.

Rapoport, S. and Guest, G. M. (1941). Distribution of acid-soluble phosphorus in the blood cells of various vertebrates. *J. Biol. Chem.*, **138**, 269–80.

Rhodes, T. and Twentyman, P. R. (1992). A study of ethacrynic acid as a potential modifier of melphalan and cisplatin sensitivity in human lung cancer parental and drug-resistant cell lines. *Br. J. Cancer*, **65**, 684–90.

Roberts, A. B. and Sporn, M. B. (1988). Transforming growth factor β. *Adv. Cancer Res.*, **51**, 107–45.

Roberts, A. B. and Sporn, M. B. (1990). The transforming growth factor-betas. *Handbook Exp. Pharmacol.*, **95**, 419–72.

Roberts, A. B. and Sporn, M. B. (1993). Physiological actions and clinical applications of transforming growth factor-β (TGF-β). *Growth Factors*, **8**, 1–9.

Roberts, A. B., Joyce, M. E., Bolander, M. E. and Sporn, M. B. (1990). Transforming growth factor-beta (TGF-β): a multifunctional effector of both soft and hard tissue regeneration. In *Growth Factors in Health and Disease*:

Basic and Clinical Aspects (ed. B. Westermark, C. Betsholtz and B. Hökfelt), pp. 89–101. Excerpta Medica, Amsterdam.

Rockwell, S., Mato, T. P., Irvin, C. G. and Nierenburg, M. (1986). Reactions of tumors and normal tissues in mice to irradiation in the presence and absence of a perfluorochemical emulsion. *Int. J. Rad. Oncol. Biol. Phys.*, **12**, 1315–8.

Rodeck, U., Bossler, A., Graeven, U. et al. (1994). Transforming growth factor β production and responsiveness in normal human melanocytes and melanoma cells. *Cancer Res.*, **54**, 575–81.

Rosbe, K. W., Brann, T. W. and Holden, S. A. (1989). Effect of lonidamine on the cytotoxicity of four alkylating agents *in vitro*. *Cancer Chemother. Pharmacol.*, **25**, 32–6.

Rose, C. M., Lustig, R., McIntosh, N. and Teicher, B. A. (1986). A clinical trial of Fluosol-DA® 20% in advanced squamous cell carcinoma of the head and neck. *Int. J. Rad. Oncol. Biol. Phys.*, **12**, 1325–7.

Ross, W. E. (1985). DNA topoisomerases as targets for cancer therapy. *Biochem. Pharmacol.*, **34**, 4191–5.

Rothwell, N. J. (1991). Functions and mechanisms of interleukin-1 in the brain. *Trends Pharmacol. Sci.*, **12**, 430–6.

Rowinsky, E. K., Grochow, L. B., Hendricks, C. B. et al. (1992). Phase I and pharmacologic study of topotecan: A novel topoisomerase I inhibitor. *J. Clin. Oncol.*, **10**, 647–56.

Rubin, P. and Casarett, G. (1966). Microcirculation of tumors part I: anatomy, function and necrosis. *Clin. Radiol.*, **17**, 220–9.

Sakiya, S., Oosaki, T., Andoh, S. et al. (1989). Mechanisms of resistance to *cis*-diamminedichloroplatinum(II) in a rat ovarian carcinoma cell line. *Eur. J. Cancer Clin. Oncol.*, **25**, 429–37.

Salo, T. and Oikarinen, J. (1985). Regulation of type IV collagen degrading enzyme by cortisol during human skin fibroblast growth. *Biochem. Biophys. Res. Commun.*, **130**, 588–95.

Samuelsson, B., Dahlén, S.-E., Lindgren, J. Å. et al. (1987). Leukotrienes and lipoxins: structures, biosynthesis, and biological effects. *Science*, **237**, 1171–6.

Sartorelli, A. C. (1988). Therapeutic attack of hypoxic cells of solid tumors: presidential address. *Cancer Res.*, **48**, 775–8.

Schwartz, G. N., Teicher, B. A., Eder, J. P. J. et al. (1993). Modulation of antitumor alkylating agents by novobiocin, topotecan and lonidamine. *Cancer Chemother. Pharmacol.*, **32**, 455–62.

Selawry, O. S. and Hansen, H. H. (1982). Lung cancer. In *Cancer Medicine* (ed. J. F. Holland and E. Frei), pp. 1735–9. Philadelphia: Lea & Febiger, Philadelphia.

Sevick, E. M. and Jain, R. K. (1989). Geometric resistance to blood flow in solid tumors perfused *ex vivo*: effects of tumor size and perfusion pressure. *Cancer Res.*, **49**, 3513–9.

Sgagias, M. K., Kasid, A. and Danforth, D. N. (1991). Interleukin-1α and tumor necrosis factor-α (TNF α) inhibit growth and induce TNF messenger RNA in MCF-7 human breast cancer cells. *Mol. Endocrinol.*, **5**, 1740–7.

Siemann, D. W. and Keng, P. C. (1988). Characterization of radiation resistant hypoxic cell subpopulations in KHT sarcomas. (ii) Cell sorting. *Br. J. Cancer*, **58**, 296–300.

Sierocki, J. S., Hilaris, B. S., Hopfan, S. et al. (1979). *cis*-Diamminedichloroplatinum(II) and VP-16-213: an active induction

regimen for small cell carcinoma of the lung. *Cancer Treat. Rep.*, **63**, 1593–7.
Skapek, S., Colvin, O. M., Griffith, O. et al. (1988). Enhanced melphalan
    cytotoxicity following butathionine sulfoximine-mediated glutathione depletion
    in a human medulloblastoma xenograft in athymic mice. *Cancer Res.*, **48**,
    2764–7.
Smith, W. L. (1989). The eicosanoids and their biochemical mechanisms of action.
    Biochem. J., **259**, 315–24.
Somfai-Relle, S., Suzukake, K., Vistica, B. P. and Vistica, D. T. (1984). Reduction
    in cellular glutathione by buthionine sulfoximine and sensitization of murine
    tumor cells resistant to L-phenylalanine mustard. *Biochem. Pharmacol.*, **33**,
    485–90.
Song, C. W., Lee, I., Hasegawa, T. et al. (1987). Increase in pO_2 and
    radiosensitivity of tumors by Fluosol-DA (20%) and carbogen. *Cancer Res.*,
    47, 442–6.
Sotomayor, E. A., Teicher, B. A., Schwartz, G. N. et al. (1992). Minocycline in
    combination with chemotherapy or radiation therapy in vitro and in vivo.
    Cancer Chemother. Pharmacol., **30**, 377–84.
Sporn, M. B. and Roberts, A. B. (1993). A major advance in the use of growth
    factors to enhance wound healing. *J. Clin. Invest.*, **92**, 2565–6.
Stewart, A. F. and Schutz, G. (1987). Camptothecin-induced in vivo topoisomerase
    I cleavages in the transcriptionally active tyrosine aminotransferase gene. *Cell*,
    50, 1109–17.
Stewart, A. F., Herrera, R. E. and Nordheim, A. (1990). Rapid induction of *c-fos*
    transcription reveals quantitative linkage of RNA polymerase II and DNA
    topoisomerase I enzyme activities. *Cell*, **60**, 141–9.
Szekely, J. G., Lobreau, A. U. and Delaney, S. (1989). Morphological effects
    of lonidamine on two human-tumor cell culture lines. *Microscopy*, **3**,
    681–93.
Tamargo, R. J., Bok, R. A. and Brem, H. (1991). Angiogenesis inhibition by
    minocycline. *Cancer Res.*, **51**, 672–5.
Tanaka, J., Teicher, B. A., Herman, T. S. et al. (1991). Etoposide with lonidamine
    or pentoxifylline as modulators of alkylating agent activity *in vivo. Int. J.
    Cancer*, **48**, 631–7.
Teicher, B. A. and Holden, S. A. (1987). Survey of the effect of adding
    Fluosol-DA 20%/O_2 to treatment with various chemotherapeutic agents.
    Cancer Treat. Rep., **71**, 173–7.
Teicher, B. A. and Frei III, E. (1988). Development of alkylating agent resistant
    human tumor cell lines. *Cancer Chemother. Pharmacol.*, **21**, 292–8.
Teicher, B. A. and Rose, C. M. (1984a). Oxygen-carrying perfluorochemical
    emulsion as an adjuvant to radiation therapy in mice. *Cancer Res.*, **44**,
    4285–8.
Teicher, B. A. and Rose, C. M. (1984b). Perfluorochemical emulsions can increase
    tumor radiosensitivity. *Science*, **223**, 934–6.
Teicher, B. A. and Rose, C. M. (1986). Effect of dose and scheduling on growth
    delay of the Lewis lung carcinoma produced by the perfluorochemical
    emulsion, Fluosol-DA. *Int. J. Rad. Oncol. Biol. Phys.*, **12**, 1331–3.
Teicher, B. A., Lazo, J. S. and Sartorelli, A. C. (1981). Classification of
    antineoplastic agents by their selective toxicities toward oxygenated and
    hypoxic tumor cells. *Cancer Res.*, **41**, 73–81.
Teicher, B. A., Holden, S. A. and Rose, C. M. (1985a). Differential enhancement
    of melphalan cytotoxicity in tumor and normal tissue by Fluosol-DA and
    oxygen breathing. *Int. J. Cancer*, **36**, 585–9.

Teicher, B. A., Holden, S. A. and Rose, C. M. (1985b). Effect of oxygen on the cytotoxicity and antitumor activity of etoposide. *J. Natl. Cancer Inst.*, **75**, 1129–33.

Teicher, B. A., Cucchi, C. A., Lee, J. B. et al. (1986a). Alkylating agents: *in vitro* studies of cross-resistance patterns. *Cancer Res.*, **46**, 4379–83.

Teicher, B. A., Holden, S. A. and Rose, C. M. (1986b). Effect of Fluosol-DA/O₂ on tumor cell and bone marrow cytotoxicity of nitrosoureas in mice bearing FSaII fibrosarcoma. *Int. J. Cancer*, **38**, 285–8.

Teicher, B. A., Lazo, J. S., Merrill, W. W. et al. (1986c). Effect of Fluosol-DA/O₂ on the antitumor activity and pulmonary toxicity of bleomycin. *Cancer Chemother. Pharmacol.*, **18**, 213–8.

Teicher, B. A., Crawford, J. M., Holden, S. A. and Cathcart, K. N. S. (1987a). Effects of various oxygenation conditions on the enhancement by Fluosol-DA of melphalan antitumor activity. *Cancer Res.*, **47**, 5036–41.

Teicher, B. A., Holden, S. A. and Jacobs, J. L. (1987b). Approaches to defining the mechanism of enhancement by Fluosol-DA 20% with carbogen of melphalan antitumor activity. *Cancer Res.*, **47**, 513–8.

Teicher, B. A., Holden, S. A., Kelley, M. J. et al. (1987c). Characterization of a human squamous carcinoma cell line resistant to *cis*-diamminedichloroplatinum(II). *Cancer Res.*, **47**, 388–93.

Teicher, B. A., Bernal, S. D., Holden, S. A. and Cathcart, K. N. S. (1988a). Effect of Fluosol®-DA/carbogen on etoposide/alkylating agent antitumor activity. *Cancer Chemother. Pharmacol.*, **21**, 281–5.

Teicher, B. A., Herman, T. S., Holden, S. A. and Cathcart, K. N. S. (1988b). The effect of Fluosol-DA and oxygenation status on the activity of cyclophosphamide *in vivo*. *Cancer Chemother. Pharmacol.*, **21**, 286–91.

Teicher, B. A., Herman, T. S. and Rose, C. M. (1988c). Effect of Fluosol-DA® on the response of intracranial 9L tumors to x-rays and BCNU. *Int. J. Rad. Oncol. Biol. Phys.*, **15**, 1187–92.

Teicher, B. A., McIntosh-Lowe, N. L. and Rose, C. M. (1988d). Effect of various oxygenation conditions and Fluosol-DA on cancer chemotherapeutic agents. *Biomat. Artif. Cells Immobiliz. Biotechnol.*, **16**, 533–46.

Teicher, B. A., Herman, T. S. and Jones, S. M. (1989a). Optimization of perfluorochemical levels with radiation therapy in mice. *Cancer Res.*, **49**, 2693–7.

Teicher, B. A., Waxman, D. J., Holden, S. A. et al. (1989b). Evidence for enzymatic activation and oxygen involvement in cytotoxicity and antitumor activity of *N,N',N''*-triethylenethiophosphoramide. *Cancer Res.*, **49**, 4996–5001.

Teicher, B. A., Herman, T. S., Holden, S. A. et al. (1990a). Tumor resistance to alkylating agents conferred by mechanisms operative only *in vivo*. *Science*, **247**, 1457–61.

Teicher, B. A., Holden, S. A., Al-Achi, A. and Herman, T. S. (1990b). Classification of antineoplastic treatments by their differential toxicity toward putative oxygenated and hypoxic tumor subpopulations *in vivo* in FSaIIC murine fibrosarcoma. *Cancer Res.*, **50**, 3339–44.

Teicher, B. A., Herman, T. S., Holden, S. A. et al. (1991a). Lonidamine as a modulator of alkylating agent activity *in vitro* and *in vivo*. *Cancer Res.*, **51**, 780–4.

Teicher, B. A., Herman, T. S., Shulman, L. et al. (1991b). Combination of etanidazole with cyclophosphamide and platinum complexes. *Cancer Chemother. Pharmacol.*, **28**, 153–8.

Teicher, B. A., Herman, T. S., Tanaka, J. et al. (1991c). Fluosol-DA/carbogen with lonidamine or pentoxifylline as modulators of alkylating agents in the FSaIIC fibrosarcoma. *Cancer Chemother. Pharmacol.*, **28**, 45–50.

Teicher, B. A., Herman, T. S., Tanaka, J. et al. (1991d). Modulation of alkylating agents by etanidazole and Fluosol-DA/carbogen in the FSaIIC fibrosarcoma and EMT6 mammary carcinoma. *Cancer Res.*, **51**, 1086–91.

Teicher, B. A., Holden, S. A., Herman, T. S. et al. (1991e). Characteristics of five human tumor cell lines and sublines resistant to *cis*-diamminedichloroplatinum(II). *Int. J. Cancer*, **47**, 252–60.

Teicher, B. A., Holden, S. A., Herman, T. S. and Frei III, E. (1991f). Strategies for increasing the efficacy of and overcoming resistance to platinum complexes *in vivo*. In *Platinum and other Metal Coordination Compounds in Cancer Chemotherapy* (ed. S. B. Howell), pp. 295–301. Plenum Press, New York.

Teicher, B. A., Alvarez Sotomayor, E. and Huang, Z. D. (1992a). Antiangiogenic agents potentiate cytotoxic cancer therapies against primary and metastatic disease. *Cancer Res.*, **52**, 6702–4.

Teicher, B. A., Herman, T. S., Hopkins, R. E. and Menon, K. (1992b). Effect of a bovine hemoglobin preparation on the response of the FSaIIC fibrosarcoma to chemotherapeutic alkylating agents. *J. Cancer Res. Clin. Oncol.*, **118**, 123–8.

Teicher, B. A., Holden, S. A., Ara, G. et al. (1992c). Effect of a bovine hemoglobin preparation (SBHS) on the response of two murine solid tumors to radiation therapy or chemotherapeutic alkylating agents. *Biomat. Artif. Cells Immobiliz. Biotechnol.*, **20**(2–4), 657–60.

Teicher, B. A., Holden, S. A., Ara, G. et al. (1992d). Etanidazole as a modulator of combined modality therapy in the rat 9L gliosarcoma. *Int. J. Oncol.*, **1**, 625–30.

Teicher, B. A., Alvarez Sotomayor, E., Robinson, M. F. et al. (1993a). Tumor oxygenation and radiosensitization by pentoxifylline and a perflubron emulsion/carbogen breathing. *Int. J. Oncol.*, **2**, 13–21.

Teicher, B. A., Chatterjee, D., Liu, J.-T. et al. (1993b). Protection of bone-marrow granulocyte-macrophage colony-forming units in mice bearing *in vivo* alkylating-agent-resistant EMT-6 tumors. *Cancer Chemoth. Pharmacol.*, **32**, 315–9.

Teicher, B. A., Holden, S. A., Ara, G. et al. (1993c). Cyclooxygenase inhibitors: *in vitro* and *in vivo* effects of antitumor alkylating agents in the EMT-6 murine mammary carcinoma. *Int. J. Oncol.*, **2**, 145–53.

Teicher, B. A., Korbut, T. T., Menon, K. et al. (1994). Cyclooxygenase and lipoxygenase inhibitors as modulators of cancer therapies. *Cancer Chemother. Pharmacol.*, **33**, 515–22.

Templeton, N. S. and Stetler-Stevenson, W. G. (1991). Identification of a basal promoter for the human Mr 72 000 type IV collagenase gene and enhanced expression in a highly metastatic cell line. *Cancer Res.*, **51**, 6190–3.

Terranova, V. P., Hujanen, E. S. and Martin, G. R. (1986). Basement membrane and the invasive activity of metastatic tumor cells. *J. Natl. Cancer Inst.*, **77**, 311–6.

Tew, K. D., Bomber, A. M. and Hoffman, S. J. (1988). Ethacrynic acid and piripost as enhancers of cytotoxicity in drug resistant and sensitive cell lines. *Cancer Res.*, **48**, 3622.

Tryggvason, K., Hoyhtya, M. and Salo, T. (1987). Proteolytic degradation of extracellular matrix in tumor invasion. *Biochim. Biophys. Acta*, **907**, 191–217.

Tsai, C., Gazdar, A. F., Venzon, D. J. et al. (1989). Lack of in vitro synergy between etoposide and *cis*-diamminedichloroplatinum(II). *Cancer Res.*, **49**, 2390–7.

Turrisi III, A. T., Glover, D. J. and Mason, B. A. (1988). A preliminary report:

concurrent twice-daily radiotherapy plus platinum-etoposide chemotherapy for limited small cell lung cancer. *Int. J. Rad. Oncol. Biol. Phys.*, **15**, 183–7.

Twentyman, P. R. (1976). Comparative chemosensitivity of exponential versus plateau-phase cells in both in vitro and in vivo model systems. *Cancer Treat. Rep.*, **60**, 1719–22.

Ueki, N., Nakazato, M., Ohkawa, T. et al. (1992). Excessive production of transforming growth factor-β1 can play an important role in the development of tumorigenesis by its action for angiogenesis: validity of neutralizing antibodies to block tumor growth. *Biochim. Biophys. Acta*, **1137**, 189–96.

Ueki, N., Ohkawa, T., Yokoyama, Y. et al. (1993). Potentiation of metastatic capacity by transforming growth factor-β1 gene transfection. *Jap. J. Cancer Res.*, **84**, 589–93.

Utsumi, H., Shibuya, M. L., Kosaka, T. et al. (1990). Abrogation by novobiocin of cytotoxicity due to the topoisomerase II inhibitor amsacrine in Chinese hamster cells. *Cancer Res.*, **50**, 2577–81.

van Maanen, V. M. S., Retel, F., de Vries, J. and Pinedo, H. M. (1988). Mechanism of action of antitumor drug etoposide: a review. *J. Natl. Cancer Inst.*, **80**, 1526–33.

Vaupel, P. (1977). Hypoxia and neoplastic tissue. *Microvasc. Res.*, **13**, 399–408.

Vaupel, P. (1990). Oxygenation of human tumors. *Strahlentherapie Onkologischen*, **166**, 377–86.

Vaupel, P. (1993). Oxygenation of solid tumors. In *Drug Resistance in Oncology* (ed. B. A. Teicher), pp. 53–85. Marcel-Dekker, New York.

Vaupel, P., Frinak, S. and Bicher, H. I. (1981). Heterogeneous oxygen partial pressure and pH distribution C3H mouse mammary adenocarcinoma. *Cancer Res.*, **41**, 2008–13.

Vaupel, P., Fortmeyer, H. P., Runkel, S. and Kallinowski, F. (1987). Blood flow, oxygen consumption and tissue oxygenation of human breast cancer xenografts in nude rats. *Cancer Res.*, **47**, 3496–503.

Vaupel, P., Kallinowski, F. and Okunieff, P. (1989). Blood flow, oxygen and nutrient supply, and metabolic microenvironment of human tumors: a review. *Cancer Res.*, **49**, 6449–65.

Vaupel, P., Schlenger, K., Knoop, C. and Höckel, M. (1991). Oxygenation of human tumors: evaluation of tissue oxygen distribution in breast cancer by computerized O_2 tension measurements. *Cancer Res.*, **51**, 3316–22.

Vlodavsky, I., Korner, G., Ishai-Michaeli, R. et al. (1990). Extracellular matrix-resident growth factors and enzymes: possible involvement in tumor metastasis and angiogenesis. *Cancer Metast. Rev.*, **9**, 203–26.

Vogelstein, B., Pardol, D. M. and Coffey, D. S. (1980). Supercoiled loops and eukaryotic DNA replication. *Cell*, **22**, 79–85.

Von Heyden, H. W., Scherpe, A. and Nagel, G. A. (1987). cis-Diamminedichloroplatinum(II) (cis-platinum) and etoposide for patients with refractory lymphomas. *Cancer Treat. Rev.*, **9**(A), 45–52.

Walker, R. A., Dearing, S. J. and Gallacher, B. (1994). Relationship of transforming growth factor β1 to extracellular matrix and stromal infiltates in invasive breast carcinoma. *Br. J. Cancer*, **69**, 1160–5.

Wang, J. C. (1985). DNA topoisomerases. *Ann. Rev. Biochem.*, **54**, 665–97.

Wang, J. C. (1987). Recent studies of DNA topoisomerase. *Biochim. Biophys. Acta*, **909**, 1–9.

Wang, Y., Teicher, B. A., Shea, T. C. et al. (1989). Cross-resistance and glutathione-S-transferase-π levels among four human melanoma cell lines selected for alkylating agent resistance. *Cancer Res.*, **49**, 6185–92.

Ward, A. and Clissold, S. P. (1987). Pentoxifylline: a review of its pharmacodynamic properties, and its therapeutic efficacy. *Drugs*, **34**, 50–97.

Watson, J. and Chuah, S. Y. (1985). Prostaglandins, steroids and human mammary cancer. *Eur. J. Cancer Clin. Oncol.*, **21**(9), 1051–5.

Weidner, N., Semple, J. P., Welch, W. R. and Folkman, J. (1991). Tumor angiogenesis and metastasis – correlation in invasive breast carcinoma. *N. Engl. J. Med.*, **324**, 1–8.

Welch, D. R., Fabra, A. and Motowo, N. (1990). Transforming growth factor β stimulates mammary adenocarcinoma cell invasion and metastatic potential. *Proc. Natl. Acad. Sci. USA*, **87**, 7678–82.

Weistler, O., Kleihues, P. and Pegg, A. E. (1984). O^6-Alkylguanine-DNA alkyltransferase activity in human brain and brain tumors. *Carcinogenesis*, **5**, 121–4.

Willis, R. A. (1953). *Pathology of Tumors*. Butterworth & Co., Ltd, London.

Wu, H.-Y., Shyy, S., Wang, J. C. and Liu, L. F. (1988). Transcription generates positively and negatively supercoiled domains in the template. *Cell*, **53**, 433–40.

Yang, L., Wold, M. S., Li, J. J. et al. (1987). Roles of DNA topoisomerases in simian virus 40 DNA replication. *Proc. Natl. Acad. Sci. USA*, **84**, 950–4.

Yarosh, D. B., Hurst-Calderone, S. and Babich, M. A. (1986). Potentiation of O^6-methylguanine-DNA methyltransferase and sensitization of human tumor cells to killing by chloroethylnitrosourea by O^6-methylguanine as a free base. *Cancer Res.*, **46**, 1663–8.

Young, M. R. and Hoover, C. S. (1986). Inhibition of spleen cell cytotoxic capacity toward tumor by elevated prostaglandin E2 levels in mice bearing Lewis lung carcinoma. *J. Natl. Cancer Inst.*, **77**, 425–9.

Young, M. R. and Knies, S. (1984). Prostaglandin E production by Lewis lung carcinoma: mechanism for tumor establishment in vivo. *J. Natl. Cancer Inst.*, **72**, 919–22.

Young, M. R. and Newby, M. (1986). Differential induction of suppressor macrophages by cloned Lewis lung carcinoma variants in mice. *J. Natl. Cancer Inst.*, **77**, 1255–60.

Young, M. R., Newby, M. and Meunier, J. (1985). Relationships between morphology, dissemination, migration, and prostaglandin E_2 secretion by cloned variants of Lewis lung carcinoma. *Cancer Res.*, **45**, 3918–23.

Young, M. R., Wheeler, E. and Newby, M. (1986). Macrophage-mediated suppression of natural killer cell activity in mice bearing Lewis lung carcinoma. *J. Natl. Cancer Inst.*, **76**, 745–50.

Young, M. R., Newby, M. and Wepsic, H. T. (1987a). Hematopoiesis and suppressor bone marrow cells in mice bearing large metastatic Lewis lung carcinoma tumors. *Cancer Res.*, **47**, 100–5.

Young, M. R., Young, M. E. and Wepsic, H. T. (1987b). Effects of prostaglandin E_2-producing nonmetastatic Lewis lung carcinoma cells on the migration of prostaglandin E_2-responsive metastatic Lewis lung carcinoma cells. *Cancer Res.*, **47**, 3679–83.

Young, M. R. I., Young, M. E. and Kim, K. (1988). Regulation of tumor-induced myelopoiesis and the associated immune suppressor cells in mice bearing metastatic Lewis lung carcinoma by prostaglandin E2. *Cancer Res.*, **48**, 6826–31.

Young, M. R. I., Duffie, G. P., Lozano, Y. et al. (1990). Association of a functional prostaglandin E_2-protein kinase A coupling with responsiveness of metastatic

Lewis lung carcinoma variants to prostaglandin E$_2$ and to prostaglandin E$_2$-producing nonmetastatic Lewis lung carcinoma variants. *Cancer Res.*, **50**, 2973–8.

Yuan, A. M., Fenselau, C., Dulik, D. M. et al. (1990). Laser desorption electron impact: application to a study of the mechanism of conjugation of glutathione and cyclophosphamide. *Anal. Chem.*, **62**, 868–70.

Zupi, G., Greco, C. and Laudino, N. (1986). In vitro and in vivo potentiation by lonidamine of the antitumor effect of adriamycin. *Anticancer Res.*, **6**, 1245–50.

Zwelling, L. A., Estey, E., Silberman, L. et al. (1987). Effect of cell proliferation and chromatin conformation on intercalator-induced, protein-associated DNA cleavage in human brain tumor cells and human fibroblasts. *Cancer Res.*, **47**, 251–7.

3

The MDR genes

LYN MICKLEY and ANTONIO TITO FOJO

Introduction

P-glycoprotein is a member of a small gene family. Humans have two genes, *MDR1* and *MDR3*, while mice and hamsters have three each, *mdr1*, *mdr2*, and *mdr3* in mice and *pgp1*, *pgp2* and *pgp3* in hamsters. Of these, only *MDR1* in humans, *mdr1* and *mdr3* (*mdr1a* and *mdr1b*) in mice and *pgp1* and *pgp2* in hamsters can confer the multidrug resistance phenotype (Chin et al., 1989; Ng et al., 1989).

P-glycoprotein is a 170–180 kDa plasma membrane phosphoprotein that mediates multidrug resistance in mammalian cells. It functions as an energy-dependent drug efflux pump, extruding a wide range of compounds from the inside of cells. Originally identified in multidrug resistant cells, expression of this protein has been demonstrated in a wide variety of cell lines and normal tissues, with a distribution that betrays a normal role in drug detoxification (Fojo et al., 1987; Thiebaut et al., 1987; Sugawara et al., 1988). Elegant studies in knockout mice have furthered our understanding of the roles of these proteins, and these will be discussed further below (Schinkel et al., 1994). The goal of exploiting our increasing understanding of this complex protein in the treatment of human cancer still remains in its infancy, a testament to the time required to translate laboratory studies to clinical practice.

Numerous reviews of P-glycoprotein deal extensively with the history of its discovery, a description of the drug resistant phenotype, its molecular characterization and preliminary clinical studies (Pastan and Gottesman, 1987; Endicott and Ling, 1989; Van der Bliek and Borst, 1989; Kane, Pastan and Gottesman, 1990; Biedler, 1992; Chin, Pastan and Gottesman, 1993; Gottesman and Pastan, 1993). Consequently, an attempt will not be made to duplicate those efforts in the current chapter, and the reader is referred to those excellent reviews for the necessary background. Instead, we will review studies dealing with evolving or controversial topics, some of which have been largely resolved, and others that are the subject of further studies. The reported data will be presented in an unbiased manner. Where appropriate, 'editorial comments' will be included, which represent the opinion of the authors, and our admitted bias. It is hoped that these will be apparent to the reader, so that fact and bias can be discriminated. The areas covered will evolve from the structure of P-glycoprotein, to structure/function correlations. This will be followed by a review of the potential role of P-glycoprotein as a mediator of chloride homeostasis, and the regulation of *MDR1* expression. Finally, we will review recent studies that demonstrate the magnitude of the pleiotropic phenotype conferred by P-glycoprotein, evidence that indicates that this is not just a protein for now, but for the future as well.

P-Glycoprotein model

Original model

The initial isolation of complete and partial cDNA sequences from both human and hamster cell lines and subsequently from mouse cells, confirmed the sequence similarity of the various P-glycoprotein genes (Chen et al., 1986; Gros et al., 1986a; Gros, Croop and Housman, 1986b; Gros et al., 1988; Van der Bliek et al., 1988; Hsu et al., 1990). Examination of the primary sequence identified in each half of the molecule a long hydrophobic region with six predicted transmembrane domains, and a hydrophilic region with consensus sequences for a nucleotide binding site. Based on hydropathy profiles of the hydrophobic regions and sequence homology of the hydrophilic areas, a structural model was proposed and widely accepted, which predicted that the two halves of *MDR1* are organized into four structural domains corresponding to their prokaryotic counterparts (Chen et al., 1986; Gros et al., 1986a, 1988; Van der Bliek et al., 1988; Hsu et al., 1990). According to this model, the two hydrophobic domains, with six membrane spanning helices, are each followed by a large hydrophilic ATP-binding domain localized in the cytosol. Each hydrophobic transmembrane segment is connected to its preceding and/or ensuing segment by an intracellular or extracellular loop. This model led to numerous artistic representations of the three-dimensional structure of the protein. Most envisioned a protein-lined channel across the lipid bilayer for solute transport, with the cytoplasmic nucleotide-binding sites providing the energy for drug binding, transport and release.

An alternate model

Although scientifically sound and intuitively attractive, the validity of this model was challenged when studies using protein chimeras in *Xenopus* oocytes, and full-length native protein in cell-free translational systems raised questions about the topology of the carboxyl-terminal half compared to the amino-terminal segment (Skach, Calayag and Lingappa, 1993). Previous studies in other models had established that integral membrane proteins are synthesized at the endoplasmic reticulum, where the correct transmembrane topology is achieved. The correct topology can be directed by discrete sequences at the time of translation, and subsequent trafficking localizes the protein to its final destination but does not change the pre-established orientation. Using artificially constructed chimeras consisting of various lengths of P-glycoprotein and a 142 amino acid passenger domain derived from prolactin, it was concluded that the peptide region between TM8 and TM9 was extracellular. Although the authors recommended that the transmembrane topology of *MDR1* should be revised, an overwhelming amount of evidence supports the original model suggesting major revisions will not be required. While the prolactin-derived reporter had been previously shown to respond faithfully to signal and stop transfer sequences without intrinsic translocation activity, it now appears that the assay has some limitations.

In support of the original model

Evidence confirming the original P-glycoprotein model has been provided by: (1) epitope mapping of specific monoclonal antibodies to P-glycoprotein; (2) studies in which a cysteine-less mutant of human P-glycoprotein had cysteine residues reintroduced into predicted extracellular or cytoplasmic loops, followed by chemical modification with membrane-permeant or impermeant thiol-specific probes to determine their sidedness; and (3) studies in which a single antigenic epitope containing part of the hemagglutinin (HA) of influenza virus was inserted at predicted intra- or extracellular locations of P-glycoprotein.

Epitope mapping studies with C219, C32 and C494 have demonstrated that the ATP-binding domains are located in the cytoplasmic face, and similar analyses of the MRK16 binding site and the epitope of the murine monoclonal antibody, MM4.17, confirmed that the loops joining TM1/TM2 and TM7/TM8 are located on the extracellular face of the protein (Georges et al., 1990; Georges, Tsuruo and Ling, 1993; Cianfriglia et al., 1994).

In addition, a cysteine-less mutant of P-glycoprotein, which retains the ability to confer multidrug resistance, has been used to localize the site of individual residues (Loo and Clarke, 1995). Cysteine residues were reintroduced into predicted extracellular or cytoplasmic loops of the cysteine-less P-glycoprotein, and the topology of the protein was determined using membrane-permeant and membrane-impermeant thiol-specific reagents. The advantage of this approach over the use of protein chimeras in *Xenopus* oocytes and cell-free translational models is that the assays are performed in functional models in intact cells. Using this approach, loops L5–6, L7–8 and L11–12 were confirmed as extracyto-plasmic, as predicted by the original model of P-glycoprotein. Specifically, biotinylation of engineered cysteine residues placed in these predicted extracellular loops was blocked by pretreatment of the cells with a membrane-impermeant maleimide, suggesting that these residues are extracellular in location. Similarly, cysteine residues introduced into cytoplasmic loops L2–3, L4–5, L8–9, L10–11, and the C-terminal region, exhibited labeling properties consistent with an intracytoplasmic location. Labeling required higher concentrations of biotin maleimide and longer incubation periods, and consistent with their cytoplasmic location, biotinylation of these residues was not blocked by pretreatment with membrane-impermeant maleimide.

More recently, tagging with a single antigenic epitope containing part of the hemagglutinin of influenza virus has located the epitopes at amino acid positions 101, 161, 320, 736, and 961 on the extracellular side and the tags at positions 161, 235, 376, 887, and 1024 on the intra-cellular side of the membrane (Kast et al., 1995). These results are consistent with the experiments introducing cysteines into the cysteine-less mutant.

Conclusion

What can be concluded at this time regarding models of P-glycoprotein structure? We believe the accumulated evidence strongly supports the original model proposed by hydropathy profiling with twelve transmembrane segments joined by extracellular and intracellular loops. While the possibility that a small fraction of P-glycoprotein exist in another 'interchangeable' form cannot be excluded, we feel that this would likely be insignificant (Zhang, Duthie and Ling, 1993).

Functional consequences of acquired or engineered mutations in P-glycoprotein

The diversity of drug resistance phenotypes described in cells expressing P-glycoprotein in vitro can be partially explained by the structural diversity of P-glycoproteins. Normal mouse *mdr1* and *mdr3*, for example, encode functionally distinct P-glycoproteins (Devault and Gros, 1990), and these in turn confer phenotypes that are different to that of human P-glycoprotein. How this diversity occurs has been the subject of extensive studies, which have broadened our comprehension of P-glycoprotein function in particular, and the ABC transporter family in general.

Experimental approaches and their limitations

Increased understanding of the transport of substrates by P-glycoprotein has been realized through the characterization of mutant P-glycoproteins isolated from human, mouse, and hamster genes. Through structure–function analyses, this approach has helped to identify residues critical for drug binding or transport. The infrequent occurrence of acquired mutations during the course of drug selections in cell lines expressing P-glycoprotein has been supplemented by extensive studies utilizing genetically altered transporters. The latter have been either products of site-directed mutagenesis with usually a single amino acid change, or *MDR1/MDR3* chimeras. The use of *MDR1/MDR3* chimeras is logical, since in man they are encoded by two genes which share 77% amino acid identity and similar topology, but only *MDR1* mediates multidrug resistance.

These studies provide the best approach to explore structure/function relationships, although they are difficult to perform, and suffer certain liabilities. These include: (1) Intrinsic clonal variability in resistance independent of the genetic manipulation, such as that mediated by differences in growth rates, a common variable of great importance for the commonly used P-glycoprotein substrates, which are generally schedule dependent. Studies reporting drug accumulations are valuable in this regard. (2) The frequent practice of normalizing resistance based on the level of P-glycoprotein, an unproven assumption, although probably a close approximation in the case of small differences. (3) The lack of documentation of post-translational modifications, which could affect transport efficiency or specificity, and which need not be homogeneous among individual clones. (4) The pitfall of concluding that a lack of effect in an engineered mutant excludes a role for a given residue in drug binding or transport. As an example, a glycine residue may line a drug channel but its importance may be overlooked if a residue of sufficient bulk or charge is not introduced to interfere with drug passage. Obviously, only a limited number of mutants can be studied. (5) The use of chimeras has unique limitations, since the effect of conserved residues is not investigated, and because interaction of various residues may confound results, thus overlooking regions of importance. As a result of the latter, the phenotype observed with specific mutations may differ from that of chimeras.

For the majority, if not all, of the studies identified to date as important

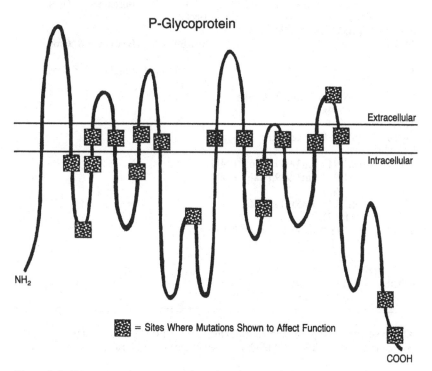

Figure 3.1. Diagrammatic representation of P-glycoprotein, indicating sites important in drug binding/transport. Sites where mutations are depicted have been shown to affect function.

Table 3.1. *Summary of acquired and engineered mutations affecting function*

	Effect on function shown	Effect on function shown
NH$_2$-end		
TM1		
TM2		
L2–3	(h)185 (Choi et al., 1988)	
	(h)165,166,168,169,183,185 (Currier et al., 1992)	
	(h)140–229 (Currier et al., 1992)	
	(h)141, 187 (Loo & Clarke, 1994a)	
TM3		(h)140–229 (Currier et al., 1992)
TM4	(h)223 (Loo & Clarke, 1993a)	
L4–5	(h)228 (Loo & Clarke, 1994a)	
TM5		(m1)307–411 (Buschman & Gros, 1991)
TM6	(r)338,339 (Devine et al., 1992)	(m1)307–411 (Buschman & Gros, 1991)
ABC/ATS	(h)536 (Hoof et al., 1994)	
TM7		(m1)693–764 (Buschman & Gros, 1991)
TM8		(m1)693–764 (Buschman & Gros, 1991)
L8–9	(h)812,830 (Loo & Clarke, 1994a)	
TM9		
TM10	(h)866 (Loo & Clarke, 1993a)	
L10–11		
TM11	(m1)941, (m3)939 (Gros, 1991)	
	(m1)941, (m3)939 (Kajiji et al., 1993)	
	(m1)941, (m3)939 (Dhir et al., 1993)	
TM12	(h)978 (Loo & Clarke, 1993b)	
	(h)975–991 (Zhang et al., 1995)	
ABC/ATS		
COOH-end	(h)1258–1280 (Currier, 1989)	
	(h)1228–1280 (Currier, 1989)	

Abbreviations: L,loop; (h),human; (m1),mouse *mdr1*; (m3), mouse *mdr3*; (r), hamster. ABC/ATS, ATP-binding cassette transporter signature.

in drug binding/transport (Table 3.1, Figure 3.1), several possibilities can be proposed: (1) the residue(s) are part of a binding site common to most or all drugs, and structural changes influence interactions with multiple substrates; (2) the residue(s) line a hydrophobic gate or channel in the cell membrane and changes in size, charge or hydrophobicity affect drug transit; or (3) the residue(s) are part of a region in the folded protein which, when altered, indirectly influences function. Indeed, while the important residues identified to date are well separated in the linear structure of the P-glycoprotein molecule, the three-dimensional structure may bring these various domains in close proximity.

MDR1/MDR3 chimeras

The results using *MDR1/MDR3* chimeras have succeeded in identifying areas of importance, albeit with varying degrees of specificity (Buschman and Gros, 1991; Currier et al., 1992; Zhang, Collins and Greenberger, 1995). The prediction that functional differences between *MDR1* and *MDR3* would be mediated by the regions of greatest amino acid diversity between these genes has been largely confirmed. Such regions are located in the transmembrane domains and the linker region connecting both halves of each protein. Consistent with this, chimeras of the human or mouse genes containing large spans of transmembrane domains have been unable to confer drug tolerance. In addition, substitution of the first intracytoplasmic or the last extracytoplasmic loops also impair drug binding or transport. In contrast, the nucleotide binding regions, which are highly conserved among all MDR genes, are interchangeable.

These studies, which were among the initial attempts to examine structure–function relationships, suffer from a lack of specificity and incomplete data, with drug-resistance profiles providing functional correlations. Because drug resistance depends on at least three P-glycoprotein mediated steps, including drug binding, transport and release, the lack of ancillary studies, in these and in other reports, precludes precise conclusions from being reached. Although there is only scant evidence identifying these three discrete steps, a general consensus might be reached in support of at least this degree of complexity. However, in many studies, these terms are used interchangeably.

Ancillary studies: photoaffinity labeling

Among ancillary studies, photoaffinity labeling has been most widely reported (Bruggemann et al., 1989; Greenberger et al., 1990, 1991; Bruggemann et al., 1992; Greenberger, 1993; Morris et al., 1994). The observation that the binding of photoaffinity probes is competitively inhibited by P-glycoprotein substrates has been accepted as indirect evidence that chemotherapeutic drugs and photoaffinity probes share a common binding region in P-glycoprotein. Photoaffinity labeling studies have been used to define the drug binding domains of P-glycoprotein. Using probes derived from anticancer drugs or chemosensitizing agents, photoaffinity labeling domains have been mapped. Peptide mapping of photoaffinity drug-binding sites indicates that there are two drug-binding sites, one each in the amino- and the carboxy-terminal half of the molecule. Azidopine, a photoactive calcium channel blocker, has been most widely utilized. Using antibodies for specific regions of P-glycoprotein, azidopine labeling of protease fragments from each half of the molecule has been shown for both the human and mouse proteins. What remains unsolved is whether these represent two distinct binding regions or whether the two regions come together to form a single independent binding site. The latter is most likely. Specifically, one drug binding site resides within or close to transmembrane segments TM4, TM5, and TM6; while the second is close to transmembrane segments TM11 and TM12. Similarly, photoaffinity analogs of forskolin and prazosin bind to small common domains that are present in both halves of P-glycoprotein. The forskolin and prazosin analogs label both halves of P-glycoprotein. Labeling in the amino-terminal half has been localized to residues 291–359, which span transmembrane regions 5 and 6. The evidence indicates both drugs label the same sites in P-glycoprotein.

That the effects of acquired or engineered mutations are mediated at least in some cases through drug binding or release and not just by interfering with drug transport is supported in part by the effects on azidopine labeling (Figure 3.2). Azidopine, a dihydropiridine derivative, is only poorly transported by P-glycoprotein. Consequently, labeling is generally assumed to reflect drug binding. The fact that some mutations alter azidopine labeling suggests that they do so by affecting drug binding.

Inspection of the data suggests that the drug-binding sites reside in part within the transmembrane domains and partly outside the membrane, albeit in likely close proximity. Residues located in the transmem-

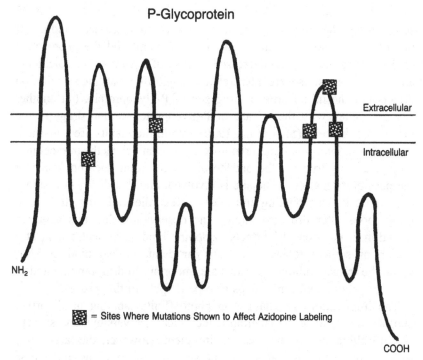

Figure 3.2. P-glycoprotein, showing sites where mutations affect azidopine labeling.

brane domains have been implicated in drug binding, since labeling studies with photoactive analogs suggest that these regions contribute to the drug-binding sites (Loo and Clarke, 1993b, 1994a; Zhang, Collins and Greenberger, 1995). Specifically, a number of engineered mutations have shown effects on azidopine binding. For example, mutation of Phe-335 to non-aromatic amino acids, such as alanine, greatly impairs P-glycoprotein mediated vinblastine and actinomycin D resistance, with retention of colchicine and adriamycin resistance. In these mutants, binding of azidopine, which is thought to bind the same binding site as vinblastine, was increased. In addition, affinity for vinblastine was also increased, as evidenced by increased vinblastine competition of azidopine labeling. Together, these results are thought to provide evidence of increased affinity for vinblastine resulting in decreased vinblastine resistance.

The properties of the Phe-335 to Ala substitution resemble those previously described for an acquired mutation in the first cytoplasmic loop (Choi et al., 1988; Safa et al., 1990). For the Gly185 to Val185 substitution, the mutant P-glycoprotein showed increased binding of photoactive analogs of vinblastine and verapamil and the photoactive compound azidopine, and decreased binding of a photoactive colchicine analog. These results were interpreted as suggesting that 'the substitution affects not the initial drug binding site of P-glycoprotein, but another site associated with the release of P-glycoprotein-bound drugs to the outside of the cell' (Safa et al., 1990). While the results are consistent with such an interpretation, it requires that one envisions the intracellular loop releasing drugs to the outside of the cell; and does not consider the possibility that only one site is involved, and that different residues participate in drug binding and release. Regardless of how changes in these loops alter drug specificity, the observation that this acquired mutation at position 185 affects azidopine binding indicates that, at a minimum, some cytoplasmic regions participate in drug binding. Thus while the transmembrane domains are important in drug binding and/or transport, the cytoplasmic loops also participate in this process.

The implications of changes in photoaffinity labeling need further substantiation, since the labeling is inefficient, irreversible, and suscep- tible to alterations in the local environment. However, the large body of available data implicates multiple sites in drug binding and release (Figure 3.2).

The effect of residue size on resistance profile

Concern that the size and charge of both the normal and the substituting residue can affect results are drawbacks to using engineered mutations to determine the importance of individual residues (Dhir et al., 1993; Kajiji et al., 1993; Loo and Clarke, 1993b, 1994a). Examples supporting this include: (1) Mutations of Ser-939 and Ser-941 in TM11, which are encoded by mouse *mdr3* and *mdr1*, respectively. Replacement of these serines by alanine, cysteine, threonine, tyrosine, tryptophan, and aspartic acid had only limited effect on vinblastine resistance. However, disparate results were observed when colchicine, adriamycin and actinomycin D resistance were analyzed. The hydroxyl group did not seem essential for activity, as evidenced by a wild type phenotype in both *mdr1* and *mdr3* mutants with alanine or cysteine substitutions; and significantly reduced resistance in threonine-bearing mutants. However, the insertion of residues with bulkier side chains had a more complex effect on the resistance profiles. The introduction of tyrosine or tryptophan caused an almost complete loss of colchicine and adriamycin resistance in both *mdr1* and *mdr3*, with opposite effects on actinomycin D resistance, causing either a 3-fold or a 4–8-fold decrease in resistance in *mdr1* and *mdr3*, respectively. (2) TM6 substitutions also suggest that colchicine resistance in part depends on the size of certain residues. In these experiments, substitution of Phe-335 or Val-338 by smaller residues increased colchicine resistance; while substitution of Gly-341 and Ala-342 by larger residues decreased resistance to colchicine. To be sure, resistance to vinblastine, doxorubicin and actinomycin D were discordant, precluding generalized conclusions, but rather suggesting a complex phenomenon involving numerous residues, as discussed below.

Grouping of substrates and diversity of the amino- and carboxy-terminal halves

While attempts have been made to classify substrates in groups, evidence from several laboratories and even from a single laboratory suggest that specificity is at best complex, and at worst very poor (Devine, Ling and Melera, 1992; Dhir et al., 1993; Kajiji et al., 1993; Loo and Clarke, 1993a, 1993b; Hoof et al., 1994; Loo and Clarke, 1994a; 1994b; Zhang et al., 1995). An abundance of evidence suggests that vinblastine and colchicine resistance are at least in part independent of each other, but which drugs segregate with either agent is less clear. The properties and phenotypes of the different mutants suggest that different residues participate in vinblastine and colchicine resistance. Biochemical evidence includes the observation that labeling of P-glycoprotein by azidopine, photoactive analogs of verapamil, or vinblastine is blocked by vinblastine but not by colchicine. However, the 'linkage' of other substrates is less straightforward. Indeed, the diversity of phenotypes observed in mutant P-glycoproteins should restrain attempts to categorize substrates as belonging to putative 'groups'. Examples of diversity in grouping abound in both human and mouse P-glycoproteins. (1) In human *MDR1/MDR3* chimeras, 'the most striking observation' was that replacement of TM12 with *MDR3* impaired resistance to vincristine and doxorubicin, but did not affect colchicine resistance. In contrast, replacement of the loop between TM11 and TM12 with *MDR3* saw the segregation of colchicine with doxorubicin, with supernormal levels of resistance for both, without enhancement of vincristine resistance. The positive and negative effects on actinomycin D resistance conferred by the loop between TM11 and TM12 and TM12 alone,

Table 3.2. *Effect of mutations on cross-resistance and azidopine labeling when mutant P-glycoprotein function is compared to wild-type P-glycoprotein*

	Pro-223 Pro-866	Phe-335	Phe-978	Gly-141 Gly-812	Gly-187 Gly 288 Gly-830
Vinblastine	no change	decreased	decreased	no change	no change
Actinomycin D	decreased	decreased	decreased	no change	decreased
Colchicine	decreased	increased	decreased	increased	increased
Adriamycin	decreased	increased	decreased	increased	increased
Azidopine labeling	no change	increased	no change	no change	no change

respectively, were shown to be additive. (2) The phenotypic expression following the replacement of Ser-939 (*mdr3*) or Ser-941 (*mdr1*) with phenylalanine was found to be complex to individual drugs. For both mouse *mdr1* and *mdr3* decreased resistance to colchicine, adriamycin, and to a lesser extent, even vinblastine, was observed; with no effect on the level of actinomycin D resistance mediated by *mdr1*, but a large decrease in that conferred by *mdr3*. (3) Mutations of human Phe-335 to Ala, or the adjacent Val-338 to Ala confer preferential resistance to colchicine but not vinblastine; but disparate resistance to actinomycin D, which is reduced in mutant Phe-335 to Ala, but not in mutant Val-338 to Ala. (4) Similar diversity observed in other reports from one laboratory are summarized in Table 3.2 (Loo and Clarke, 1993a,b, 1994b).

The discrepancies may be explained in part by the fact that drug resistance is influenced by drug binding, transport and release. For example, two drugs with disparate binding sites may share a common channel, and thus the sensitivity profiles may differ depending on whether the acquired or engineered mutation affects the drug-binding site, or the drug channel. Thus there may be distinct binding sites, and certain substrates might have a preference for one over the other. However, the evidence suggests a greater degree of complexity.

Also to be considered, are the drugs examined in the majority of these studies. The frequent observation of 'linkage' between colchicine (M_r 399) and adriamycin (M_r 580), compared to vinblastine (M_r 909) and actinomycin (M_r 1256) may be explained in part by size differences. However, where size is not a significant factor, adriamycin may segregate away from colchicine (neutral at physiologic pH), and instead form a group consisting of adriamycin, vinblastine and actinomycin D (charged compounds). The limited number of compounds examined could be expanded to include some of the many P-glycoprotein substrates discussed below.

Similarly, while it is generally assumed that the two halves of P-glycoprotein are highly homologous, the data suggests that this similarity has its limits (Devine et al., 1992; Loo and Clarke, 1993b; Zhang et al., 1995). For example, the double mutation identified in the sixth transmembrane domain of a hamster P-glycoprotein was shown to enhance actinomycin D resistance; while replacement of TM 12 of human *MDR 1* with *MDR 3* sequences resulted in a P-glycoprotein with impaired actinomycin D resistance. Four additional mutations in human TM 6 had either no effect or reduced actinomycin D resistance. More importantly, mutation of homologous phenylalanines in TM 6 and TM 12 to alanines (Phe-335 and Phe-978) yielded disparate transporters. The Phe-335 mutant conferred little resistance to vinblastine or actinomycin D but retained ability to confer resistance to colchicine and adriamycin. By contrast, the Phe-978 mutant conferred little or no resistance to colchicine or adriamycin, while its ability to confer resistance to vinblastine or actinomycin D was retained, albeit considerably reduced. Similarly, studies examining the role of proline residues suggest that residues in one half of the tandemly duplicated molecule that are important are likely to be important at the equivalent position in the other half of the molecule, although their roles and contribution to transport function may be different.

Mutations affecting synthesis and processing of P-glycoprotein

While the above discussion has largely centered on the effect of mutations on the drug resistant phenotype, numerous mutations with effects on processing and temperature sensitivity have also been described (Hoof et al., 1994; Loo and Clarke, 1993b, 1994b, 1995). Residues identified as critical for normal biosynthesis and processing include: (1) Gly-251, Gly-268, Gly-269 and Gly-781, which are predicted to be in cytoplasmic loops, have been shown to have profound effects on protein structure, with a 150 kDa product observed in transfectants. These smaller proteins were sensitive to endoglycosidase H digestion, indicating a probable localization to the endoplasmic reticulum, presumably as a consequence of a mechanism that prevents the transport of misfolded proteins that would otherwise be destined for further processing. The latter was supported by the lack of degradation products. Two of these mutants (Gly-269, Gly-781) resulted in temperature-sensitive processing of the protein to the fully mature, 170 kDa form. Full processing increased dramatically when the cells were incubated at 26°C. The latter suggests that at the permissive, lower temperature, mutant protein was able to leave the endoplasmic reticulum and proceed to the Golgi apparatus, where more extensive glycosylation occurred. (2) Phe-777, which in a manner similar to the glycine substitutions described above resulted in predominance of a 150 kDa product when replaced by an alanine residue. As with the glycine substitutions, the 150 kDa product was found to be sensitive to endoglycosidase H treatment, indicating that the product was a partially glycosylated intermediate localized in the endoplasmic reticulum, which had not been further processed through the Golgi apparatus (3) Lys-272, Ser-795, Asn-809 and Tyr-853, which when substituted by a cysteine in a cysteine-less P-glycoprotein mutant affected biosynthesis, resulting in a protein of apparent mass 150 kDa, which was most likely retained in the endoplasmic reticulum due to misfolding. (4) The introduction of cystic fibrosis type mutations has also been shown to result in defective processing. Specifically, the phenotype of missense substitutions in P-glycoprotein analogous to mutations in the CFTR gene have been characterized. Mutagenesis was performed in the center region and the 'signature sequence' (dodecapeptide or linker peptide) of the first nucleotide-binding fold. These motifs are universally conserved in ABC transporters but unlike Walker A and B motifs are not shared with other nucleotide-binding proteins. Replacement of Tyr-490 from the center region resulted in a severe processing defect, without detectable protein (Figure 3.3).

Conclusion

While the evidence indicates that only a percentage of residues are important in determining substrate specificity and activity, it is not yet clear how many residues are so involved. Both random and directed mutations have been performed, and consequently an accurate percentage cannot be determined. The evidence does indicate that a large number of residues are involved, and as summarized in Table 3.1 and Figures 3.1 and 3.2, that these are widely distributed throughout the protein. As discussed above, a negative result may not be indicative of a lack of importance, since the engineered residue may lack sufficient

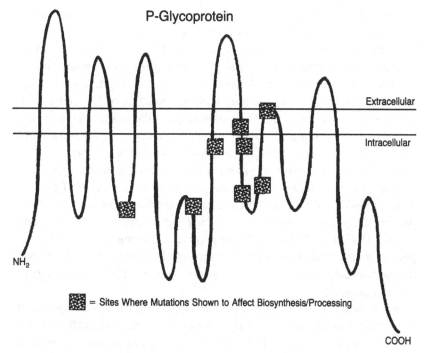

Figure 3.3 P-glycoprotein, showing sites where mutations affect biosynthesis/ processing.

bulk or charge to effect a significant change in specificity or activity. This is well demonstrated by the studies examining TM6 and TM11 substitutions, which suggest that drug resistance in part depends on the size of certain residues.

In addition to the overwhelming evidence implicating the transmembrane segments in drug binding and/or transport, the results suggest that changes in the cytoplasmic loops may have complex effects on both initial drug binding and subsequent release, possibly to a drug channel. While such a hypothesis is attractive if one envisions the transmembrane segments lining a channel and the cytoplasmic loops 'scavenging' for drugs intracellularly, it must be reconciled with the 'vacuum cleaner' hypothesis where drugs are removed from the plasma membrane. It may be that drugs can enter a channel by either of two pathways, or that the cytoplasmic loops deliver drug to the membrane and that in turn the drug then enters the putative channel. In accordance with this view, the mutation at position 185 would affect the delivery of drug to the membrane compartment and not to the outside of the cell.

Furthermore, the introduction of amino acid substitutions in the ATP-binding cassette transporter signature (linker peptide or dodecapeptide) has been shown to alter the drug-resistance profile, suggesting that this region is also involved in the drug transport function of P-glycoprotein. According to one view, 'for P-glycoprotein . . . the linker peptide would both transmit the signal of nucleotide binding and hydrolysis and modify its selectivity for drug transport function' (Hoof et al., 1994).

How such a diversity of sites could be involved in drug transport awaits further clarification. It has been suggested that Gly-185 (loop 2–3) and Phe-335 (TM6) 'are in close proximity to each other and participate in drug–protein interactions during the transport cycle' (Loo and Clarke, 1993b); and that 'the linker peptide . . . interacts with the hydrophobic transport domain' (TM6) (Hoof et al., 1994). While these may not be mutually exclusive, such 'crowding' around TM6 may be physically impossible.

What then can be concluded at this time regarding the regions of P-glycoprotein important for drug transport? Actually, we prefer to leave that conclusion to the critical reader of the literature and this review. Our own bias is that the present data strongly suggests that nearly all regions of P-glycoprotein are involved in drug binding or transport and that future studies will identify additional areas and crucial residues. Specifically, we would expect data demonstrating a role for all transmembrane domains in drug transport and all intracellular 'loops' in drug binding or transport, as well as data implicating the ABC 'signature' sequence in the second half of the molecule in drug resistance. To be sure, only a limited number of mutations are expected to influence activity. For some residues that are not critical, such changes are inconsequential. For critical residues, some changes are tolerable, or can be adapted to, but others will alter the phenotype. Furthermore, as discussed above, not all possible mutations can be examined.

The chloride channel controversy

ABC proteins

P-glycoprotein belongs to the family of ABC (*A*TP-*b*inding *c*assette) proteins, which contain six transmembrane α-helices and an ATP-binding motif per cassette. In common with many ABC transporters,

P-glycoprotein contains and requires two cassettes to form a functional unit. ABC transporters are involved in the movement of a variety of small molecules across membranes including Cl^- (the cystic fibrosis transmembrane regulator), peptides associated with antigen processing (TAP proteins), and hydrophobic anticancer drugs (P-glycoprotein and the multidrug resistance-associated protein, MRP) (Higgins, 1995). While the function of P-glycoprotein in normal tissues has not been fully clarified, its distribution and its role in multidrug resistance strongly support a role in drug disposition (Fojo et al., 1987; Thiebaut et al., 1987; Sugawara et al., 1988; Thiebaut et al., 1989). Initial studies with knockout mice lacking the *mdr1a* gene has demonstrated the importance of this protein in the blood–brain barrier and drug disposition (Schinkel et al., 1994). In this context, it was somewhat surprising when initial studies reported a function for P-glycoprotein in Cl^- transport (Gill et al., 1992; Valverde et al., 1992). These studies purported to show that expression of P-glycoprotein was associated with a cell volume-regulated chloride channel.

Chloride channels

Demonstration of severely reduced chloride permeability in cystic fibrosis has been the principal catalyst for studies examining the plasma membrane chloride permeability of epithelial cells. While the intricacies of chloride flux have not been fully elucidated, studies in epithelia have identified chloride currents following exposure to a variety of stimuli (Krouse et al., 1994). Included among these are (1) Swelling activated chloride currents that result in loss of KCl, effecting a regulatory volume decrease which helps to re-establish homeostasis. These swelling-activated chloride currents have been demonstrated by whole-cell patch recordings of cultured epithelial cells. They are large, outwardly rectifying chloride channels (ORCC) that show inactivation at positive voltages. (2) Depolarization-induced chloride currents, observed when plasma membranes from a variety of cells are excised and depolarized. These currents identified as outwardly rectifying, depolarization induced chloride currents (ORDIC currents) are most commonly generated following depolarization. However, it is well known that many other factors influence the appearance of these channels although their physiologic significance has not been established. (3) Chloride currents have also been described in response to cAMP elevating agents. These have been shown to be linear without obvious voltage-dependent properties, and more permeable to chloride than to iodide. (4) Chloride currents have also been described after exposure to Ca^{2+} ionophores. These are voltage dependent and more permeable to iodide than to chloride.

Since the channels responsible for these currents have not been conclusively identified, it has not been possible to establish if these different currents are generated by different channel proteins or from altered states of a common-channel protein, or for that matter a protein with diverse functions. The cystic fibrosis gene product, CFTR, is thought to be both a chloride channel itself and a regulator of the activity of several other ion channels (Higgins, 1995). The concept of CFTR as a multi-functional protein is suggested by evidence that an outwardly rectifying chloride channel (ORCC), which is abnormally regulated in cystic fibrosis cells, and CFTR are distinct channel proteins; and recent studies have been interpreted as showing CFTR as a cAMP-dependent negative regulator of Na channels. The latter establishes a central role for CFTR as the 'switch' that balances the rates of Na absorption and Cl⁻ secretion to properly hydrate airway secretions in normal airway epithelia.

Chloride currents in P-glycoprotein expressing cells

Initial studies reported increases in the magnitude of cell swelling activated Cl⁻ currents in cells expressing P-glycoprotein and led to the proposal, now abandoned even by its proponents, that P-glycoprotein was bifunctional, with both transport and channel activities. The failure of others to duplicate these findings led to a modification of this hypothesis, and the currently advanced view that P-glycoprotein is not a channel, but that it regulates an endogenous channel protein (Altenberg et al., 1994a,b; Luckie et al., 1994; Rasola et al., 1994; Wang et al., 1994; De Greef et al., 1995; Hardy et al., 1995; Higgins, 1995). According to this view, P-glycoprotein alters the sensitivity of an as yet unidentified channel to osmotic gradients and imposes protein kinase C dependency on channel activation.

The need to revise the original hypothesis and the inability of other investigators to duplicate the original findings raises questions as to the significance of these findings. In a number of different cell lines, an association between expression of P-glycoprotein and chloride channel activity has not been demonstrated, or has been calculated to be insufficient to cause a significant chloride efflux (Altenberg et al., 1994a,b; Luckie et al., 1994; Rasola et al., 1994; Wang et al., 1994; De Greef et al., 1995). While proteins with diverse functions are well described in other biological systems, a function in chloride transport for a protein with the distribution described for P-glycoprotein seems to some of uncertain importance.

Conclusions

What can be concluded from the increasing, albeit conflicting, evidence regarding P-glycoprotein and chloride transport? It seems safe to neglect the original thesis that suggested that P-glycoprotein had dual functions as a drug transporter and a chloride channel. Whether P-glycoprotein has a more limited role as a regulator of channel function is in doubt, but we would advise that this thesis be approached with skepticism, pending the presentation of more convincing evidence. The latter should be possible, given the plethora of well-defined models. Specifically, it should be possible in one model to establish a direct correlation between P-glycoprotein expression and substantive effects on chloride currents. These effects should not be present, or be considerably diminished in control cells, or drug-sensitive revertants. An effect of protein kinase modulators should be accompanied by demonstration of changes in P-glycoprotein phosphorylation, or ideally, should be addressed directly with the use of available mutants, avoiding the myriad of effects these agents have. And most importantly, the potential role in normal tissues should be addressed. While P-glycoprotein is expressed in what can be considered to be 'classical epithelial cells', any hypothesis must address why Cl⁻ transport would be so critical in the blood–testis and blood–brain barriers, and in the adrenal gland?

The regulation of *MDR1* expression

Increased expression of P-glycoprotein is almost invariably observed in cell culture models of multidrug resistance and is frequently found in clinical samples obtained from refractory patients. Thus, it is surprising that until recently, more studies have not focused on the regulation of P-glycoprotein expression. While progress is slowly being made, the mechanisms of regulation of P-glycoprotein are not fully understood.

Modulation of MDR1 RNA expression

Published studies have demonstrated modulation of *MDR1* RNA expression by a variety of compounds including carcinogens, differentiating agents, estrogen, progesterone, arsenite, cadmium, chemotherapeutic agents and P-glycoprotein antagonists (Fairchild et al., 1987; Thorgeirsson et al., 1987; Bates et al., 1989; Mickley et al., 1989; Arceci et al., 1990; Chin et al., 1990a, 1990b; Chin et al., 1993; Herzog et al., 1993; Hu et al., 1995). (1) In rat liver, *MDR1* RNA expression has been shown to increase following exposure to toxic insults including carcinogens, heat shock and partial hepatectomy. (2) In four human colon carcinoma and two neuroblastoma cell lines, increased expression of *MDR1* has been reported following treatment with differentiating agents. (3) The observation that one of the mouse *mdr1* genes is expressed at high levels in the secretory epithelium of the endometrium during pregnancy, led to the demonstration that mouse *mdr1b* RNA levels are increased by estrogen and progesterone in the secretory glands of the mouse uterus. (4) In a human kidney cell line, arsenite and cadmium have been shown to increase *MDR1* expression, and this increase has been shown to correlate with a transient increase in drug resistance. (5) Increased expression of *MDR1* RNA has been reported in rodent cells following exposure to either chemotherapeutic agents known to be substrates for P-glycoprotein or topoisomerase inhibitors. Recently 'rapid up-regulation of *mdr1* expression by anthracyclines' was reported in a 'variant human multidrug resistant cell line' (Hu et al., 1995). (6) Increased *MDR1* expression following treatment of a human colon carcinoma cell line with a variety of P-glycoprotein antagonists has also been observed.

In addition to these agents, other factors have been shown to influence *MDR1* expression in select models (Fairchild et al., 1987; Thorgeirsson et al., 1987; Abraham et al., 1990; Scala et al., 1995). In rat liver, *MDR1* RNA expression has been shown to increase in regenerating liver following partial hepatectomy. Heat shock led to increased *MDR1* RNA expression in a human kidney cell line, and in several models, modulation of protein kinase activity (PKA) has been implicated in regulating *MDR1* expression. In human breast cancer cells, increased expression of *MDR1* was observed following exposure to 8-Cl-cAMP, suggesting a role for PKA. Additionally, a cAMP-dependent PKA mutant and a transfectant Chinese hamster ovary cell line expressing the defective regulatory subunit (RI) for PKA from this mutant were sensitive to multiple P-glycoprotein substrates. This sensitivity was shown to be secondary to decreased P-glycoprotein expression in these cells. Together, these studies support a regulatory role for PKA in the expression of the *MDR1* genes that remains undefined.

Promoter and transcription factors

While these studies underscore the complexity of the regulation of *MDR1* expression, more recent efforts have attempted to define the promoter elements and transcription factors involved (Kohno et al., 1989; Chin et al., 1990b; Kohno et al., 1992). The identification of heat shock consensus elements in the promoter region of *MDR1* led to the subsequent documentation that its expression could be regulated by heat shock, arsenite and cadmium in a human kidney cell line. While this study represented a logical test of the role of a putative element, the role of other putative elements present in the *MDR1* promoter should be interpreted with caution, since functional correlations have not yet been established for most of these regulatory elements. For example, an inverted Y-box consensus element has been shown to be essential for CAT activity, but its role in regulating *MDR1* expression awaits further studies (Goldsmith et al., 1993).

Similarly, the role of transcription factors in regulating *MDR1* expression is not fully understood. Early studies reported increased CAT activity in co-transfection experiments of both mouse and hamster *mdr1a* promoters with expression vectors encoding the c-*jun* and c-*fos* proteins, which interact with AP-1 sites (Chin et al., 1993). Recent reports have identified the transcriptional regulator nuclear factor for interleukin-6 (NF-IL6), and the tumor suppressor *p53* as potential candidates (Chin et al., 1992; Cohen et al., 1994; Combates et al., 1994; Goldsmith et al., 1995). For NF-IL6, co-transfection of an NF-IL6 expression vector with a chloramphenicol acetyltransferase reporter gene driven by 1018 base pairs of *MDR1* 5'-flanking sequences demonstrated that NF-IL6 transactivated the *MDR1* promoter. This trans-activation was significantly reduced when the NF-IL6 element in the reporter gene construct was deleted or mutated. For *p53*, conflicting reports have been observed in different models. The initial study sought to implicate *ras* and *p53* in the expression of *MDR1* during tumor progression. Expression of *MDR1* can occur in tumors in the absence of drug treatment and a hypothesis that links this expression to tumor progression is attractive. To explore this possibility, NIH3T3, KNIH and SW13 cells were co-transfected with several promoter–CAT constructs and the expression vectors for c-Ha-*ras*-1. Measurement of CAT activity confirmed that the promoter of the human *MDR1* gene was a target for the c-Ha-*ras*-1 oncogene and the *p53* tumor suppressor gene product, both of which are associated with tumor progression. Whereas c-Ha-*ras*-1 enhanced the activity of four additional promoters, suggesting the effect on *MDR1* was not specific, the effects of *p53* and its mutant were more specific. Wild-type *p53* had no significant effect on five promoters, whereas mutant *p53* enhanced only *MDR1*-CAT expression. The authors concluded that 'the results imply that the *MDR1* gene could be activated during tumor progression associated with mutations in *ras* and *p53*', but cautioned that 'an alternative model . . . is that both wild type and mutant *p53* can activate or repress transcription in a promoter and cell-type specific manner' (Chin et al., 1992). This latter explanation now appears to be accurate. When similar studies were performed in H358 human lung carcinoma cells, which are *p53* negative, the opposite results were obtained. In contrast to the results in NIH3T3 cells, in the H358 lung carcinoma cells, and three other cell lines, co-transfection with a wild-type *p53* expression vector stimulated *MDR1*-CAT activity, while co-transfection with mutant *p53* expression vectors altered at amino acid positions 181, 252, 258, or 273 failed to stimulate expression. 'Although the bases for the apparently opposite results are unclear, the cell lines, *p53* expression vectors, the *MDR1* reporter constructs, the methods of transfection, and the time of analyses . . . were different . . . (making) a direct comparison (of) studies difficult' (Goldsmith et al., 1995). Additional studies will be needed to determine the significance of these conflicting observations. Interestingly, clinical studies have not documented an association between wild-type or mutant *p53* and *MDR1* expression (Renninson et al., 1994; Schneider et al., 1994).

Conclusions

What can be concluded about the regulation of *MDR1* expression? The available information indicates that regulation is complex, and under the control of a variety of stimuli. The diversity of results can be explained in part by the diversity of models used in published studies. There is a broad range of *MDR1* RNA expression in different human tissues, and similar results have been observed in rodents. These differences most likely reflect a tissues' differential mRNA transcription, processing and stability, although the mechanisms responsible have not been fully identified. Some of the discrepancies between human and rodent cell lines may eventually be traced to their respective promoters. While some of the reported differences in promoter regions may not be functionally significant, others are likely to influence gene regulation. In this regard, our bias is to consider studies that only report increased expression of transfected reporter genes as preliminary observations. The modest changes observed in CAT activity in some experiments, often coupled with a lack of internal and reference controls, preclude final conclusions from being drawn. Only when regulation of the endogenous *MDR1* gene can be demonstrated in more than one model, should full credence be given to a proposed mechanism. Reflecting our own bias, a key question remains unanswered: is expression in drug-selected cell lines and refractory tumors under similar regulatory control as that in normal tissues, unselected cell lines and untreated human tumors? While the answer to this question is likely to be complex, preliminary results indicate that gene rearrangement with capture of *MDR1* by an active promoter can bring about transcriptional activation during the course of drug selection. This in turn could influence the modulation of expression in different models, so that for example, induction by chemotherapeutic agents is observed only in select cell lines.

Transport diversity: the broad range of substrates

The multidrug resistance phenotype

The literature generally recognizes a multidrug resistance phenotype that consists of resistance to colchicine, the anthracyclines, the vinca alkaloids, actinomycin D, and paclitaxel. These compounds are generally hydrophobic and possess a positive charge at physiologic pH. The drugs enter cells by passive diffusion through the plasma membrane and are subsequently extruded from cells, either by removal from the plasma membrane, the cytosol or both.

The diversity of drugs transported by P-glycoprotein necessitates structural compromise in drug binding and drug transport sites. A compromise that retains the ability to bind many compounds, but binds none optimally, could explain the broad range of transport efficiency. In this view, the alteration of a given site might enhance the recognition of some compounds but only at the expense of a diminished ability to recognize others. While this still remains speculative, the recurrent observation that alterations in P-glycoprotein invariably confer increased resistance to one or more drugs at the expense of others is strongly supportive of this.

An even more pleiotropic phenotype

Also in accord with this are recent findings which have enormously expanded the list of P-glycoprotein substrates (Butryn et al., 1994; Lee et al., 1994; Toppmeyer et al., 1994; Zhang et al., 1994; Alvarez et al., 1995; Russo et al., 1995). With the identification of new substrates the structural diversity of compounds transported by P-glycoprotein has been increased further; and the observation that cross-resistance to these new substrates varies enormously, is consistent with a broad range of transport efficiency. Individual studies have identified homoharringtonine, bisantrene, dolastatin 10, and bizelesin as P-glycoprotein substrates. (1) Homoharringtonine, a cephalotaxine alkaloid, showed low efficiency in refractory and relapsed leukemia and in the blastic phase of chronic myeloid leukemia (CML). These diseases are frequently characterized by high levels of expression of P-glycoprotein. This led to the postulate of a relationship between the poor antileukemic effect of homoharringtonine and the expression of P-glycoprotein, a thesis that led to its confirmation as a P-glycoprotein substrate. (2) Bisantrene, which like mitoxantrone and other anthracyclines is an anthracene derivative, was shown to be an excellent substrate for P-glycoprotein with numerous P-glycoprotein expressing cells demonstrating 10-fold greater resistance to bisantrene compared to vinblastine, doxorubicin or colchicine. (3) Dolastatin 10, a cytotoxic pentapeptide, was also identified as a P-glycoprotein substrate, leading the authors to conclude that P-glycoprotein might also function as a peptide transporter. (4) Bizelesin, a synthetically derived analog of the highly potent, alkylating, antitumor antibiotic, CC1065, was used in the selection of drug-resistant cell lines. The resultant cells exhibited a multidrug resistant phenotype and genotype, suggesting that this agent was a P-glycoprotein substrate. In addition, multidrug resistant cells were shown to be cross-resistant to bizelesin, and several of its analogs, adding to the multidrug resistant phenotype a new class of compounds.

Predicting P-glycoprotein substrates

The above compounds were predicted to be P-glycoprotein substrates using the large database of the NCI Anticancer Drug Screen and a modified version of the COMPARE program (Lee et al., 1994; Alvarez et al., 1995). The studies were performed in one of two ways: The first generated a 'Drug Resistance Profile' by measuring the level of *MDR1* mRNA in the sixty cell lines of the Anticancer Drug Screen. The second generated a P-glycoprotein activity profile using rhodamine-123 efflux as a functional assay. As expected, there was a significant correlation between *MDR1* expression and rhodamine efflux. These profiles were then used as 'seeds', for the COMPARE analysis with over 30 000 compounds in the Anticancer Drug Screen database. Hundreds of compounds with activity patterns inversely correlated with the level of *MDR1* expression, or rhodamine 123 efflux, were identified as likely P-glycoprotein substrates. Evidence that these compounds are P-glycoprotein substrates includes: (a) enhancement of cytotoxicity by verapamil; (b) demonstration of cross-resistance in multidrug resistant cell lines; (c) ability to antagonize P-glycoprotein, increasing vinblastine accumulation by decreasing efflux; (d) inhibition of photoaffinity labeling by azidopine; and (e) ability to lead to the isolation of multidrug resistant cell lines expressing P-glycoprotein when used as selecting agents.

Compared to the 30 000 compounds in the database, the putative P-glycoprotein substrates varied from the norm in several ways. Most importantly, over 40% were clearly of natural origin, 10 times the percentage of purified natural products in the NCI chemical database, and an additional percentage were semisynthetic in origin. The molecular weights of the putative P-glycoprotein substrates appeared to be distributed differently according to their net charge. Neutral molecules had an average molecular weight of 861 compared to 517 for those with a cationic charge or basic side chain. The majority of compounds identified were heretofore not regarded as P-glycoprotein substrates. Furthermore, this analysis can now be used prospectively to identify whether a drug is a likely P-glycoprotein substrate. Although for some, one might have made such a prediction, for others their identification broadened the spectrum of P-glycoprotein substrates.

Conclusions

Realization that such a broad range of compounds are P-glycoprotein substrates has implications for future clinical trials. It is reasonable to predict that many new drugs entering future clinical trials will be P-glycoprotein substrates. Although the incidence of 'significant' P-glycoprotein expression in clinical samples remains unclear, in virtually every tumor type, expression at some level has been reported, and since many of the new substrates identified are transported to a greater degree than drugs used clinically, it is possible that even low levels of P-glycoprotein could confer resistance, precluding clinical efficacy. Indeed, clinical studies with homoharringtonine, bisantrene and olivomycin, three excellent P-glycoprotein substrates, were terminated after they failed to show significant activity. Because the addition of a P-glycoprotein antagonist could enhance activity, one could argue that such substrates should not be developed without the addition of a P-glycoprotein antagonist. Or we can leave that argument for others to make.

We wonder how many investigators or pharmaceutical companies will forgo years of study and monetary investment without trying a promising drug that is known to be an excellent P-glycoprotein substrate without a suitable antagonist in a clinical trial?

References

Abraham, I., Chin, K.-V., Gottesman, M. M. et al. (1990). Transfection of a mutant regulatory subunit gene of cAMP-dependent protein kinase causes increased drug sensitivity and decreased expression of P-glycoprotein. *Exp. Cell. Res.*, **189**, 133–41.

Altenberg, G., Vanoye, C. G., Hans, E. S. et al. (1994a). Relationship between rhodamine-123 transport, cell volume, and ion-channel function of P-glycoprotein. *J. Biol. Chem.*, **269**, 7145–9.

Altenberg, G. A., Deitmer, J. W., Glass, D. C. and Reuss, L. (1994b). P-glycoprotein-associated Cl⁻ currents are activated by cell swelling but do not contribute to cell volume regulation. *Cancer Res.*, **54**, 618–22.

Alvarez, M., Paull, K., Monks, A. et al. (1995). Generation of a drug resistance profile by quantitation of mdr-1/P-glycoprotein in the cell lines of the National Cancer Institute Anticancer Drug Screen. *J. Clin. Invest.*, **95**, 2205–14.

Arceci, R. J., Baas, F., Raponi, R. et al. (1990). Multidrug resistance gene expression is controlled by steroid hormones in the secretory epithelium of the uterus. *Mol. Reprod. Dev.*, **25**, 101–9.

Bates, S. E., Mickley, L. A., Chen, Y.-N. et al. (1989). Expression of a drug resistance gene in human neuroblastoma cell lines: modulation by retinoic acid-induced differentiation. *Molec. Cell. Biol.*, **9**, 4337–44.

Biedler, J. L. (1992). Genetic aspects of multidrug resistance. *Cancer*, **70**, 1799–809.

Bruggemann, E. P., Germann, U. A., Gottesman, M. M. and Pastan, I. (1989). Two different regions of phosphoglycoprotein are photoaffinity labeled by azidopine. *J. Biol. Chem.*, **264**, 15483–8.

Bruggemann, E. P., Currier, S. J., Gottesman, M. M. and Pastan, I. (1992). Characterization of the azidopine and vinblastine binding sites of P-glycoprotein. *J. Biol. Chem.*, **267**, 21020–6.

Buschman, E. and Gros, P. (1991). Functional analysis of chimeric genes obtained by exchanging homologous domains of the mouse *mdr1* and *mdr2* genes. *Molec. Cell. Biol.*, **11**, 595–603.

Butryn, R. K., Smith, K. S., Adams, E. G. et al. (1994). V79 Chinese hamster lung cells resistant to the bis-alkylator bizelesin are multidrug-resistant. *Cancer Chemother. Pharmacol.*, **34**, 44–50.

Chen, C. J., Chin, J. E., Ueda, K. et al. (1986). Internal duplication and homology with bacterial transport proteins in mdr-1 (P-glycoprotein) gene from multidrug-resistant human cells. *Cell*, **47**, 371–80.

Chin, J. E., Soffir, R., Noonan, K. E. et al. (1989). Structure and expression of the human MDR (P-glycoprotein) gene family. *Molec. Cell. Biol.*, **9**, 3808–20.

Chin, K.-V., Chauhan, S. S., Pastan, I. and Gottesman, M. M. (1990a). Regulation of mdr RNA levels in response to cytotoxic drugs in rodent cells. *Cell Growth Differ.*, **1**, 361–5.

Chin, K.-V., Tanaka, S., Darlington, G. et al. (1990b). Heat shock and arsenite increase expression of the multidrug resistance (MDR1) gene in human renal carcinoma cells. *J. Biol. Chem.*, **265**, 221–6.

Chin, K.-V., Ueda, K., Pastan, I. and Gottesman, M. M. (1992). Modulation of activity of the promoter of the human MDR1 gene by Ras and p53. *Science*, **255**, 459–62.

Chin, K.-V., Pastan, I. and Gottesman, M. M. (1993). Function and regulation of the human multidrug resistance gene. *Adv. Cancer Res.*, **60**, 157–80.

Choi, K., Chen, C. J., Kriegler, M. and Roninson, I. B. (1988). An altered pattern of cross-resistance in multidrug resistant human cells results from spontaneous mutations in the *mdr-1* (P-glycoprotein) gene. *Cell*, **53**, 519–29.

Cianfrigilia, M., Willingham, M. C., Tombesi, M. et al. (1994). P-glycoprotein epitope mapping. I. Identification of a linear human-specific epitope in the fourth loop of the P-glycoprotein extracellular domain by MM4.17 murine monoclonal antibody to human multidrug resistant cells. *Int. J. Cancer*, **56**, 153–60.

Cohen, D., Yu, L., Rzepka, R. W. and Horwitz, S. B. (1994). Identification of two nuclear protein binding sites and their role in the regulation of the murine multidrug resistance *mdr*1a promoter. *DNA Cell Biol.*, **13**, 641–9.

Combates, N. J., Rzepka, R. W., Pan Chen, Y.-N. and Cohen, D. (1994). NF-IL6, a member of the C/EBP family of transcription factors binds and *trans*-activates the human MDR1 gene promoter. *J. Biol. Chem.*, **269**, 29715–19.

Currier, S. J., Kane, S. E., Willingham, M. C. et al. (1992). Identification of residues in the first cytoplasmic loop of P-glycoprotein involved in the function of chimeric human MDR1-MDR2 transporters. *J. Biol. Chem.*, **25153–9**.

De Greef, C., Sehrer, J., Viana, F. et al. (1995). Volume-activated chloride currents are not correlated with P-glycoprotein expression. *Biochem. J.*, **307**, 713–18.

Devault, A. and Gros, P. (1990). Two members of the mouse mdr gene family confer multidrug resistance with overlapping but distinct drug specificities. *Molec. Cell. Biol.*, **10**, 1652–63.

Devine, S. E., Ling, V. and Melera, P. W. (1992). Amino acid substitutions in the sixth transmembrane domain of P-glycoprotein alter multidrug resistance. *Proc. Natl. Acad. Sci. USA*, **89**, 4564–8.

Dhir, R., Grizzuti, K., Kajiji, S. and Gros, P. (1993). Modulatory effects on substrate specificity of independent mutations at the Ser$^{939/941}$ position in predicted transmembrane domain 11 of P-glycoproteins. *Biochemistry*, **32**, 9492–7.

Endicott, J. A. and Ling, V. (1989). The biochemistry of P-glycoprotein-mediated multidrug resistance. *Annu. Rev. Biochem.*, **58**, 137–71.

Fairchild, C. R., Ivy, S. P., Rushmore, T. et al. (1987). Carcinogen-induced mdr overexpression is associated with xenobiotic resistance in rat preneoplastic liver nodules and hepatocellular carcinomas. *Proc. Natl. Acad. Sci. USA*, **84**, 7701–5.

Fojo, A. T., Ueda, K., Slamon, D. J. et al. (1987). Expression of a multidrug resistance gene in human tumors and tissues. *Proc. Natl. Acad. Sci. USA*, **84**, 265–9.

Georges, E., Bradley, G., Garipey, J. and Ling, V. (1990). Detection of P-glycoprotein isoforms by gene-specific monoclonal antibodies. *Proc. Natl. Acad. Sci.*, **87**, 152–6.

Georges, E., Tsuruo, T. and Ling, V. (1993). Topology of P-glycoprotein as determined by epitope mapping of MRK-16 antibody. *J. Biol. Chem.*, **268**, 1792–8.

Gill, D. R., Hyde, S. C., Higgins, C. F. et al. (1992). Separation of drug transport and chloride channel functions of the human multidrug resistance P-glycoprotein. *Cell*, **71**, 23–32.

Goldsmith, M. E., Madden, M. J., Morrow, C. S. and Cowan, K. H. (1993). A Y-box consensus sequence is required for basal expression of the human multidrug resistance (*mdr1*) gene. *J. Biol. Chem.*, **268**, 5856–60.

Goldsmith, M. E., Gudas, J. M., Schneider, E. and Cowan, K. H. (1995). Wild type p53 stimulates expression from the human multidrug resistance promoter in a p53-negative cell line. *J. Biol. Chem.*, **270**, 1894–8.

Gottesman, M. M. and Pastan, I. (1993). Biochemistry of multidrug resistance mediated by the multidrug transporter. *Annu. Rev. Biochem.*, **62**, 385–427.

Greenberger, L. M. (1993). Major photoaffinity drug labeling sites for iodoaryl azidoprazosin in P-glycoprotein are within or immediately C-terminal to transmembrane domains 6 and 12. *J. Biol. Chem.*, **268**, 11417–25.

Greenberger, L. M., Huang Yang, C.-P., Gindin, E. and Horwitz, S. B. (1990). Photoaffinity probes for the yy_1-adrenergic receptor and the calcium channel bind to a common domain in P-glycoprotein. *J. Biol. Chem.*, **265**, 4394–401.

Greenberger, L. M., Lisanti, C. J., Silva, J. T. and Horwitz, S. B. (1991). Domain mapping of the photoaffinity drug-binding sites in P-glycoprotein encoded by mouse mdr1b. *J. Biol. Chem.*, **266**, 20744–51.

Gros, P., Ben Neriah, Y., Croop, J. M. and Housman, D. E. (1986a). Isolation and expression of a complimentary DNA that confers multidrug resistance. *Nature*, **323**, 728–31.

Gros, P., Croop, J. and Housman, D. (1986b). Mammalian multidrug resistance gene: complete cDNA sequence indicates strong homology to bacterial transport proteins. *Cell*, **47**, 371–80.

Gros, P., Raymond, M., Bell, J. and Housman, D. (1988). Cloning and characterization of a second member of the mouse mdr gene family. *Molec. Cell. Biol.*, **8**, 2770–8.

Hardy, S. P., Goodfellow, H. R., Valverde, M. A. et al. (1995). Protein kinase C-mediated phosphorylation of the human multidrug resistance P-glycoprotein regulates cell volume-activated chloride channels. *EMBO J.*, **14**, 68–75.

Herzog, C. E., Tsokos, M., Bates, S. E. and Fojo, A. T. (1993). Increased mdr-1/P-glycoprotein expression after treatment of human colon carcinoma cells with P-glycoprotein antagonists. *J. Biol. Chem.*, **268**, 2946–52.

Higgins, C. F. (1995). The ABC of channel regulation. *Cell*, **82**, 693–6.

Hoof, T., Demmer, A., Hadam, M. R. et al. (1994). Cystic fibrosis-type mutational analysis in the ATP-binding cassette transporter signature of human P-glycoprotein MDR1. *J. Biol. Chem.*, **269**, 20575–83.

Hsu, S. I., Cohen, D., Kirschner, L. S. et al. (1990). Structural analysis of the mouse mdr1a (p-glycoprotein) promoter reveals the basis for differential transcript heterogeneity in multidrug-resistant J774.2 cells. *Molec. Cell. Biol.*, 10(7), 3596–606.

Hu, X. F., Slater, A., Wall, D. M. et al. (1995). Rapid up-regulation of mdr1 expression by anthracyclines in a classical multidrug-resistant cell line. *Br. J. Cancer*, 71, 931–6.

Kajiji, S., Talbot, F., Grizzuti, K. et al. (1993). Functional analysis of P-glycoprotein mutants identified predicted transmembrane domain 11 as a putative drug binding site. *Biochemistry*, 32, 4185–94.

Kane, S. E., Pastan, I. and Gottesman, M. M. (1990). Genetic basis of multidrug resistance of tumor cells. *J. Bioenergetics Biomembranes*, 22, 593–618.

Kast, C., Canfield, V. A., Levnson, R. and Gros, P. (1995). Topology of intact P-glycoprotein in mammalian cells. *AACR Special Conference, Novel Strategies*, B-19 (Abstract).

Kohno, K., Sato, S.-I., Takano, H. et al. (1989). The direct activation of human multidrug resistance gene (mdr1) by anticancer agents. *Biochem. Biophys. Res. Comm.*, 165, 1415–21.

Kohno, K., Sato, S., Uchiumi, T. et al. (1992). Activation of the human multidrug resistance 1 (MDR1) gene promoter in response to inhibitors of DNA topoisomerases. *Int. J. Oncol.*, 1, 73–7.

Krouse, M. E., Haws, C. M., Xia, Y. et al. (1994). Dissociation of depolarization-activated and swelling-activated Cl⁻ channels. *Am. J. Physiol.*, 267, C642–9.

Lee, J. S., Paull, K., Alvarez, M. et al. (1994). Rhodamine efflux patterns predict P-glycoprotein substrates in the National Cancer Institute drug screen. *Molec. Pharmacol.*, 46, 627–38.

Loo, T. W. and Clarke, D. M. (1993a). Functional consequences of proline mutations in the predicted transmembrane domain of P-glycoprotein. *J. Biol. Chem.*, 268, 3143–9.

Loo, T. W. and Clarke, D. M. (1993b). Functional consequences of phenylalanine mutations in the predicted transmembrane domain of P-glycoprotein. *J. Biol. Chem.*, 268, 19965–72.

Loo, T. W. and Clarke, D. M. (1994a). Mutations to amino acids located in predicted transmembrane segment 6 (TM6) modulate the activity and substrate specificity of human P-glycoprotein. *Biochemistry*, 33, 14049–57.

Loo, T. W. and Clarke, D. M. (1994b). Functional consequences of glycine mutations in the predicted cytoplasmic loops of P-glycoprotein. *J. Biol. Chem.*, 269, 7243–8.

Loo, T. W. and Clarke, D. M. (1995). Membrane topology of a cysteine-less mutant of human P-glycoprotein. *J. Biol. Chem.*, 270, 843–8.

Luckie, D. B., Krouse, M. E., Harper, K. L. et al. (1994). Selection for MDR1/ P-glycoprotein enhances swelling activated K⁺ and Cl⁻ currents in NIH/3T3 cells. *Am. J. Physiol.*, 267, C650–8.

Mickley, L. A., Bates, S. E., Richert, N. D. et al. (1989). Modulation of the expression of a multidrug resistance gene (*mdr-1*/P-glycoprotein) by differentiating agents. *J. Biol. Chem.*, 264, 18031–40.

Morris, D. I., Greenberger, L. M., Bruggemann, E. P. et al. (1994). Localization of the forskolin labeling sites to both halves of P-glycoprotein: similarity of the sites labeled by forskolin and prazosin. *Molec. Pharmacol.*, 46, 329–37.

Ng, W. F., Sarangi, F., Zastawny, R. L. et al. (1989). Identification of members of the P-glycoprotein multigene family. *Molec. Cell. Biol.*, 9, 1224–32.

Pastan, I. and Gottesman, M. (1987). Multiple-drug resistance in human cancer. *N. Engl. J. Med.*, **316**, 1388–93.

Rasola, A., Galietta, J. V., Gruenert, D. C. and Simmons, N. L. (1994). Volume-sensitive chloride currents in four epithelial cell lines are not directly correlated to the expression of the MDR-1 gene. *J. Biol. Chem.*, **209**, 1432–6.

Renninson, J., Baker, B. W., McGown, A. T. et al. (1994). Immunohistochemical detection of mutant p53 protein in epithelial ovarian cancer using polyclonal antibody CMI: correlation with histopathology and clinical features. *Br. J. Cancer*, **69**, 609–12.

Russo, D., Michelutti, A., Melli, C. et al. (1995). MDR-related P170-glycoprotein modulates cytotoxic activity of Homoharringtonine. *Leukemia*, **9**, 513–16.

Safa, A., Stern, R. K., Choi, K. et al. (1990). Molecular basis of preferential resistance to colchicine in multidrug-resistant human cells conferred by Gly-185–Val-185 substitution in P-glycoprotein. *Proc. Natl. Acad. Sci.*, **87**, 7225–9.

Scala, S., Budillon, A., Zhan, Z. et al. (1995). Downregulation of *mdr*-1 expression by 8-Cl-cAMP in multidrug resistant MCF-7 human breast cancer cells. *J. Clin. Invest.*, **96**, 1026–34.

Schinkel, A. H., Smit, J. J., van Tellingen, O. et al. (1994). Disruption of mouse mdr-1a p-glycoprotein gene leads to a deficiency in the blood-brain barrier and to increased sensitivity to drugs. *Cell*, **77**, 491–502.

Schneider, J., Rubio, M.-P., Barbazan, M.-J. et al. (1994). P-glycoprotein, HER-2/neu, and mutant p53 expression in human gynecologic tumors. *J. Natl. Cancer Inst.*, **86**, 850–5.

Skach, W. R., Calayag, M. C. and Lingappa, V. R. (1993). Evidence for an alternate model of human P-glycoprotein structure and biogenesis. *J. Biol. Chem.*, **268**, 6903–8.

Sugawara, I., Kataoka, I., Morishita, Y. et al. (1988). Tissue distribution of P-glycoprotein encoded by a multidrug-resistant gene as revealed by a monoclonal antibody, MRK 16. *Cancer Res.*, **48**, 1926–9.

Thiebaut, F., Tsuruo, T., Hamada, H. et al. (1987). Cellular localization of the multidrug resistance gene product P-glycoprotein in normal human tissues. *Proc. Natl. Acad. Sci. USA*, **84**, 7735–8.

Thiebaut, F., Tsuruo, T., Hamada, H. et al. (1989). Immunohistochemical localization in normal tissues of different epitopes in the multidrug transport protein P170: evidence for localization in brain capillaries and cross reactivity of one antibody with muscle protein. *J. Histochem. Cytochem.*, **37**, 159–64.

Thorgeirsson, S. S., Huber, B. E., Sorrell, S. et al. (1987). Expression of the multidrug-resistant gene in hepatocarcinogenesis and regenerating rat liver. *Science*, **236**, 1120–2.

Toppmeyer, D. H., Slapak, C. A., Croop, J. and Kufe, D. W. (1994). Role of P-glycoprotein in dolastatin 10 resistance. *Biochem. Pharmacol.*, **48**, 609–12.

Valverde, M. A., Diaz, M., Sepulveda, F. V. et al. (1992). Volume-regulated chloride channels associated with the human multidrug-resistance P-glycoprotein. *Nature*, **355**, 830–3.

Van der Bliek, A. M. and Borst, P. (1989). Multidrug resistance. *Adv. Cancer Res.*, **52**, 165–203.

Van der Bliek, A. M., Kooiman, P. M., Schneider, C. and Borst, P. (1988). Sequence of mdr3 cDNA encoding a human P-glycoprotein. *Gene*, **71**, 401–11.

Wang, X., Wall, D. M., Parkin, J. D. et al. (1994). P-glycoprotein expression in classical multidrug resistant leukemia cells does not correlate with enhanced chloride channel activity. *Clin. Exp. Pharmacol. Physiol.*, **21**, 101–8.

Zhang, J.-T., Duthie, M. and Ling, V. (1993). Membrane topology of the N-terminal half of the hamster P-glycoprotein molecule. *J. Biol. Chem.*, **268**, 15101–10.

Zhang, X., Collins, K. I. and Greenberger, L. M. (1995). Functional evidence that transmembrane 12 and the loop between transmembrane 11 and 12 form part of the drug binding domain in P-glycoprotein encoded by MDR1. *J. Biol. Chem.*, **270**, 5441–8.

Zhang, X. P., Ritke, M. K., Yalowich, J. C. et al. (1994). P-glycoprotein mediates profound resistance to bisantrene. *Oncol. Res.*, **6**, 291–301.

4

Topoisomerase genes and resistance to topoisomerase inhibitors

GIUSEPPE GIACCONE

DNA topoisomerase genes and their functions

DNA topoisomerases are vital enzymes present in all living cells, and essential to the resolution of DNA topology. They modify the topological structure of DNA, leaving intact its nucleotide sequence. The activity of topoisomerases is required in order to separate the two intertwined chains of DNA, and allow several important physiological steps such as DNA replication and transcription. In eukaryotic cells there are essentially two types of DNA topoisomerases: DNA topoisomerase I (topo I) and DNA topoisomerase II (topo II).

Several steps are performed by topoisomerases in their dynamic interaction with DNA: DNA binding, DNA cleavage, DNA strand passage (single-strand for topo I and double-strand for topo II), religation, and enzyme turnover (Osheroff, 1989). Topo I determines one strand break at a time, followed by passage of the other strand of the double-stranded DNA helix and by religation. Topo II cuts both strands of DNA, and forms a gap through which a whole DNA double strand can pass, followed by religation.

Both type topoisomerases interact with the DNA through a tyrosine residue, by forming an enzyme–DNA ester bond; after the strand passage the deoxyribose hydroxyl group at the broken end reforms the DNA phosphodiester linkage and frees the enzyme for the next round of reactions.

There are essentially three major activities that are catalyzed by topoisomerases: relaxation of supercoiled DNA, knotting/unknotting of DNA, and catenation/decatenation. The first two reactions can be catalyzed by both type topoisomerases; the third type of reaction can only be catalyzed by topo II in mammalian cells.

In addition to chromosomal DNA, double-stranded circular genome is also present in mitochondria, and encodes the RNAs exclusively utilized for mitochondrial translation. Some mitochondrial transcription products are essential components of the respiratory chain and the ATP-generating apparatus. A mitochondrial topo I present in human platelets has been immunologically identified (Kosovsky and Soslau, 1993), and a mitochondrial DNA topo II has also been described (Osheroff, 1989).

In this chapter the recent knowledge on DNA topoisomerases will be discussed, with particular reference to human topoisomerase genes, and their involvement in anticancer therapy and drug resistance.

Topoisomerase I

Type I topoisomerases catalyze the breakage/reunion of the DNA double helix by introducing transient single-strand breaks, and change the DNA linking number in steps of one (Wang, 1985). The linking number describes the number of times two DNA strands cross each other when projected onto a plane.

Single-strand breaks caused by topo I help to remove excessive positive as well as negative DNA supercoils arising during DNA replication and transcription. Roles for topo I in human cells are thought to include the initiation and elongation phases of DNA transcription and DNA replication (Watt and Hickson, 1994). In the absence of topo I, replication fork movement would be arrested by the accumulation of torsional strain in the DNA template (Gupta, Fujimori and Pommier, 1995). Eukaryotic topo I can also promote illegitimate DNA recombination.

Activity of topo I does not require a high energy cofactor (i.e. ATP), and although this enzyme can work in the absence of a divalent cation, the presence of magnesium, calcium, or manganese, can stimulate the activity 2–25 fold (Osheroff, 1989). Under optimal conditions eukaryotic topo I acts via a processive reaction mechanism, whereby the enzyme relaxes all supercoils in a DNA molecule, before dissociation.

The enzyme binds to approximately 15–25 nucleotides of DNA (Osheroff, 1989), and is attached to the 3'-phosphate of the broken DNA strand, via an *O4*-phosphotyrosine bridge. The cleavable complex is formed by a reversible transesterification reaction in which a 5' oxygen of a phosphodiester bond is exchanged for a tyrosine hydroxyl group (Tyr-723 for human topo I). Only weak consensus sequences have been identified for interaction of topo I with DNA. Approximately 90% of topo I sites have a T at position ×1, both in the absence and presence of the topo I inhibitor camptothecin. The site-specific action of the enzyme is governed solely by the DNA sequence within a minimal 16 bp core duplex, whereas contacts in the flanking regions may influence the DNA binding affinity of the enzyme or may be critical for activation or enzyme-mediated DNA scission (Andersen, Svejstrup and Westergaard, 1994).

Genetic studies in unicellular organisms, including eubacteria and yeasts, indicate that topo I is not essential for viability, whereas in multicellular organisms, such as *Drosophila*, topo I is essential for the growth and development of the fruit fly (Lee et al., 1993). Topo I has been estimated to be present in approximately 2×10^4 to 10^5 copies per cell in HeLa and rat liver, and associates preferentially with transcriptionally active loci (Hwang and Hwong, 1994).

Unlike topo II, topo I cellular levels in normal tissue are relatively independent of cell cycle phases. Topo I is present in normal lymphocytes, cells confined to G_0/G_1 phase, while topo II is undetectable in such cells (Potmesil, 1994). However, following phytohemagglutinin stimulation of T lymphocytes, a rapid increase in topo I mRNA was observed, corresponding to the entry of cells into S phase. The increase in protein expression was much lower than that of mRNA, due to a reduced half-life of the protein in proliferating T cells (9 h instead of 36 h in resting lymphocytes) (Hwong et al., 1993). This suggests that topo I protein levels remain relatively constant due to changing of protein stability during the different phases of the cell cycle.

The human genome contains three loci hybridizing with topoisomerase I-derived cDNA probes; two of these are truncated processed pseudogenes (retrosequences), whereas the third locus, on chromosome 20q12–13.2, contains the functional topoisomerase I gene (Juan et al., 1988). The topo I gene is a single-copy gene. Recently the whole exon/intron structure and the promoter region have also been clarified (Kunze et al., 1991): the gene consists of 21 exons distributed over at least 85 kb of human genomic DNA and the size of the introns varies widely between 0.2 and at least 30 kb. The gene encoding topo I specifies a 4 kb mRNA, and the human topo I protein is a phosphoprotein monomer of approximately 100 kDa molecular weight. The recent clarification of the three-dimensional structure of the 67 kDa N-terminal fragment of *E. coli* topo I confirmed that the four domains fold in a way to form a large hole that may accommodate a double-stranded DNA (Lima, Wang and Mondragon, 1994). The active site Tyr-319 is located deep in the complex structure, and conformational changes have been proposed to expose this active site, during the strand-passage activity.

There are extensive similarities between the human topo I and the type I topoisomerases from the yeasts *Saccharomyces cerevisiae* and *Schizosaccharomyces pombe*. Whereas the former does not contain introns, the latter has two small introns, in positions similar to human introns 1 and 3. However, the human protein is rather different from *E. coli* DNA topo I or III (Wang, 1987).

The promoter region, a few hundred nucleotides upstream of exon 1, has features of promoter regions of constitutively expressed genes (Kunze et al., 1991); in particular the upstream region conspicuously lacks TATA box and CCAAT box elements, which are common sequence motifs of promoters in regulated genes. Moreover, there is a high percentage of GC base pairs (67%), with a high percentage of CpG dinucleotides, and multiple closely spaced transcriptional start sites located in a region 200–250 bp upstream of the translational initiation codon; two potential binding sites of the transcriptional factor Sp1, two variants of the octamer motif, and one cAMP-responsive element (Kunze et al., 1991). At the transcriptional activation level topo I is regulated by a complex network of negatively and positively acting transcription factors, including members of the Myc-related family of basic/helix-loop-helix/leucine-zipper proteins (Heiland, Knippers and Kunze, 1993).

The homology comparison of eukaryotic topo I with other species allows its division into domains. At least six domains have been identified: domains II, III, IV, and VI are regions with extensive identities, usually higher than 50% of amino acids. Domain I is variable in length among species and is dispensable for the catalytic activity; however, it may play a role in protein–protein and protein–nucleic acid interactions. Furthermore, one phosphorylation site has been mapped to a serine residue near the N-terminus (Hwang and Hwong, 1994). Domain I may have a regulatory role for the enzymatic activities; moreover a nuclear localization sequence also appears to be present in domain I.

Among the possible post-translational modifications, only phosphorylation and poly(ADP-ribosylation) have been described for the topoisomerases. For topo I, three serine and threonine residues were identified as the major phosphorylation sites. Whereas phosphorylation in tyrosine inactivates calf thymus topo I, phosphorylation at serine residues enhances topo I activity (Gupta et al., 1995). Casein kinase II-like protein kinase and protein kinase C may be the physiological regulators of topo I (Gupta et al., 1995).

Poly(ADP-ribosylation) of DNA topoisomerases has been shown to occur in vitro, this modification is carried out by a nuclear enzyme, poly(ADP-ribose) synthetase, capable of ribosylating both topo I and II. Ribosylation results in inactivation of these enzymes. Since the activity of poly(ADP-ribose) synthetase is stimulated by a variety of DNA-damaging agents, including alkylators and ionizing radiation, the ribosylation of eukaryotic topoisomerases has raised questions regarding its possible involvement in DNA repair (Hwang and Hwong, 1994).

Topoisomerase II

Type II topoisomerases catalyze the topological crossing of two double helices of DNA by introducing transient double-strand breaks and change the DNA linking number in steps of 2 (Wang, 1985). Human topo II, like other eukaryotic type II DNA topoisomerases, catalyzes relaxation of positive and negative DNA supercoils, but is unable to supercoil DNA (Chen and Liu, 1994). Mammalian topo II is a homo-dymer protein that produces DNA double-strand breaks with the two subunits covalently linked to the 5'-phosphoryl ends; the 3'-hydroxyl ends are recessed by four base pairs.

In addition to transcription and DNA replication, topo II has also been implicated in DNA recombination and chromosomal segregation (Wang, 1985, 1987; Wang and Giaever, 1988; Adachi, Luke and Laemmli, 1991), condensation and decondensation of chromosomes during mitosis and probably also meiosis (Wang, 1994). Furthermore, there are also indications that topo II may be implicated in DNA repair mechanisms (Tan et al., 1987) and in the promotion of illegitimate recombination.

Topo II is a vital enzyme for replication and mitosis, as yeast temperature-sensitive mutants are unable to complete mitosis (Wang, 1994).

Expression and replication of genes lying ahead of a tracking complex appear to be dependent on the presence of a DNA-relaxing activity, that could be provided by either topo I or II. One or the other enzyme is sufficient to stop the build-up of supercoils during the elongation phase of DNA replication in yeast; however, in the absence of topo I the chain extension is somewhat delayed. On the other hand, mutations in topo II enzymes have little effect on the rate of chain elongation, supporting the idea that topo I is the normal replication swivel, at least in yeast (Watt and Hickson, 1994). Topo II is only crucial for the separation of newly replicated chromosomes. Eukaryotic topoisomerases appear however to have some ability to substitute for each other in many cellular processes.

The role of topo II in chromosomal segregation is quite complex. Topo II is localized in the chromosomal scaffold or nuclear matrix (what is left of chromosomes or nuclei after extraction of histones and treatment with DNase) (Watt and Hickson, 1994). Topo II constitutes the major component of metaphase scaffolds, and the requirement for topo II for chromosome condensation in mitotic extracts has been demonstrated, suggesting that topo II might function both catalytically in regulating the DNA conformation and structurally in maintaining chromosomal organization. The most recent data, however, suggest that topo II may not play a specific scaffolding role.

AT-rich consensus sites are a common feature of DNA sequences that specifically bind to the scaffold (SARs – scaffold-associated regions). Chromosomal organization has been suggested to be regulated by attachment of the basis of the chromatin loops to the scaffold, through SARs. SAR attachment is topo II-mediated. Localization of topo II has been studied in living *Drosophila melanogaster* embryos; the enzyme is not restricted to a central chromosomal axis, but is uniformly distributed throughout the chromosome. About 70% of the enzyme leaves the nucleus and localizes in the cytoplasm during mitosis (Swedlow, Sedat and Agard, 1993).

DNA topo II has been estimated to be present at about 10^5–10^6 copies per cell in HeLa and human skin fibroblasts, and is found upstream and downstream of transcribed regions and also near regulatory regions, including enhancers (Hwang and Hwong, 1994).

The physical question of how topo II can be linked to one strand of DNA, cut it and let another strand go through the break, has been a matter of lengthy debate, and two major theories have been proposed: the one-gate theory and the two-gate theory. Recent results directly demonstrated the validity of the two-gate theory (Figure 4.1). DNA topo II molecule is a homodymer that acts as an ATP-dependent molecular clamp that is in open state when ATP is absent; the clamp closes upon binding of ATP and opens up again upon ATP hydrolysis and dissociation of the products. When the two jaws of the enzyme bound to the broken DNA close, then a free DNA strand can be captured and transported through the DNA gate and exit from the other side of the gate (Roca and Wang, 1994). The transported duplex DNA segment is

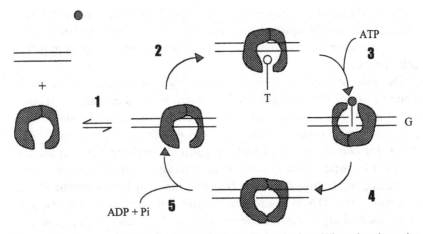

Figure 4.1. Two-gate model for topo II strand passing action. When the clamp is open (2), a new DNA strand can enter the hole formed by the enzyme and pass through the gate opened in the DNA strand attached to the enzyme (3), on the other side of the complex. T-segment is the transported duplex DNA segment; G-segment has the topo II-mediated gate through which the T-segment passes.

called 'T-segment', whereas the other DNA segment, linked to topo II, through which a gate is formed, is called 'G-segment'. The recent investigation of the crystal structure of a 92 kDa fragment of yeast topo II has allowed the identification of a heart-shaped dimeric protein with a large central hole of 55 Å at its base (Berger et al., 1996). This study provides a molecular model of the enzyme as an ATP-modulated clamp with two sets of jaws at opposite ends, connected by multiple joints. This protein structure with bound DNA can admit a second DNA duplex through one set of jaws, and expel it through the other set (Berger et al., 1996). Similar observations on the human topo II enzyme have been done by scanning transmission electron microscopy (Schultz et al., 1996). A major conformational change has been shown with this technique when the ATP binding site is occupied. The two-gate theory has been demonstrated by inserting reversible disulfide links across the dimer interface, which allowed dissection of subsequent steps of the strand passage. The second DNA enters the enzyme through the gate formed in the N-terminal parts of the enzyme and leaves it through the gate close to the C-termini (Roca et al., 1996).

Topo II–DNA interactions are very sensitive to salt concentrations. The reaction of topo II with DNA requires the presence of a divalent cation (such as magnesium, calcium, cobalt, copper, manganese, mercury, nickel, or zinc), and ATP in order to perform a covalent bond with DNA during the catalytic strand-passage. No energy source is, however, required for the binding of eukaryotic topo II to DNA, although omission of ATP results in a 30% lower level of binding (Osheroff, 1989). Binding also decreases by approximately 50% when salt is increased from 100 to 250 nM. The enzyme is attached to the 5'-termini of the cleaved DNA. The religation process in vitro requires the presence of divalent cations, but takes place in the absence of an energy source. After religation, topo II remains noncovalently bound to DNA, until topo II itself hydrolyzes the bound ATP molecule to ADP and inorganic phosphate (see also Figure 4.1). The enzyme turnover absolutely requires ATP hydrolysis (Osheroff, 1989).

Kinetic studies performed with eukaryotic topo II have shown that the single cleaved molecules are intermediates, indicating that topo II cleaves DNA by making two single-stranded breaks rather than a concerted double-stranded break, in which each single-stranded break is mediated by a separate enzyme subunit (Andersen et al., 1994). It is still unclear whether the two subunits are coordinated in the cleavage reaction.

Eukaryotic topo II acts at preferred sites on the DNA and shows some nucleotide sequence specificity, although consensus sequences are rather weak. At least four different consensus sequences have been reported, but no one consensus fits all of the known sequences (Osheroff, Corbett and Robinson, 1994).

Two isoenzymes of topo II are present in murine and human cells, called DNA topo IIα and DNA topo IIβ, of 170 and 180 kDa molecular weight, respectively, and the cDNA sequences of both genes have also been identified (Tsai-Pflugfelder et al., 1988; Chung et al., 1989; Drake et al., 1989). Extraction of the topo IIβ form requires higher salt concentrations, suggesting a tighter association with chromatin or the nuclear matrix (Drake et al., 1989). All known topoisomerases II are ATP dependent, and extensive analysis of their sequences shows that they are evolutionary and structurally related. Unlike topo I, topo II enzymes share significant homology from prokaryotes to eukaryotes. However, analysis of Southern blotting revealed that the topo IIβ, unlike the topo IIα form, was present in the mouse but not in yeast or *Drosophila* (Austin et al., 1993).

The two mammalian isoenzymes are coded by different genes, localized on different chromosomes (Tan et al., 1992): while the topo IIα gene is localized on chromosome 17q21−22 (Tsai-Pflugfelder et al.,

1988), the topo IIβ gene has been localized on chromosome 3p24 (Jenkins et al., 1992). However, the complete exon/intron structure of these genes remains largely unknown. In addition to the cDNA sequence of topo IIβ reported by Jenkins et al. (1992), a second form (designated topoisomerase IIβ-2) has been identified, which encodes a protein with five additional amino acids; the two forms are produced by differential splicing and are both widely distributed in human cell lines and tissues (Davies, Jenkins and Hickson, 1993); the significance of this finding is still unclear.

The structure of a 2.5 kb region encompassing the translation start of the topo IIα gene has been elucidated (Hochauser et al., 1992). The promoter was identified and it shows similarity with promoters of a number of 'housekeeping' genes, in being moderately GC rich and lacking a TATA box; it also contains a high frequency of CpG dinucleotides, potential acceptor sites for methylation, involved in control of topo IIα expression. In the absence of a TATA box, other alternative recognition sequences must direct binding of RNA polymerase II. A number of potential transcription-factor-binding sites were also identified in the 650 bp region upstream of the translation start site, for example two Sp1 factor-binding sites, and an inverted CCAAT box, which is recognized specifically by the DNA-binding protein YB1.

The two human topo II are highly homologous, with a degree of homology of 72%. The proposed coding region of the topo IIβ protein is 4863 nucleotides long and encodes a polypeptide of M_r 182 705. The greatest divergences in the sequences lie at the extreme N-terminus and over a C-terminal domain, which comprises 25% of the whole protein (Jenkins et al., 1992). However, the homology is higher between the two human topo II enzymes than between the human topo IIβ and the non-human topo II enzymes (Jenkins et al., 1992).

The first domain (N-terminal ATPase domain) is predicted to span the first 450 residues of topo IIβ. The central domain (involved in DNA breakage/reunion) is predicted to span residues 451 to 1200 approximately and include the putative active site Tyr-821; this region has been reported to contain a leucine zipper motif, however this is not conserved in topo IIβ (Austin et al., 1993). The third domain (the C-terminal domain) spans from approximately residue 1200 to the C-terminus, and this sequence consists of an alternation of basic and acid amino acids; because this is the least conserved sequence, it may be important in determining and regulating unique cellular roles for the two topo isoforms. Within this domain there are a number of sequences that closely match the consensus for sites of phosphorylation catalyzed by casein kinase II, protein kinases A and C, and p34[cdc2] kinase (Jenkins et al., 1992). By comparison with the other topo II enzymes, it is predicted that Tyr-821 would be the active site residue forming the covalent phosphotyrosil linkage when topo IIβ transiently breaks DNA (Jenkins et al., 1992).

Based on the overall homology of all topo II genes in different species, the large eukaryotic peptyde can be divided into four domains:

1. the N-terminal 400 amino acids covering the ATP domain and involved in ATP hydrolysis (homologous to the *E. coli* gyrase B subunit);
2. a linker region of about 130 amino acids, which interacts with the second half of the molecule;
3. the DNA cutting–rejoining reactions domain of about 400 amino acids (homologous to the *E. coli* gyrase A subunit) and
4. a more variable C-terminal region of 300–400 amino acids, disposed in clusters of charged amino acids.

Although ATP binding sites have not been conclusively identified for topo II, the cDNA sequence of the human enzyme reveals three conserved nucleotide binding domains, and the suggested consensus sequence for ATP binding of topo II is composed of motif A, motif B, and DNBS. The N-terminal fragment of Gyr B, protein subunit of a bacterial topo II, contains an ATP binding site at amino acids 103 through 126. This sequence corresponds, in the human topo IIα, to amino acids 149–172 (reviewed by Capranico et al., 1994a).

Tyr-122 of the *Escherichia coli* DNA gyrase A subunit and Tyr-783 of the single subunit *Saccharomyces cereviesiae* DNA topoisomerase II are the respective active site tyrosine residues. The DNA-stimulated ATPase site is located near the amino terminus of the B subunit of bacterial gyrase; from the sequence comparisons, it can be readily inferred that the ATPase site is located near the amino end of eukaryotic DNA topo II. The location of the active-site Tyr has been mapped to position 804 in human topo IIα.

The putative leucine zipper may be important either for dimerization of the individual topo II promoters or for interactions with other proteins. The C-terminal domain includes a signal that is necessary for nuclear localization, but at least another site must be present in the molecule to direct efficient nuclear localization (Watt and Hickson, 1994).

In a number of cell lines examined, there was no obvious relationship in terms of levels of expression between the topo IIα and β genes (Jenkins et al., 1992), the expression of both genes being readily detectable. The two isoenzymes display differences in nuclear localization (Negri et al., 1992; Zini et al., 1992; Zini et al., 1994), with topo IIα mainly localized in the nucleoplasm, whereas topo IIβ is mainly localized in the nucleolus. Based on this differential nuclear localization, a function mainly limited to transcription has been proposed for the β isoform. However, using other specific polyclonal antibodies for the two topo II isoforms, both were shown in the nucleoplasm and in the nucleolus (Petrov et al., 1993), at the periphery of heterochromatic regions in the nucleoplasm and in the fibrillar regions in the nucleus, where transcription of ribosomal RNA takes place.

During the cell cycle there is a differential expression of the two isoforms, also indicating different functions. It appears that these two forms of topoisomerase II are differently regulated (Hsiang, Wu and Liu, 1988; Woessner et al., 1990, 1991; Zwelling et al., 1990). The level of topo IIα is highest during rapid proliferation (in G_2/M phases), whereas that of topo IIβ is highest in cells that are in the plateau phase of growth (Drake et al., 1989). In other cells, levels of p180 did not change depending on phase of cell cycle, whereas p170 was higher in exponentially growing cells (Kimura et al., 1994). Topo IIα expression was shown to be highest in bone marrow cells enriched in promyelocytes and myelocytes and undetectable in mature granulocytes (Kauffman et al., 1991). Topo IIα was higher in *ras*-transformed NIH-3T3 cells, which were also more sensitive to topo II inhibitors (Woessner et al., 1990).

Moreover, a different tissue specificity has been found for the two isoforms (Capranico et al., 1992; Juenke and Holden, 1993), being the α form more highly expressed in proliferating tissues, whereas the β form is more widely expressed, including non-proliferating terminally differentiated tissues.

Phosphorylation of topo II has been the subject of some controversy. In Swiss 3T3 cells a high level of topo II phosphorylation was observed in proliferating cells, while no or low levels were seen in quiescent cells (Saijo, Ui and Enomoto, 1992). The amino acid that was phosphorylated on the topo II protein was a serine. Upon stimulation of growth by serum, the phosphorylation increased to a maximum at 28 h and then decreased, and was sensitive to inhibitors of DNA synthesis, whereas the synthesis of the enzyme was not. This suggests that the regulation of phosphorylation of topo II differs from that of the expression of the enzyme. In Chinese hamster ovary cells, higher topo II protein expression was observed in G_2-phase cells, whereas maximum phosphorylation was seen in M-phase cells. Topo II activity, measured by etoposide-induced DNA double-strand breaks, was maximal in the M phase (Burden, Goldsmith and Sullivan, 1993), further indicating that phosphorylation is cell-cycle dependent and critical in determining catalytic and cleavage activity.

Phosphorylation can occur in a number of potential sites in the C terminal domain; phosphorylation at these sites may allow differential control of isozyme activity, direct nuclear localization, influence of enzyme stability, and control the extent of interactions of topo II with DNA and other nuclear proteins. Two major sites of phosphorylation of human topo II have been identified on serine residues 1524 and 1376 (Wells et al., 1994). Specific sites of phosphorylation were identified for interphase and mitosis on topo IIα, along with a mobility shift caused by phosphorylation of topo IIβ in mitosis; this demonstrates that there are qualitative differences between interphase and mitosis in the phosphorylation state of both topo II isoforms (Burden and Sullivan, 1994). The catalytic activity of topo II is stimulated about 2- to 3-fold following phosphorylation by either protein kinase C or casein kinase II; both kinases regulate the catalytic function of topo II by a common mechanism and the ATP hydrolysis step is the control point for activation of topo II (Corbett, Fernald and Osheroff, 1993).

Other topoisomerases

More topoisomerases have been described in other organisms. In the yeast *Saccharomyces cerevisiae*, the *TOP3* gene has been identified, which encodes for topoisomerase III, an ATP-independent relaxing topoisomerase, homologous to topoisomerase I (Wang, 1991). Recently, a human homologous cDNA sequence has been described, as a single-copy gene localized on chromosome 17p11.2–12 (Hanai, Caron and Wang, 1996). The protein has been denoted DNA topoisomerase III. The yeast gene *HPR1* may encode yet another topoisomerase. In *E. coli*, the two genes *parC* and *parE* code for topoisomerase IV; the amino acid sequences of *parC* and *parE* are homologous respectively to the subunits A and B of DNA gyrase, the bacterial DNA topoisomerase II. The functions of this additional topo II may be to anchor chromosomes on membranes, a function previously attributed to eukaryotic topo II (Kato, Suzuki and Ikeda, 1992). Recently a topoisomerase with similar characteristics to topo I has been discovered in a hyperthermophilic prokaryote, and has been called topoisomerase V (Slesarev et al., 1993), which shows that eukaryotic transcription–translation and replication machineries existed before the emergence of eukaryotes, and suggests that the closest living relatives to eukaryotes may be hyperthermophiles.

Topoisomerases as targets of anticancer drugs

In analogy to bacterial gyrases, which have been shown to be inhibited by coumarin and quinolone antibiotics (e.g. norfloxacin, nalidixic acid), topoisomerases have been recognized as major targets of a number of antitumor agents (D'Arpa and Liu, 1989; Liu, 1989). Inhibitors of topo I and topo II are known (Table 4.1). Based on the type of interaction with the enzyme and DNA, the topoisomerase drugs can be further subdivided into two classes: the class I drugs, including the bacterial gyrase quinolone antibiotics and the topoisomerase I drug camptotecin, and the topoisomerase II drugs doxorubicin, amsacrine, etoposide, which all act through stabilization of the covalent ternary complex formed between topoisomerase, DNA and drug (cleavable complex). This class of drugs has also been called topoisomerase poisons, as they convert a latent single- or double-strand break into an irreversible double-stranded DNA break, which is toxic for the cell. The class II drugs interfere with the catalytic function of topoisomerases, but do not trap the cleavable complex; this class includes topoisomerase II inhibitors such as suramin, merbarone and others, in addition to the coumermycin family of antibiotics. For this class of drugs, information of the exact mechanism of action is less complete, and it may involve inhibition of topo II-catalyzed reactions, such as interference with the ATPase activity, or with the DNA breakage and rejoining steps, or involving allosteric changes that normally accompany the reactions catalyzed by the enzymes (Wang, 1994). Among the catalytic inhibitors that do not stabilize the cleavable complex are the bis(2,6-dioxopiperazine) derivatives ICRF-159 and ICRF-193. Furthermore, novobiocin, in use as antibiotic, acts on the ATPase domain, by inhibiting the ATPase reaction.

Topoisomerase poisons are thought to act through the formation of the ternary complex DNA–enzyme–drug, which results in the inhibition of the resealing of the transient DNA break induced by the enzyme. DNA single- or double-strand breaks can be recovered by addition of SDS (sodium dodecyl sulfate) or strong alkali. The stabilization of the cleavable complex most likely starts a cascade of events, one of which

Table 4.1. *Topoisomerase targeted anticancer drugs*

topo I drugs

Non-DNA binders
camptothecin, topotecan, CPT-11 (irinotecan), 9-amino-camptothecin.
indolocarbazoles

DNA binders
actinomycin D[a]
saintopin[a,b]
intoplicine[a,b]
morpholinyldoxorubicin

minor-groove binders
Hoecht 33342
distamycin[b]
neutropsin[b]

topo II drugs

Intercalaters and DNA binders	
anthracyclines	e.g. doxorubicin, epirubicin
ellipticines	e.g. 2-methyl-9-hydroxyellipticinium
aminoacridines	e.g. CI-921, amsacrine
anthracenediones	e.g. mitoxantrone
anthrapyrazoles	
actinomycin D[a]	
amonafide[b]	
streptonigrin[b]	
saintopin[a,b]	
intoplicine[a,b]	

Non-intercalaters	
epipodophyllotoxins	e.g. etoposide and teniposide
thiobarbituric acid derivatives	e.g. merbarone
bis(dioxo)piperazines	e.g. ICRF-159 and 187
suramin[b]	
novobiocin	
genistein	
fostriecin[b]	
terpenoids	

[a] Dual topo I and II drugs.
[b] Topo inhibitors (non-cleavable complex stabilizers).

might be the block of replication forks, ultimately leading to cell death (D'Arpa and Liu, 1989; Kyprianou, Alexander and Isaacs, 1991). For topoisomerase I–DNA cleavable complexes it has been demonstrated that the interaction with camptothecin leads to irreversible arrest of the replication fork and the formation of double-strand DNA breaks at the fork (Tsao et al., 1993). Exposure of cells to camptothecin produces protein-linked DNA breaks (PLDB), which are reversible upon drug removal, within 15 minutes. A model has been proposed by which the collision of the replicating fork (Liu, 1989) with the reversible PLDB induces DNA double-strand breaks, which are not rapidly reversible but persist within the cell (Ryan et al., 1991). This ultimately leads to conversion of the cleavable complexes into complexes that are 'cleaved' and to G_2 arrest and cell death.

Among the topo II inhibitors, anthracyclines and epipodophyllotoxins are widely used anticancer drugs both for the treatment of hematological malignancies and widespread solid tumors, such as breast and lung cancers. Other drugs of this group, such as mitoxantrone, and amsacrine have a more restricted application to the clinic. Between the two topo II isoforms, it is still unclear which isoform is more important for the interaction with cytotoxic drugs. Topo IIβ is 3–4-fold less sensitive to inhibition by intercalating agents and epipodophyllotoxins than the α form (Drake et al., 1989).

Most of these agents intercalate into DNA (anthracyclines, anthracenediones, ellipticines, amsacrine), but some do not (epipodophyllotoxins) (Chen et al., 1984; Ross et al., 1984). Intercalation is not essential for stabilization of the cleavable complex; epipodophyllotoxins are potent topo II inhibitors that bind only weakly to DNA and do not intercalate. Like many DNA-damaging agents, these topo II inhibitors also induce sister chromatide exchange, chromosomal recombination and chromosomal aberrations, and are associated with a significant risk of secondary leukemia. Recently, chromosome band 11q23, involved in reciprocal translocation, which occurs frequently in secondary leukemias, was found to contain translocation breakpoints that are topo II cleavage sites, strongly suggesting this enzyme involvement in the development of secondary leukemias (Felix et al., 1995). In a recent report, amsacrine was shown to induce megabase pair deletions, and it was suggested that amsacrine-induced deletions be mediated by a series of subunit exchanges between overlapping topo II dimers (Shibuya et al., 1994).

Antibacterial quinolones (nalidixic acid, ciprofloxacin and derivatives) are DNA gyrase inhibitors with no or very limited effect on the human topo II enzyme (Gupta et al., 1995). Interestingly, the new anthracycline derivative morpholinyldoxorubicin is not a topo II drug but is a topo I inhibitor.

Actinomycin D (Chen and Liu, 1994) and several new anticancer agents (Capranico and Zunino, 1992; Swaffar, Ireland and Barrows, 1994) possess both topo I and II inhibiting activities (Riou et al., 1991).

The ability of topo II inhibitors to make double-strand breaks, also allowed the recent development of screening methods to identify new topo II anticancer agents (Swaffar et al., 1994), by using a DNA double-strand break repair-deficient CHO line. The ratio of double- and single-strand breaks varies between topo II drugs: anthracyclines and ellipticine produce almost exclusively double-strand breaks, while VP16 and amsacrine produce 10–20 times more single-strand than double-strand breaks.

Direct evidence that inhibition of topo II results in resistance to topo II-interactive drugs, has been provided recently by the isolation of genetic suppressor elements encoding antisense RNA (Gudkov et al., 1993). Interestingly, this new method provided evidence that only topo II poisons were affected, but not drugs that do not interact with topo II. Studies in yeast have firmly demonstrated that at least in yeast topo II is the only significant target of amsacrine (Wasserman and Wang, 1994).

Camptothecin, the first known topo I inhibitor (Wall et al., 1966), was dismissed in the early seventies when it was found to be too toxic in patients (Gottlieb, Guarino and Call, 1970); however, after the discovery that topo I is the specific target of this drug, new research has brought to the discovery of potent and more water-soluble analogues (Avemann et al., 1988; Giovannella et al., 1989), two of which have already undergone extensive clinical investigation, especially in lung and colon cancer where they have shown definite activity (reviewed by Slichenmeyer et al., 1993). Nowadays, camptothecin and its analogues (Liu et al., 1989) are no longer the only available agents that specifically inhibit topoisomerase I; newer agents have in fact been discovered that are not structurally related to camptothecins, some of which also inhibit topo II (see Table 4.1).

Camptothecin is highly S-phase specific; this specificity is due to a lethal interaction between the moving replication fork and the reversible topo I–camptothecin–DNA cleavable complex (Chen and Liu, 1994). Differences in potency and cleavable complex formation between camptothecin analogues are dependent on the stability of the complex (i.e., less rapidly reversible) (Tanizawa et al., 1995).

DNA minor groove-binders have recently been shown to have topoisomerase I as a target; the cleavage sites of these new agents are distinctly different from those induced by camptothecins and no correlation was found between DNA binding and cleavage efficiency (Chen et al., 1993). Like camptothecin, minor groove-binders abort topo I reactions by trapping reversible cleavable complexes.

Unlike topo I inhibitors such as camptothecin, topo II inhibitors do not exhibit a high degree of S-phase specificity. Studies with inhibitors of nucleic acid synthesis have suggested that both replication and transcription are involved in the cytotoxic mechanisms of topo II inhibitors (reviewed by Chen and Liu, 1994). It also appears that the DNA of actively transcribed genes may be more vulnerable to the action of these drugs on topoisomerases (Fleischmann et al., 1984). For the class I drugs (trapping the cleavable complex), a major determinant of their cytotoxicity is the conversion of a latent single- or double-stranded DNA break into an irreversible double-stranded DNA break. Replication appears to be a key cellular function that drives this conversion in topoisomerase I inhibitors, whereas processes other than replication may also be important for topoisomerase II inhibitors; in particular the cell killing by topoisomerase II and I drugs necessitates the progression of the cell cycle through mitosis.

DNA breakage patterns differ from drug to drug and special nucleotide requirements are needed in order for the ternary complex to form (Yang et al., 1985; Kjeldsen et al., 1988a; Capranico and Zunino, 1990; Capranico, Kohn and Pommier, 1990a; Capranico et al., 1990b; Fosse et al., 1991; Jaxel et al., 1991; Pommier et al., 1991). For instance, camptothecin has a strong preference for a G in position 1 relative to the break, whereas doxorubicin has a preference for A in position −1. Drugs that inhibit the religation reaction of topo II can dramatically modify the pattern and sites of topo II cleavage. Moreover, drugs structurally very dissimilar, such as bisantrene and mAMSA have been shown to have the same sequence specificity (Capranico et al., 1994b). These findings suggest that the sequence specificities may be due to specific interactions with DNA bases immediately adjacent to the cleavage site, and that different drugs may share common steric and electronic features that may constitute a specific pharmacophore (Capranico et al., 1994b).

All these findings strongly suggest that inhibitors interact directly with the DNA bases at the cleavage site, placing the inhibitor binding site precisely at the site of DNA cleavage (Freudenreich and Kreuzer, 1993). The amino acid sequence PLRGK of topo II has been implicated in the covalent binding of drugs to the DNA−enzyme complex. This knowledge may be of help in designing new drugs with topo inhibiting action.

There are not many structural similarities among the topoisomerase inhibitors, but most of them have an aromatic polycyclic structure (Figure 4.2), with a planar ring system that could intercalate between

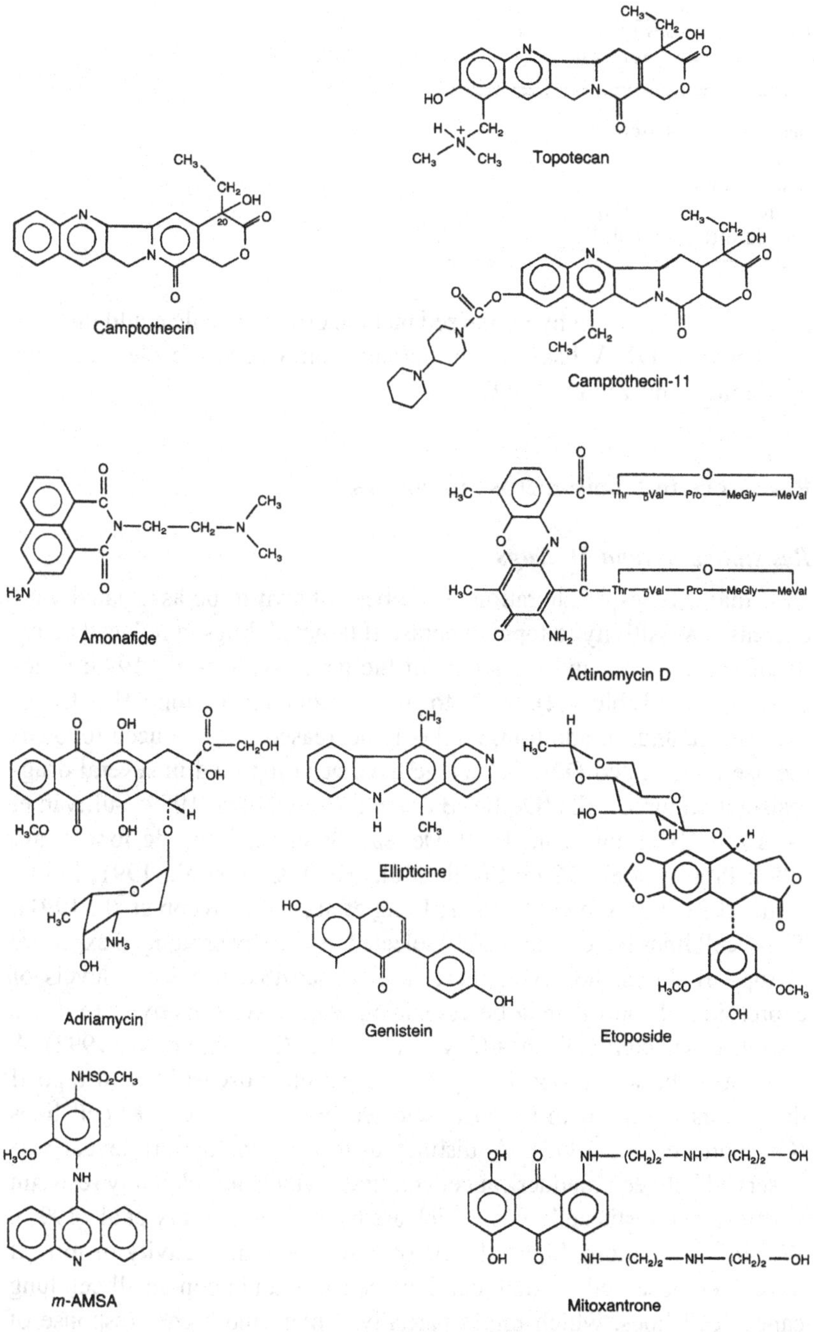

Figure 4.2. Structure of topoisomerase inhibitors.

Table 4.2. *Causes of reduced topo*
activity and/or expression

Decreased transcription
Gene mutations
Gene methylation
Altered phosphorylation
Altered mRNA stability

base pairs. It has been hypothesized that the drug molecule could intercalate between DNA bases in the ternary complex at the cleavage site
(Capranico and Zunino, 1992).

Resistance to topoisomerase inhibitors

Resistance to topo II drugs

Two major types of alterations have been shown to be associated with
decreased sensitivity to topoisomerase II targeted drugs: a reduced activity of the enzyme, and mutations of the gene (Beck et al., 1993; Giaccone, 1994) (Table 4.2). A 2- to 4-fold reduction of topo II activity/
expression, and, in addition, markedly decreased drug-induced topoisomerase II-mediated DNA cleavage have been reported in several drug-
resistant cultured cells (Deffie, Batra and Goldenberg, 1989; Sullivan et
al., 1989; Zwelling et al., 1989; De Isabella et al., 1990; de Jong et al.,
1990; Pratesi et al., 1990; Smith et al., 1990; Cole et al., 1991; Friche
et al., 1991; Lefevre et al., 1991; Long et al., 1991; Webb et al., 1991).
These cell lines have been mainly selected in vitro by prolonged exposure
to topo II drugs; however, there is evidence that decreased levels of
expression of topo II may be associated with lower sensitivity to drugs
also in unselected cell lines (Fry et al., 1991; Giaccone et al., 1992). A
correlation between topo II expression and chemosensitivity to topo II
drugs was observed in seven unselected human lung cancer cell lines
(Giaccone et al., 1992). A distinct difference in topo II levels was
observed between bladder cancer cell lines, which are relatively resistant
to drugs, and testis cell lines, which are hypersensitive (Fry et al., 1991).
Within lung tumors, higher levels of expression and activity of topo II
have been observed in small cell lung cancer than in non-small cell lung
cancer cell lines, which might partially explain the higher response of
the former to etoposide and doxorubicin (Kasahara et al., 1992). As

an additional mechanism of resistance, in this study Kasahara et al. also reported a lower etoposide uptake in non-small cell lung cancer cells.

Using yeast as a model, the induced overexpression of topo II led to hypersensitivity to the topo II inhibitors amsacrine and etoposide (Nitiss et al., 1992), indicating that topo II is the cellular target for these drugs, and that modulation of topo II expression may offer a way to increase activity of topo II drugs.

A relative resistance during quiescence phases has been shown for several cell lines, human lymphocytes and murine tissues (Zwelling et al., 1987; Heck and Earnshaw, 1986; Markovits et al., 1987), and this is in agreement with the low topo IIα expression in slowly proliferating cells (Heck, Hittelman and Earnshaw, 1988; Hwang et al., 1989).

Very little is known of the mechanism of reduced expression of topoisomerase genes. One mechanism that has been shown as possibly responsible for reduced expression is the hypermethylation of one allele of the topoisomerase II gene (Tan et al., 1989). In general DNA methylation is deregulated during oncogenesis; methylation can interfere with transcription and may have profound effects on the activity of both topoisomerase types and may alter the distribution of cleavage sites produced by anticancer drugs in chromatin (Leteurtre et al., 1994).

In KB cells, resistant to etoposide and teniposide, a 5-fold reduction of transcriptional activity of topo IIα was observed, which was in agreement with the 5-fold reduced mRNA level of this gene. In these cell lines a 3-fold increase of expression of S3 was observed (Kubo et al., 1995). S3 belongs to the superfamily of transcription factors, for which the promotor of topo IIα has consensus sequences for recognition. Instead of S1 and S2, which stimulate transcription, S3 inhibits transcription.

A diminished activity can also be due to post-translational modifications of the protein (Heck et al., 1988). Still a controversial issue is the influence of phosphorylation state of topo II on sensitivity to drugs (Kroll and Rowe, 1991; Takano et al., 1991; Ganapathi et al., 1993). In etoposide-resistant KB cell lines there was a reduced expression of topo II, but also a greatly increased relative specific phosphorylation (Takano et al., 1991). Furthermore, in an etoposide-resistant leukemia cell line, a 2-5-fold reduction in phosphorylation was observed, in the absence of mutations (Ritke et al., 1994).

Phosphorylation of the enzyme induced a significant reduction in the ability of topo inhibitors to stabilize the cleavable complexes (DeVore,

Corbett and Osheroff, 1992). Interestingly, no cross-resistance was seen between topo II inhibitors that induce DNA cleavage and newer topo II inhibitors that do not cause DNA breaks, such as merbarone, aclarubicin, fostriecin (Chen and Beck, 1993), providing additional evidence of a different mechanism of action of these two types of topo II drugs.

Among topo II inhibitors several (e.g. anthracyclines and epipodo-phyllotoxins) are substrates for drug membrane transporters, such as P-glycoprotein and the more recently described MRP (multidrug resist-ance associated protein). Therefore, it may well be that for one drug several mechanisms of resistance are active. For example, overexpres-sion of MRP and altered topo II sensitivity was reported in etoposide-resistant human breast carcinoma cells (Schneider et al., 1994).

During the cell cycle, not only modifications in topo II expression has been seen, but also of *MDR1* expression, in a study of P388 doxorubicin resistant cells (P388/R-84) (Ramachandran et al., 1995). Whereas $GST\pi$ mRNA remained constant during cell cycle phases, *mdr1* mRNA increased 3-fold in cells in S phase and topo IIα mRNA peaked in G_2/M cells. This indicates that not only topo IIα but also other resistance markers may modify during the cell cycle and this may have therapeutic implications, depending on the proliferation characteristics of the tumor.

Several different mechanisms may, however, simultaneously play roles in the same cells (Hoban et al., 1992; de Jong et al., 1993), which may explain particular sensitivity patterns observed in some cell lines. In CHO-K1 cells resistant to doxorubicin, a cross-resistance was observed to mitomycin C, which was probably explained by the over-expression of α class glutathione S-transferase (Hoban et al., 1992).

Collateral sensitivity to topoisomerase inhibitors has been described in a number of cell lines that have been selected in vitro for resistance to alkylating agents. Increased cellular sensitivity to cisplatin was shown to parallel the increased resistance to etoposide and teniposide (Takano et al., 1991). Increased expression of topo IIα induced by transfection of full-length Chinese hamster ovary topo IIα into EMT6 mouse mammary carcinoma cells was associated with 5–10-fold increased resistance to cisplatin. This suggests that topo IIα may have a role in cisplatin resist-ance, possibly involving an increased repair of cisplatin-induced DNA damage (Eder et al., 1995). A rhabdomyosarcoma xenograft resistant to melphalan displayed a 2-fold increase in topo II and 2-fold decrease in topo I activity/expression, explaining the augmented sensitivity to etoposide and the cross-resistance to the topo I inhibitor topotecan (Friedman et al., 1994).

Among mechanisms by which transcription can be regulated is through gene amplification, although this does not appear to be a frequent phenomenon (Coutts et al., 1993). Co-amplification of topo IIα with c-*erb*-B2 has been shown in 12% of breast cancer samples and cell lines, with no signs of isolated amplification of topo IIα (Smith et al., 1993).

It remains rather unclear whether both topo II isoforms are equally important as targets of topo II drugs. While abundant evidence is available to link the topo IIα isoform to sensitivity and resistance of topo II drugs, far less clear is the implication of topo IIβ (Hochhauser and Harris, 1993). In general the expression of topo IIβ is not reduced in resistant cells. However, in the HL-60 cell line, resistant to mitoxantrone (Harker et al., 1991), and in Susa testicular cell lines, with a moderate degree of resistance to etoposide (Hosking et al., 1994), reduced topo IIα expression and very low expression of topo IIβ were observed. Interestingly, in human leukemic cell lines made resistant to the topo II inhibitor genistein, a marked reduction of expression of topo IIβ was observed, with no apparent modification of the α isoform (Markovits et al., 1995). These findings indicate that topo IIβ also may have an active role in drug resistance to topo II inhibitors.

Also of interest is that modifications of topo II expression appear to precede P-glycoprotein overexpression in etoposide-resistant cell lines, and to represent the predominant mechanism underlying low levels (< 10-fold) resistance (Hosking et al., 1994).

Resistance to topo I drugs

Mechanisms of resistance similar to those observed in cell lines resistant to topo II inhibitors have been described for camptothecin-resistant cell lines, where reduced topo I expression and activity, and mutations have been observed (Andoh et al., 1987; Gupta et al., 1988; Kjeldsen et al., 1988b; Tan et al., 1989; Eng et al., 1990; Sugimoto et al., 1990a; Tamura et al., 1991). In several unselected cell lines of different histological origin, however, no correlation was found between topoisomerase mRNA expression and chemosensitivity to camptothecin and also no correlation was seen with the percentage of cells in S phase (Perego et al., 1994). Moreover, also in another study of pancreatic cell lines, no correlation was observed between cytotoxicity and topo I mRNA levels in unselected cell lines, whereas a good correlation was found only in cell lines selected for resistance to CPT-11 in vitro (Takeda et al., 1992).

Upon prolonged exposure to camptothecin, a reduction of protein-linked DNA breaks was observed, which was due to a reduction of topo I protein expression, transcription remaining the same, suggesting that continued exposure determines post-transcriptional modification in topo I. This in turn may reduce the activity of camptothecin when prolonged exposures are used (Beidler and Cheng, 1995).

Although much less is known about phosphorylation of topo I, compared to topo II, there is some evidence that a reduced level of topo I phosphorylation may be implicated in resistance to camptothecin (Staron et al., 1995).

Accumulation defects have also been described as responsible for reduced activity of topo I inhibitors (reviewed by Potmesil, 1994). Topo I inhibitors are in general poor substrates of P-glycoprotein, although highly charged drugs such as topotecan appear to be more in vitro sensitive to the overexpression of this membrane protein than other camptothecin analogues (Hendricks et al., 1992). This defect can be restored by verapamil co-treatment (Chen et al., 1991). The cross-resistance of certain camptothecin analogues with typical *MDR1* substrates in P-glycoprotein overexpressing cells was, however, not observed in vivo (Mattern et al., 1993).

In a panel of seven unselected colon carcinoma cell lines, topo I expression did not predict sensitivity to camptothecin, and differences in accumulation were also minor (less than 3-fold). The cleavable complex formation appeared to more accurately predict sensitivity, although large differences were observed in sensitivity despite a small difference in cleavable complex formation for some cell lines, suggesting that parameters downstream from the formation of the cleavable complex may also be critical for camptothecin action (Goldwasser et al., 1995).

In three unselected brain tumor cell lines, the relative resistance to etoposide could not be explained by altered etoposide uptake or altered topo II. *Bcl*-2 overexpression or mutant *p53*, both present in these cell lines, could have been implicated in the prevention of etoposide-mediated apoptosis (Herzog et al., 1995).

Since camptothecin cytotoxicity is highly dependent on the fraction of cells that are in the S phase of the cell cycle, any deregulation of cyclins, cell-cycle regulated kinases and phosphatases may have a key role in the cytotoxicity of topo I inhibitors (Gupta et al., 1995).

Cell lines deficient of topo I expression/activity have been shown to be hypersensitive to topo II inhibitors (Sugimoto et al., 1990b; Woessner et al., 1992), following an increased topo II activity. The lack of topo I activity is probably being partially compensated by topo II function. In this respect one may suggest that resistance to camptothecin may be overcome by administration of topo II inhibitors.

An increase in topo I mRNA expression with increased sensitivity to camptothecin has been described in a cisplatin-resistant bladder cancer cell line (Kotoh et al., 1994); a possible enhanced DNA repair of the DNA damage caused by cisplatin has been hypothesized to be mediated by topo I. In addition, the radiosensitization properties of camptothecin have been proposed to be mediated by topo I, supporting a role for this enzyme in DNA repair (Boothman et al., 1992).

A mechanism of resistance typically developing only for CTP-11 is the reduced metabolic activation to SN-38. In a human ovarian cancer cell line resistant to cisplatin, a cross-resistance to CPT-11 was observed, and this was due to decreased conversion of the prodrug CPT-11 into the active metabolite SN-38, which occurs via a carboxyl-esterase (Niimi et al., 1992).

Mutations

The role of mutations of the topo II genes, which lead to a mutated enzyme and cellular resistance to topoisomerase II inhibitors, remains to be firmly established in human tumor cells. Mutations of the topo genes have been proposed as a possible mechanism of drug resistance in model tumor lines. For some cell lines detailed information on the altered base sequence has been obtained and is summarized in Table 4.3 (Bugg et al., 1991; Hinds et al., 1991; Lee, Wang and Beran, 1992; Chan et al., 1993; Patel and Fisher, 1993; Campain, Gottesman and Pastan, 1994; Hashimoto et al., 1995). For other cell lines there is less precise information on the nature of the mutations, in the absence of sequencing data. Mutations have been described as ranging from discrete or single base pair changes to large rearrangements of the gene.

In an unselected human small cell lung cancer cell line, relatively resistant to a wide array of anticancer drugs, including topo II inhibitors, a gross rearrangement in the topo IIα gene was described (Binaschi et al., 1992), leading to a larger 7.4 kb transcript in addition to the normal topo IIα transcript. The mutated mRNA lacked a substantial part of the 3'-terminal of the gene, and the extractability of topo II in this

Table 4.3. *Amino acid mutations in the DNA topo IIα gene of drug-resistant cell lines*

Reference	Cell line	Selecting drug	Cell type	Amino acid change
Lee et al., 1992	KBM-3/AMSA	mAMSA	Human leukemia	Lys^{479} to Glu Arg^{486} to Lys Lys^{519} to stop codon
Hinds et al., 1991	HL60/AMSA	mAMSA	Human leukemia	Arg^{486} to Lys
Bugg et al., 1991	CEM/VM-1	VM-26	Human leukemia	{Arg^{449} to Gln
Danks et al., 1993	CEM/VM-1-5	VM-26		{Pro^{802} to Ser
Chan et al., 1993	VpmR-5/VP-16	VP-16	Hamster ovary	Arg^{493*} to Gln
Patel and Fisher, 1993	CEM/VP-1	VP-16	Human leukemia	Lys^{797} to Asn
Hashimoto et al., 1995	V513	VP-16	Chinese hamster	Gly^{851*} to Asp
Campain et al., 1994	FVP3	VP-16	Human melanoma	Ala^{428} deletion

* Equivalent human amino acid number. The Chinese hamster enzyme has two additional lysines at positions 39 and 40 compared to the human enzyme. This table only includes the naturally occurring mutations, in resistant cell lines selected by drugs. Only published reports (no abstracts) are presented.

cell line was more easily detected and measured at relatively lower salt concentrations, suggesting a lower affinity of the enzyme for DNA.

Another gross rearrangement has been described in a doxorubicin-resistant P388 murine leukemia cell line (McPherson, Brown and Goldenberg, 1993). The rearrangement has been identified as a fusion with part of the murine retinoic acid receptor α gene; both genes (topo IIα and RARα) map to band q21 on chromosome 17. Interestingly, topo IIβ also maps in close proximity with the RARβ to band p24 on chromosome 3. The significance of this is unclear.

Particular functional areas of the topo II sequence have been identified that are possibly also important for the induction of drug resistance: Motif A, Motif B, and DNBS, which are putative ATP binding sites, the Tyr-804, and the leucine-zipper. The direct evidence identifying the functional ATP-binding site in the human topo II is still lacking, and the putative sites are inferred from analogies with other proteins (Figure 4.3). So far mutations have been described in resistant cell lines in the Motif B and in the DNBS site, and around the tyrosine-binding site (Table 4.3).

A recent deletion of 3 bp has been shown in a human melanoma cell line made resistant to VP-16 (Campain et al., 1994). This led to the deletion of Ala-429, which might be implicated in inducing the resistance pattern. Because the sensitivity of topo IIα in nuclear extracts was the same as the parental cell line, but the resistant cells were much less sensitive to the drug-induced cleavable complex formation, it was also

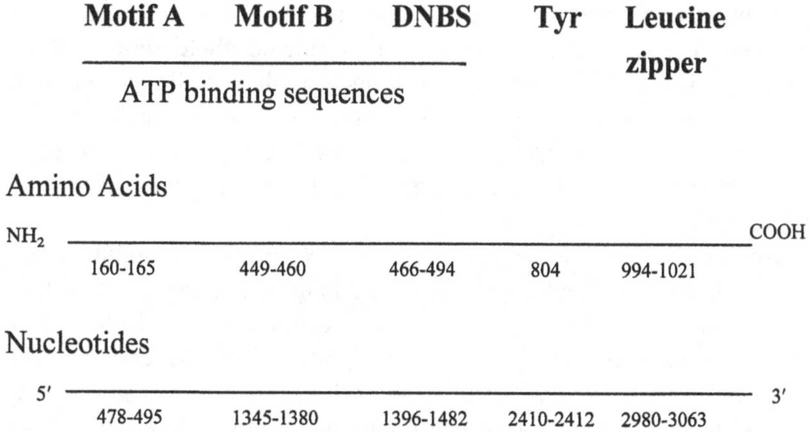

Motif A	**Motif B**	**DNBS**	**Tyr**	**Leucine zipper**

ATP binding sequences

Amino Acids

NH$_2$ ————————————————————————————COOH

160-165	449-460	466-494	804	994-1021

Nucleotides

5' ———————————————————————————— 3'

478-495	1345-1380	1396-1482	2410-2412	2980-3063

Figure 4.3. Functional regions of topo II.

hypothesized that this alteration may modify the intracellular localization of the enzyme or change its interaction with other factors.

Recently the same base pair change in the topo II gene has been described in two human leukemia cell lines resistant to m-AMSA (Hinds et al., 1991; Lee et al., 1992). In CCRF-CEM cells resistant to VM26 two point mutations were observed, one thought to involve the ATP-binding site (Bugg et al., 1991), and the other around the Tyr-804 site (Danks et al., 1993). By functional expression of mutated human topo IIα in yeast, both mutations described in these cell lines have been shown to confer drug resistance to topo II agents (Hsiung et al., 1996). The simultaneous presence of both mutations could induce a higher level of drug resistance than single mutations separately.

A point mutation has been described in the DNA-binding domain of topo IIα in Chinese hamster cells resistant to etoposide (Hashimoto et al., 1995). This is associated to a reduced etoposide-induced cleavable complex in the absence of uptake deficiencies for this drug. The point mutation was found at a position that may interfere with enzyme–DNA binding.

In the human leukemic cell line CEM/VP-1, resistant to etoposide, a single base pair mutation was observed at position 2391, which led to a Lys^{797}–Asn substitution at the protein level. This change was already visible at early resistance steps (Patel and Fisher, 1993). In this cell line also gross modifications of the chariotype were seen, compared to the parental cell line.

Yeast has been extensively used as a model to investigate the role of topo gene mutants. A temperature-sensitive mutant in the yeast *TOP2* gene has shown resistance to amsacrine and etoposide (Jannatipour, Liu and Nitiss, 1993). The sequence of the mutated allele showed three different amino acid changes; it is still unclear whether all three changes are important; however the cluster of mutations are in a region that is conserved among eukaryotic topoisomerases. Yeast topo II mutants have been investigated and three classes of mutants have been identified (Wasserman and Wang, 1994).

Another possible mechanism of resistance to topo II inhibitors has been described in H209/V6, a small cell lung cancer cell line resistant to etoposide, in which an aberrant topo II cytoplasmic localization was found (Mirski and Cole, 1995). A new topo II of 160 kDa, derived from a 4.8 kb mRNA, was present in this cell line, in which a 988 amino acid sequence from the 3'-coding region and 3'-noncoding region was absent. This probably led to the loss or disruption of three putative bipartite nuclear localization signals, which caused the cytoplasmic localization of the 160 kD topo II.

Another cell line independently characterized was also reported to have a 160 kDa cytoplasmic topo IIα-related protein. In this HL60/ MX2 cell line (mitoxantrone resistant), very low levels of topo IIβ were found, compared to the parental cell line, in the absence of structural gene alterations. An additional 4.8 kb transcript of the topo IIα gene was observed (Harker et al., 1995a), which was shown to be due to the replacement of 1321 nucleotides missing in the 3' terminus, by 122 nucleotides, which contain an inframe stop codon, originated from an adjacent intron as a result of altered RNA processing. The disruption of the topo IIα gene carboxy-terminus in this cell line, which contains putative nuclear targeting sequences, may have caused the cytoplasmic distribution of the 160 kDa protein and be responsible for the growth advantage of this cell line in the presence of mitoxantrone (Harker et al., 1995b).

Scarce information is available on the importance of mutations in clinical material. Mutations have so far been described in only one patient out of 13 examined with small cell lung cancer, by SSPC screening followed by sequencing (Kubo et al., 1996). Interestingly, this patient had received etoposide-containing chemotherapy. The gene contained two mutations: at codons 486 and 494, resulting in two mis-sense mutations (Arg to Lys, and Glu to Gly, respectively). The first of these two mutations has also been reported in two amsacrine-resistant human leukemia cell lines (Hinds et al., 1991; Lee et al., 1992). In a study of 15 relapsed ALL patients (Danks et al., 1993), and in samples from 23 patients with untreated AML (Kaufmann et al., 1994), no mutations could be identified by PCR-based SSCP screening analysis in both isoforms of topo II, in the regions in which mutations had been described in cell lines.

At least four domains can be identified in the topo I eukaryotic enzymes, since most of the mutations and conserved amino acids fall within these domains (Gupta et al., 1995). Several point mutations have been described in the topo I gene of cell lines selected in vitro for resistance to topo I inhibitors (Table 4.4) (Tamura et al., 1991; Kubota et al., 1992; Tanizawa et al., 1993; Rubin et al., 1994; Fujimori et al., 1995).

Two point mutations in the topo I gene have been described in a human leukemia cell line resistant to camptothecin (Fujimori et al., 1995). The mutation at 722 is very close to the Tyr-723 region, which

Table 4.4. *Amino acid mutations in the DNA topo I gene of drug-resistant cell lines*

Reference	Cell line	Selecting drug	Cell type	Amino acid change
Kubota et al., 1992	PC-7/CPT	CPT-11	Human lung cancer	Thr^{729} to Ala
Tamura et al., 1991	CPT-K5	CPT-11	Human leukemia	$Asp^{533, 583}$ to Gly
Rubin et al., 1994	U-937	9N-CPT	Human leukemia	Phe^{361} to Ser
Tanizawa et al., 1993	DC3F/C-10	CPT	Chinese hamster	Gly^{505*} to Ser
Fujimori et al., 1995	CEM/C2	CPT	Human leukemia	Met^{370} to Thr
				Asn^{722} to Ser

CPT, camptothecin; CPT-11 irinotecan; 9N-CPT, 9-nitro-camptothecin.
* Equivalent human amino acid number. This table only includes the naturally occurring mutations, in resistant cell lines selected by drugs.

is highly conserved among type I topoisomerases in eukaryotes. In yet another cell line resistant to camptothecin, another single point mutation was found, probably responsible for the altered topo I catalytic activity, in the absence of alterations in transcription (Tanizawa et al., 1993).

In human U-937 myeloid leukemia cells a point mutation was discovered at residue 361. Partial purification of this mutated topo I demonstrated resistance of this enzyme to 9-nitro-camptothecin in catalytic assays (Rubin et al., 1994). No difference in RNA or protein expression was seen, and also no difference in catalytic activity in absence of the drug was observed.

In the human lung cancer cell line PC-7/CPT, 10-fold resistant to CPT-11, a base substitution was discovered (Kubota et al., 1992).

Two point mutations (Tamura et al., 1991) were observed in a human leukemia cell line resistant to camptothecin. When the resistant topo I was expressed in *E. coli* as a fusion protein with Staphylococcal Protein A fragment, the activity was resistant to camptothecin, indicating that either or both amino acid changes may be responsible for the resistance. In this cell line, the mutation might have caused the reduced topo I activity. In this topo I mutant, a higher cleavage/religation activity was found, with as a result improved binding and a concomitant shift in the equilibrium between cleavage and religation towards the religation step (Gromova et al., 1993).

Topo I mutants with substitutions of Arg and Ala for the amino acid residues immediately N-terminal to the active site tyrosine in human DNA topo I vac mutants, led to broad resistance to camptothecin and a broad spectrum of camptothecin derivatives (Knab, Fentala and Bjornsti, 1995). This has been demonstrated by exploiting the yeast *Saccharomyces cerevisiae*, as carrier of mutated human topo I genes. Using a similar method other important sites of mutations, possibly involved in the interaction of topo I with the DNA, were described (Benedetti et al., 1993). This approach is also feasible with yeast cells expressing heterologous topos, e.g. human DNA topo IIα.

In conclusion, the information on the expression of topoisomerase genes and its regulation, and the presence of gene mutations, is scarce in human tumors. It is still unclear what might be the role of topoisomerases in resistance to chemotherapy in human malignancies, and the way that it may develop.

Studies in human tissues

Studies in human material is nowadays readily feasible due to the availability of probes and antibodies that specifically recognize the topoisomerases. Panels of resistance markers in addition to topoisomerases may
be investigated in the same sample (Efferth, Mattern and Volm, 1992).
A large panel of topo monoclonals has been developed (Negri et al.,
1992), which may help in immunohistochemistry studies.

Whereas a fair amount of information is available on the RNA or
protein expression levels of the topoisomerase genes in cell lines, relatively few studies have been performed on human tumors; moreover,
the activity of topoisomerase II on tumors and normal tissues (Holden,
Rolfson and Wittwer, 1990), does not appear to correlate well with
protein expression (Holden, Rolfson and Wittwer, 1992). Furthermore,
large heterogeneity in activity of topo I and II was observed in different
tumor types (McLeod et al., 1994).

The two topo II isoforms have different patterns of expression in
tissues; in fact, in contrast to the α form, the β form is also expressed
in non-proliferating tissues. Tumor cells from surgical biopsies, mainly
in G_0/G_1 phase, exhibited 95% topo IIβ versus 5% of the α isoform
(Prosperi et al., 1992).

Topo IIα is in general more expressed in human cancers with high
percentages of cycling cells (Holden et al., 1992). In clinically resistant
CLL no topoisomerase II could be detected, while by Western blotting
it was possible to detect topoisomerase II in malignant lymphomas
(Potmesil et al., 1988).

In non-small cell lung cancer a clear differential expression of topo
II genes was present. The mRNA expression of the two topo II isoforms
in non-small cell lung cancer tissues was lower than in cancer cell lines,
which are much more rapidly proliferating than typical solid tumors
(Giaccone et al., 1995). Similar findings were obtained in AML samples,
as compared to HL-60 cells (Kaufmann et al., 1994). Although virtually
absent in normal lung parenchyma and stromal cells, topo IIα was
expressed in most tumors. In contrast, similar levels of topo IIβ were
expressed in normal lung and non-small cell lung cancer (Giaccone et
al., 1995). Topo IIα was also higher in ovarian tumors than normal
ovary (van der Zee et al., 1991). Topo IIα was expressed in 65% of 54
ovarian tumors, at higher levels in stage IV and grade III (van der Zee
et al., 1994); in contrast, topo IIβ and I were expressed in all ovarian
tumors examined. However, in superficial bladder cancer mRNA,

expression of both topo II genes was lower in tumor tissues than in normal bladder (Davies et al., 1996).

In non-small cell lung cancer, there was no obvious relationship in terms of level of expression between topo IIα and IIβ genes (Giaccone et al., 1995), as was also observed in a number of cell lines (Jenkins et al., 1992). However, in AML, a strong correlation of expression of the two topo II isoforms has been shown (Kaufmann et al., 1994), whereas no correlation was found in a number of solid tumors (D'Andrea, Farber and Foglesong, 1994), indicating possible differences between tumor types. A much stronger correlation was found between Ki-67 staining (a proliferation marker) and topo IIα than topo IIβ (D'Andrea et al., 1994), indicating once again that the α isoform is a proliferation marker. In non-small cell lung cancer, higher expression levels of topo IIα were in general associated with higher expression of Ki-67 (Giaccone et al., 1995). In contrast, no correlation was present between expressions of Ki-67 and topo IIβ or topo I. A similar correlation between topo IIα expression and Ki-67 has been shown in a number of solid tumors (D'Andrea et al., 1994).

The staining with the antibody Ki-S1, found to recognize topo IIα (Boege et al., 1995), had prognostic value in mammary carcinomas (Kreipe et al., 1993). This antibody was developed in order to detect proliferating cells. Similar results were found in another study, where a higher percentage of topo IIα-staining cells, with a polyclonal antibody, in breast tumors was associated with a poorer prognosis (i.e. higher grade, larger tumor size, higher nodal status, and presence of distant metastases at diagnosis), suggesting a possible role as prognostic factor (Hellemans et al., 1995). Similar results were obtained with a topo IIα monoclonal antibody and the proliferation marker MIBI (Ki-67 in paraffin-embedded material) in non-Hodgkin's lymphomas (Holden et al., 1995), with higher expression in high grade tumors.

Topo I expression was higher in colon (Giovannella et al., 1989), lung (Giaccone et al., 1995), ovary (van der Zee et al., 1991), and prostate (Husain et al., 1994) tumors than normal counterparts, but no difference was found in kidney tumors versus normal kidney, indicating that topo I expression may be tumor-type specific, and suggesting that increase in topo I levels are either due to increased topo I transcription or increased mRNA stability (Husain et al., 1994). Interestingly, the topo I protein expression was higher in more advanced stages of colon cancer (Giovannella et al., 1989).

The results of expression of topo I in non-small cell lung cancer, prostate and colon cancer would indicate an advantage in using topo I inhibitors in these malignancies. Strikingly, CPT-11, a novel camptothecin derivative, has recently shown remarkable antitumor activity in advanced lung and colorectal cancers (Slichenmayer et al., 1993).

Topo II expression and response to chemotherapy

Reduced levels of topo genes appear to be the most common mechanism of cellular resistance to topo inhibitors in vitro, and the quantification of expression and/or activity of topoisomerases would be desirable to identify patients' sensitivity to treatment. Interestingly, lower levels of topo II expression were present in ovarian cancer patients resistant to a topo II unrelated chemotherapy (cisplatin–cyclophosphamide) (van der Zee et al., 1991).

In a recent study, no correlation was found between topo II expression and resistance to doxorubicin as determined by a short term in vitro cytotoxicity test, in 48 surgically resected squamous cell carcinomas of the lung (Volm and Mattern, 1992). However, in this study, immuno-histochemistry was performed using a polyclonal antibody that does not distinguish between the two topo II isoforms.

In AML patients (Kaufmann et al., 1994) no correlation was found between topo IIα expression, as assessed by Western blotting, and patient response to induction chemotherapy.

Similarly, in childhood ALL no correlation was found between topo IIα expression, as assessed by RNase protection assay, and in vitro sensitivity to topo inhibitors of fresh leukemic cells, and no difference in levels of expression were seen between newly diagnosed patients and relapsing patients (Klumper et al., 1995). However, in a study on six human acute lymphoblastic leukemia cell lines a direct correlation was found between expression of topo IIβ and cytotoxicity to doxorubicin and etoposide, but not with topo IIα (Brown et al., 1995). This indicates that the exact role of the two topo II isoforms in drug sensitivity to topo II inhibitors is still not settled, and suggests that, at least in ALL, topo IIβ may be more important than the α isoform in relation to drug resistance.

In 15 myeloma cases no correlation was observed between expression of topo I and II or other resistance genes and clinical response to chemo-therapy. However, Northern blotting was used in this study (Ishikawa et al., 1993), which resulted in only one case positive. This method has been shown to be insufficiently sensitive in solid tumors such as lung cancer (Giaccone et al., 1995).

In a study of 15 fresh tumor specimens, of which 11 were breast cancer specimens, a significant correlation ($P < 0.01$) was found between topo II expression detected by RNA dot blot and clinical response to doxorubicin (Kim et al., 1991).

A recent study found no correlation between response to epirubicin instillation and topo IIα, topo IIβ-1 or IIβ-2, in superficial bladder carcinoma; unexpectedly topo IIβ-1 mRNA levels were higher in unresponsive tumors (Davies et al., 1996).

Once that topo II can be established as a good marker for sensitivity to topo II inhibitors, one may try to stimulate topo II expression/activity. This has been accomplished in vitro with G-CSF in leukemia cell lines (Towatari et al., 1990), where mRNA levels increased by about 2-fold. GM-CSF was given in a clinical protocol for AML 3 days preceding the chemotherapy and the increased expression was also confirmed in the clinical setting (Kaufmann et al., 1994). Whether this approach will prove more effective than standard treatment is still not known.

Another way of stimulating expression/activity of topo II has been shown to be pretreatment with a topo I inhibitor: pretreatment of human xenografts with CPT-11 induced an increase in the S-phase cell population with an increase in topo II mRNA expression after 24–48 hours. This may be clinically exploited while investigating combinations of topo I and topo II inhibitors (Kim et al., 1992), keeping in mind the possible antagonistic effect of this type of combination (Kaufmann, 1991).

References

Adachi, Y., Luke, M. and Laemmli, U. K. (1991). Chromosome assembly *in vitro*: topoisomerase II is required for condensation. *Cell*, **64**, 137–48.

Andersen, A. H., Svejstrup, J. Q. and Westergaard, O. (1994). The DNA binding, cleavage, and religation reactions of eukaryotic topoisomerases I and II. In *Advances in Pharmacology*, Volume 29A (ed. L. F. Liu), pp. 83–101.

Andoh, T., Ishii, K., Suzuki, Y. et al. (1987). Characterization of a mammalian mutant with a camptothecin resistant DNA topoisomerase I. *Proc. Natl. Acad. Sci. USA*, **84**, 5565–9.

Austin, C. A., Sng, J.-H., Patel, S. and Fisher, L. M. (1993). Novel HeLa topoisomerase II is the IIβ isoform: complete coding sequence and homology with other type II topoisomerases. *Biochim. Biophys. Acta*, **1172**, 283–91.

Avemann, K., Knippers, R., Koller, T. and Sogo, J. M. (1988). Camptothecin, a specific inhibitor of type I DNA topoisomerase, induces DNA breakage at replication forks. *Mol. Cell. Biol.*, **8**, 3026–34.

Beck, W. T., Danks, M. K., Wolverton, J. S. et al. (1993). Drug resistance
    associated with altered DNA topoisomerase II. *Adv. Enzyme Regul.*, **33**,
    113–27.
Beidler, D. R. and Cheng, Y.-C. (1995). Camptothecin induction of a time- and
    concentration-dependent decrease of topoisomerase I and its implication in
    camptothecin activity. *Mol. Pharmacol.*, **47**, 907–14.
Benedetti, P., Fiorani, P., Capuani, L. and Wang, J. C. (1993). Camptothecin
    resistance from a single mutation changing glycine 63 of human DNA
    topoisomerase I to cysteine. *Cancer Res.*, **53**, 4343–8.
Berger, J. M., Gamblin, S. J., Harrison, S. C. and Wang, J. C. (1996). Structure and
    mechanism of DNA topoisomerase II. *Nature*, **379**, 225–32.
Binaschi, M., Giaccone, G., Supino, R. et al. (1992). Characterization of a
    topoisomerase II gene rearrangement in a human small-cell lung cancer cell
    line. *J. Natl. Cancer Inst.*, **84**, 1710–16.
Boege, F., Andersen, A., Jensen, S. et al. (1995). Proliferation-associated nuclear
    antigen Ki-S1 is identical with topoisomerase IIα. Delineation of a
    carboxyl-terminal epitope with peptide antibodies. *Am. J. Pathol.*, **146**,
    1302–8.
Boothman, D. A., Wang, M., Schea, R. A. et al. (1992). Posttreatment exposure to
    camptothecin enhances the lethal effects of X-rays on radioresistant human
    malignant melanoma cells. *Int. J. Rad. Oncol. Biol. Phys.*, **24**, 939–48.
Brown, G. A., McPherson, J. P., Gu, L. et al. (1995). Relationship of DNA
    topoisomerase IIα and β expression to cytotoxicity of antineoplastic agents in
    human acute lymphoblastic leukemia cell lines. *Cancer Res.*, **55**, 78–82.
Bugg, D. Y., Dank, M. K., Beck, W. T. and Suttle, D. P. (1991). Expression of a
    mutant DNA topoisomerase II in CCRF-CEM human leukemic cells
    selected for resistance to teniposide. *Proc. Natl. Acad. Sci. USA*, **88**, 7654–8.
Burden, D. A. and Sullivan, D. M. (1994). Phosphorylation of the α- and
    β-isoforms of DNA topoisomerase II is qualitatively different in interphase
    and mitosis in Chinese hamster ovary cells. *Biochemistry*, **33**, 14651–5.
Burden, D. A., Goldsmith, L. J. and Sullivan, D. M. (1993). Cell-cycle-dependent
    phosphorylation and activity of Chinese-hamster ovary topoisomerase II.
    Biochem. J., **293**, 297–304.
Campain, J. A., Gottesman, M. M. and Pastan, I. (1994). A novel mutant
    topoisomerase IIα present in VP-16 resistant human melanoma cell lines has a
    deletion of alanine 429. *Biochemistry*, **33**, 11327–32.
Capranico, G. and Zunino, F. (1990). Structural requirements for DNA
    topoisomerase II inhibition by anthracyclines. In: *Molecular Basis of
    Specificity in Nucleic Acid–Drug Interactions* (ed. B. Pullman and J. Jortner),
    pp. 167–75. Kluwer Academic Publishers, Netherlands.
Capranico, G. and Zunino, F. (1992). DNA topoisomerase-trapping antitumor
    drugs. *Eur. J. Cancer*, **28A**, 2055–60.
Capranico, G., Kohn, K. W. and Pommier, Y. (1990a). Local sequence
    requirements for DNA cleavage by mammalian topoisomerase II in the
    presence of doxorubicin. *Nucl. Acids Res.*, **18**, 6611–19.
Capranico, G., Zunino, F., Kohn, K. W. and Pommier, Y. (1990b). Sequence
    selective topoisomerase II inhibition by anthracycline derivatives in SV40
    DNA: relationship with DNA binding affinity and cytotoxicity. *Biochemistry*,
    29, 562–9.
Capranico, G., Tinelli, S., Austin, C. A. et al. (1992). Different patterns of gene
    expression of topoisomerase II isoforms in differentiated tissues during murine
    development. *Biochim. Biophys. Acta*, **1132**, 43–48.

Capranico, G., Giaccone, G., Zunino, F. et al. (1994a). DNA topoisomerase inhibitors. In *Cancer Chemotherapy and Biological Response Modifiers, Annual 15* (ed. H. M. Pinedo, D. L. Longo and B. A. Chabner), pp. 67–86. Elsevier Science, B.V.

Capranico, G., Palumbo, M., Tinelli, S. et al. (1994b). Conformational drug determinants of the sequence specificity of drug-stimulated topoisomerase II DNA cleavage. *J. Mol. Biol.*, **235**, 1218–30.

Chan, V. T. W., Ng, S.-W., Eder, J. P. and Schnipper, L. E. (1993). Molecular cloning and identification of a point mutation in the topoisomerase II cDNA from an etoposide-resistant Chinese hamster ovary cell line. *J. Biol. Chem.*, **268**, 2160–5.

Chen, A. Y. and Liu, L. F. (1994). Mechanisms of resistance to topoisomerase inhibitors. In *Anticancer Drug Resistance: Advances in Molecular and Clinical Research* (ed. L. J. Goldstein and R. F. Ozols), pp. 263–81. Kluwer Academic Publishers.

Chen, A. Y., Yu, C., Potmesil, M. et al. (1991). Camptothecin overcomes MDR1-mediated resistance in human KB carcinoma cells. *Cancer Res.*, **51**, 6039–44.

Chen, A. Y., Yu, C., Gatto, B. and Liu, L. F. (1993). DNA minor groove-binding ligands: a different class of mammalian DNA topoisomerase I inhibitors. *Proc. Natl. Acad. Sci. USA*, **90**, 8131–5.

Chen, G. L., Yang, L., Rowe, R. C. et al. (1984). Nonintercalative antitumor drugs interfere with the breakage-reunion reaction of mammalian DNA topoisomerase II. *J. Biol. Chem.*, **259**, 13560–6.

Chen, M. and Beck, W. T. (1993). Teniposide-resistant CEM cells, which express mutant DNA topoisomerase IIα, when treated with non-complex-stabilizing inhibitors of the enzyme, display no cross-resistance and reveal aberrant functions of the mutant enzyme. *Cancer Res.*, **53**, 5946–53.

Chung, T. D., Drake, F. H., Tan, K. B. et al. (1989). Characterization and immunological identification of cDNA clones encoding two human DNA topoisomerase II isoenzymes. *Proc. Natl. Acad. Sci. USA*, **86**, 9431–5.

Cole, S. P. C., Chanda, E. R., Dicke, F. P. et al. (1991). Non-P-glycoprotein-mediated multidrug resistance in a small cell lung cancer cell line: evidence for decreased susceptibility to drug-induced DNA damage and reduced levels of topoisomerase II. *Cancer Res.*, **51**, 3345–52.

Corbett, A. H., Fernald, A. W. and Osheroff, N. (1993). Protein kinase C modulates the catalytic activity of topoisomerase II by enhancing the rate of ATP hydrolysis: evidence for a common mechanism of regulation of phosphorylation. *Biochemistry*, **32**, 2090–7.

Coutts, J., Plumb, J. A., Brown, R. and Keith, W. N. (1993). Expression of topoisomerase II alpha and beta in an adrenocarcinoma cell line carrying amplified topoisomerase II alpha and retinoic acid receptor alpha genes. *Br. J. Cancer*, **68**, 793–800.

D'Andrea, M. R., Farber, P. A. and Foglesong, P. D. (1994). Immunohistochemical detection of DNA topoisomerase IIα and IIβ compared with detection of Ki-67, a marker of cellular proliferation, in human tumors. *Appl. Immunhist.*, **2**, 177–85.

Danks, M. K., Warmoth, M. R., Friche, E. et al. (1993). Single-strand conformational polymorphism analysis of the Mr 170 000 isozyme of DNA topoisomerase II in human tumor cells. *Cancer Res.*, **53**, 1373–9.

D'Arpa, P. and Liu, L. F. (1989). Topoisomerase-targeting antitumor drugs. *Biochim. Biophys. Acta*, **989**, 163–77.

Davies, S. L., Jenkins, J. R. and Hickson, I. D. (1993). Human cells express two differentially spliced forms of topoisomerase IIβ mRNA. *Nucl. Acids Res.*, **21**, 3719–23.

Davies, S. L., Popert, R., Coptcoat, M. et al. (1996). Response to epirubicin in patients with superficial bladder cancer and expression of the topoisomerase IIα and β genes. *Int. J. Cancer*, **65**, 63–6.

Deffie, A. M., Batra, J. K. and Goldenberg, G. J. (1989). Direct correlation between DNA topoisomerase II activity and cytotoxicity in adriamycin-sensitive and resistant P388 leukemia cell lines. *Cancer Res.*, **49**, 58–62.

De Isabella, P., Capranico, G., Binaschi, M. et al. (1990). Evidence of topoisomerase II-dependent mechanisms of multidrug resistance in P388 leukemia cells. *Mol. Pharmacol.*, **37**, 11–16.

de Jong, S., Zijlstra, J. G., de Vries, E. G. E. and Mulder, N. H. (1990). Reduced DNA topoisomerase II activity and drug-induced DNA cleavage activity in an adriamycin-resistant human small cell lung carcinoma cell line. *Cancer Res.*, **50**, 304–9.

de Jong, S., Kooistra, A. J., de Vries, E. G. E. et al. (1993). Topoisomerase II as a target of VM-26 and 4'-(9-acridinylamino)methanesulfon-m-aniside in atypical multidrug resistant human small cell lung carcinoma cells. *Cancer Res.*, **53**, 1064–71.

DeVore, R. F., Corbett, A. H. and Osheroff, N. (1992). Phosphorylation of topoisomerase II by casein kinase II and protein kinase C: effects on enzyme-mediated DNA cleavage/religation and sensitivity to the antineoplastic drugs etoposide and 4'-(9-acridinylamino)methane-sulfon-m-anisidide. *Cancer Res.*, **52**, 2156–61.

Drake, P. H., Hofmann, G. A., Bartus, H. F. et al. (1989). Biochemical and pharmacological properties of p170 and p180 isoforms of topisomerase II. *Biochemistry*, **28**, 8154–60.

Eder, J. P., Chan, V. T.-V., Ng, S.-W. et al. (1995). DNA topoisomerase IIα expression is associated with alkylating agent resistance. *Cancer Res.*, **55**, 6109–16.

Efferth, T., Mattern, J. and Volm, M. (1992). Immunohistochemical detection of P glycoprotein, glutathione S transferase and DNA topoisomerase II in human tumors. *Oncology*, **49**, 368–75.

Eng, W. K., McCabe, F. L., Tan, K. B. et al. (1990). Development of a stable camptothecin-resistant subline of P388 leukemia with reduced topoisomerase I content. *Mol. Pharmacol.*, **38**, 471–80.

Felix, C. A., Lange, B. J., Hosler, M. R. et al. (1995). Chromosome band 11q23 translocation breakpoints are DNA topoisomerase II cleavage sites. *Cancer Res.*, **55**, 4287–92.

Fleischmann, G., Pflugfelder, G., Steiner, E. K. et al. (1984). Drosophila DNA topoisomerase I is associated with transcriptionally active regions of the genome. *Proc. Natl. Acad. Sci. USA*, **81**, 6958–62.

Fosse, P., Rene, B., Le Bret, M. et al. (1991). Sequence requirements for mammalian topoisomerase II mediated DNA cleavage stimulated by an ellipticine derivative. *Nucl. Acids Res.*, **19**, 2861–8.

Freudenreich, C. H. and Kreuzer, K. N. (1993). Mutational analysis of a type II topoisomerase cleavage site: distinct requirements for enzyme and inhibitors. *EMBO J.*, **12**, 2085–97.

Friche, E., Danks, M. K., Schmidt, C. A. and Beck, W. T. (1991). Decreased DNA topoisomerase II in daunorubicin-resistant Ehrlich ascites tumor cells. *Cancer Res.*, **51**, 4213–18.

Friedman, H. S., Dolan, M. E., Kaufmann, S. H. et al. (1994). Elevated polymerase α, DNA polymerase β, and DNA topoisomerase II in a melphalan-resistant rhabdomyosarcoma xenograft that is cross-resistant to nitrosoureas and topotecan. *Cancer Res.*, **54**, 3487–93.

Fry, A. M., Chresta, C. M., Davies, S. M. et al. (1991). Relationship between topoisomerase II level and chemosensitivity in human tumor cell lines. *Cancer Res.*, **51**, 6592–5.

Fujimori, A., Harker, G., Kohlhgen, G. et al. (1995). Mutation at the site of topoisomerase I in CEM/C2, a human leukemia cell line resistant to camptothecin. *Cancer Res.*, **55**, 1339–46.

Ganapathi, R., Zwelling, L., Constantinou, A. et al. (1993). Altered phosphorylation, biosynthesis and degradation of the 170 kDa isoform of topoisomerase II in amsacrine-resistant human leukemia cells. *Biochem. Biophys. Res. Comm.*, **192**, 1274–80.

Giaccone, G. (1994). DNA topoisomerases and topoisomerase inhibitors. *Pathol. Biol.*, **4**, 346–52.

Giaccone, G., Gazdar, A. F., Beck, H. et al. (1992). The multidrug sensitivity phenotype of human lung cancer cells associated with topoisomerase II expression. *Cancer Res.*, **52**, 1666–74.

Giaccone, G., van Ark-Otte, J., Scagliotti, G. et al. (1995). Differential expression of DNA topoisomerases in non-small cell lung cancer and normal lung. *Biochim. Biophys. Acta*, **1264**, 337–46.

Giovanella, B. C., Stehlin, J. S., Wall, M. E. et al. (1989). DNA topoisomerase I targeted chemotherapy of human colon cancer in xenografts. *Science*, **246**, 1046–8.

Goldwasser, F., Bae, I., Valenti, M. et al. (1995). Topoisomerase I-related parameters and camptothecin activity in the colon carcinoma cell lines from the National Cancer Institute anticancer screen. *Cancer Res.*, **55**, 2116–21.

Gottlieb, J. A., Guarino, A. M. and Call, J. B. (1970). Preliminary pharmacologic and clinical evaluation of camptothecin (NSC-100880). *Cancer Chemother. Rep.*, **54**, 461.

Gromova, I. I., Kjeldsen, E., Svejstrup, J. Q. et al. (1993). Characterization of an altered DNA catalysis of a camptothecin-resistant eukaryotic topoisomerase I. *Nucl. Acids. Res.*, **21**, 593–600.

Gudkov, A. V., Zelnick, C. R., Zakarov, A. R. et al. (1993). Isolation of genetic suppressor elements, inducing resistance to topoisomerase II-interactive cytotoxic drugs, from human topoisomerase II cDNA. *Proc. Natl. Acad. Sci. USA*, **90**, 3231–5.

Gupta, M., Fujimori, A. and Pommier, Y. (1995). Eukaryotic DNA topoisomerase I. *Biochim. Biophys. Acta.*, **1262**, 1–14.

Gupta, R. S., Gupta, R., Eng, B. et al. (1988). Camptothecin-resistant mutants of Chinese hamster ovary cells containing a resistant form of topoisomerase I. *Cancer Res.*, **48**, 6404–10.

Hanai, R., Caron, P. R. and Wang, J. C. (1996). Human TPO3: a single copy gene encoding DNA topoisomerase III. *Proc. Natl. Acad. Sci. USA*, **93**, 3653–7.

Harker, W. G., Slade, D. L., Drake, F. H. et al. (1991). Mitoxantrone resistance in HL-60 leukemia cells: reduced nuclear topoisomerase II catalytic activity and drug-induced DNA cleavage in association with reduced expression of the topoisomerase IIβ isoform. *Biochemistry*, **30**, 9953–61.

Harker, W. G., Slade, D. L., Parr, R. L. et al. (1995a). Alterations in the topoisomerase IIα gene, messenger RNA, and subcellular protein distribution as well as reduced expression of the DNA topoisomerase IIβ enzyme in a mitoxantrone-resistant HL-60 human leukemia cell line. *Cancer Res.*, **55**, 1707–16.

Harker, W. G., Slade, D. L., Parr, R. L. and Holguin, M. H. (1995b). Selective use of an alternative stop codon and polyadenylation signal within intron sequences leads to a truncated topoisomerase IIα messenger RNA and protein in human HL-60 leukemia cells selected for resistance to mitoxantrone. *Cancer Res.*, **55**, 4962–71.

Hashimoto, S., Danks, M. K., Chatterjee, S. et al. (1995). A novel point mutation in the 3' flanking region of the DNA-binding domain of topoisomerase IIα associated with acquired resistance to topoisomerase II active agents. *Oncol. Res.*, **7**, 21–9.

Heck, M. M. S. and Earnshaw, W. C. (1986). Topoisomerase II: a specific marker for cell proliferation. *J. Cell. Biol.*, **103**, 2569.

Heck, M. M. S., Hittelman, W. N. and Earnshaw, W. C. (1988). Differential expression of DNA topoisomerase I and II during the eukaryotic cell cycle. *Proc. Natl. Acad. Sci. USA*, **85**, 1086–90.

Heiland, S., Knippers, R. and Kunze, N. (1993). The promoter region of the human type-I-DNA topoisomerase gene. Protein-binding sites and sequences involved in transcriptional regulation. *Eur. J. Biochem.*, **217**, 813–22.

Hellemans, P., van Dam, P. A., Geykens, M. et al. (1995). Immunohistochemical study of topoisomerase II-α expression in primary ductal carcinoma of the breast. *J. Clin. Pathol.*, **48**, 147–50.

Hendricks, C. B., Rowinsky, E. K., Grochow, L. B. et al. (1992). Effect of P-glycoprotein on the accumulation and cytotoxicity of topotecan (SK&F 104864), a novel camptothecin analogue. *Cancer Res.*, **52**, 2268–78.

Herzog, C. E., Zwelling, L. A., McWatters, A. and Kleinerman, E. S. (1995). Expression of topoisomerase II, Bcl-2, and p53 in three human brain tumor cell lines and their possible relationship to intrinsic resistance to etoposide. *Clin. Cancer Res.*, **1**, 1391–7.

Hinds, M., Deisseroth, K., Mayes, J. et al. (1991). Identification of a point mutation in the topoisomerase II gene from a human leukemia cell line containing an amsacrine-resistant form of topoisomerase II. *Cancer Res.*, **51**, 4729–31.

Hoban, P. R., Robson, C. N., Davies, S. M. et al. (1992). Reduced topoisomerase II and elevated α class glutathione S-transferase expression in a multidrug resistant CHO cell line highly cross-resistant to mitomycin C. *Biochem. Pharmacol.*, **43**, 685–93.

Hochhauser, D. and Harris, A. L. (1993). The role of topoisomerase IIα and β in drug resistance. *Cancer Treat. Rev.*, **19**, 181–94.

Hochhauser, D., Stanway, C. A., Harris, A. L. and Hickson, I. D. (1992). Cloning and characterization of the 5'-flanking region of the human topoisomerase IIα gene. *J. Biol. Chem.*, **267**, 18961–5.

Holden, J. A., Rolfson, D. H. and Wittwer, C. T. (1990). Human DNA topoisomerase II: evaluation of enzyme activity in normal and neoplastic tissues. *Biochemistry*, **29**, 2127–34.

Holden, J. A., Rolfson, D. H. and Wittwer, C. T. (1992). The distribution of immunoreactive topoisomerase II protein in human tissues and neoplasms. *Oncol. Res.*, **4**, 157–66.

Holden, J. A., Perkins, S. L., Snow, G. W. and Kjeldsberg, C. R. (1995). Immunohistochemical staining for DNA topoisomease II in non-Hodgkin's lymphomas. *Am. J. Clin. Pathol.*, **104**, 54–9.

Hosking, L. K., Whelan, R. D. H., Shellard, S. A. et al. (1994). Multiple mechanisms of resistance in a series of human testicular teratoma cell lines selected for increasing resistance to etoposide. *Int. J. Cancer*, **57**, 259–67.

Hsiang, Y. H., Wu, H. Y. and Liu, L. F. (1988). Proliferation-dependent regulation of DNA topoisomerase II in cultured human cells. *Cancer Res.*, **48**, 3230–5.

Hsiung, Y., Jannatipour, M., Rose, A. et al. (1996). Functional expression of human topoisomerase IIα in yeast: mutations at amino acids 450 and 803 of topoisomerase IIα result in enzymes that can confer resistance to anti-topoisomerase II agents. *Cancer Res.*, **56**, 91–9.

Husain, I., Mohler, J. L., Seigler, H. F. et al. (1994). Elevation of topoisomerase I messenger RNA, protein, and catalytic activity in human tumors: demonstration of tumor-type specificity and implications for cancer chemotherapy. *Cancer Res.*, **54**, 539–46.

Hwang, J. and Hwong, C.-L. (1994). Cellular regulation of mammalian DNA topoisomerases. In *Advances in Pharmacology*, Volume 29A (ed. L. F. Liu), pp. 167–89. Academic Press.

Hwang, J., Shyy, S., Chen, A. Y. et al. (1989). Studies of topoisomerase-specific antitumor drugs in human lymphocytes using rabbit antisera against recombinant human topoisomerase II polypeptide. *Cancer Res.*, **49**, 958–62.

Hwong, C.-L., Chen, C.-Y., Shang, H.-F. and Hwang, J. (1993). Increased synthesis and degradation of DNA topoisomerase I during the initial phase of human T lymphocyte proliferation. *J. Biol. Chem.*, **268**, 18982–6.

Ishikawa, H., Kawano, M. M., Okada, K. et al. (1993). Expressions of DNA topoisomerase I and II genes and the genes possibly related to drug resistance in human myeloma cells. *Br. J. Haematol.*, **83**, 68–74.

Jannatipour, M., Liu, Y.-X. and Nitiss, J. L. (1993). The top2-5 mutant of yeast topoisomerase II encodes an enzyme resistant to etoposide and amsacrine. *J. Biol. Chem.*, **268**, 18585–92.

Jaxel, C., Capranico, G., Kerrigan, D. et al. (1991). Effect of local DNA sequence on topoisomerase I cleavage in the presence or absence of camptothecin. *J. Biol. Chem.*, **266**, 20418–23.

Jenkins, J. R., Ayton, P., Jones, T. et al. (1992). Isolation of cDNA clones encoding the β isozyme of human DNA topoisomerase II and localization of the gene to chromosome 3p24. *Nucl. Acids Res.*, **20**, 5587–92.

Juan, C. C., Hwang, J., Liu, A. A. et al. (1988). Human DNA topoisomerase I is encoded by a single-copy gene that maps to chromosome region 20q12-13.2. *Proc. Natl. Acad. Sci. USA*, **85**, 8910–13.

Juenke, J. E. M. and Holden, J. A. (1993). The distribution of DNA topoisomerase II isoforms in differentiated adult mouse tissues. *Biochim. Biophys. Acta*, **1216**, 191–6.

Kasahara, K., Fijiwara, Y., Sugimoto, Y. et al. (1992). Determinants of response to the DNA topoisomerase II inhibitors doxorubicin and etoposide in human lung cancer cell lines. *J. Natl. Cancer Inst.*, **84**, 113–18.

Kato, J.-I., Suzuki, H. and Ikeda, H. (1992). Purification and characterization of DNA topoisomerase IV in *Escherichia coli*. *J. Biol. Chem.*, **267**, 25676–84.

Kaufmann, S. H. (1991). Antagonism between camptothecin and topoisomerase II-directed chemotherapeutic agents in a human leukemia cell line. *Cancer Res.*, **51**, 1129–36.

Kaufmann, S. H., McLaughlin, S. J., Kastan, M. B. et al. (1991). Topoisomerase II levels during granulocytic maturation *in vitro* and *in vivo*. *Cancer Res.*, **51**, 3534–43.

Kaufmann, S. H., Karp, J. E., Jones, R. J. et al. (1994). Topoisomerase II levels and drug sensitivity in adult acute myelogenous leukemia. *Blood*, **83**, 517–30.

Kim, R., Hirabayashi, N., Nishiyama, M. et al. (1991). Expression of MDR1, GST-π and topoisomerase II as an indicator of clinical response to adryamicin. *Anticancer Res.*, **11**, 429–32.

Kim, R., Hirabayashi, N., Nishiyama, M. et al. (1992). Experimental studies on biochemical modulation targeting topoisomerase I and II in human tumor xenografts in nude mice. *Int. J. Cancer*, **50**, 760–6.

Kimura, K., Saijo, M., Ui, M. and Enomoto, T. (1994). Growth state- and cell cycle-dependent fluctuation in the expression of two forms of DNA topoisomerase II and possible specific modification of the higher molecular weight forms in the M phase. *J. Biol. Chem.*, **269**, 1173–6.

Kjeldsen, E., Mollerup, S., Thomsen, B. et al. (1988a). Sequence-dependent effect of camptothecin on human topoisomerase I DNA cleavage. *J. Mol. Biol.*, **202**, 333–42.

Kjeldsen, E., Bonven, B. J., Andoh, T. et al. (1988b). Characterization of a camptothecin-resistant human DNA topoisomerase I. *J. Biol. Chem.*, **263**, 3912–16.

Klumper, E., Giaccone, G., Pieters, R. et al. (1995). Topoisomerase IIα gene expression in childhood lymphoblastic leukemia. *Leukemia*, **9**, 1653–60.

Knab, A. M., Fentala, J. and Bjornsti, M.-A. (1995). A camptothecin-resistant DNA topoisomerase I mutant exhibits altered sensitivities to other DNA topoisomerase poisons. *J. Biol. Chem.*, **270**, 6141–8.

Kosovsky, M. J. and Soslau, G. (1993). Immunological identification of human platelet mitochondrial DNA topoisomerase I. *Biochem. Biophys. Acta*, **1164**, 101–7.

Kotoh, S., Naito, S., Yokomizo, A. et al. (1994). Increased expression of DNA topoisomerase I gene and collateral sensitivity to camptothecin in human cisplatin-resistant bladder cancer cells. *Cancer Res.*, **54**, 3248–52.

Kreipe, H., Alm, P., Olsson, H. et al. (1993). Prognostic significance of a formalin-resistant nuclear proliferation antigen in mammary carcinomas as determined by the monoclonal antibody Ki-S1. *Am. J. Pathol.*, **152**, 651–7.

Kroll, D. J. and Rowe, T. C. (1991). Phosphorylation of DNA topoisomerase II in a human tumor cell line. *J. Biol. Chem.*, **266**, 7957–61.

Kubo, T., Kohno, K., Ohga, T. et al. (1995). DNA topoisomerase IIα gene expression under transcriptional control in etoposide/teniposide-resistant human cancer cells. *Cancer Res.*, **55**, 3860–4.

Kubo, A., Yoshikawa, A., Hirashima, T. et al. (1996). Point mutations of the topoisomerase IIα gene in patients with small cell lung cancer treated with etoposide. *Cancer Res.*, **56**, 1232–6.

Kubota, N., Kanzawa, F., Nishio, K. et al. (1992). Detection of topoisomerase I gene point mutation in CPT-11 resistant lung cancer cell line. *Biochem. Biophys. Res. Comm.*, **188**, 571–7.

Kunze, N., Yang, G. C., Dolberg, M. et al. (1991). Structure of the human type I DNA topoisomerase gene. *J. Biol. Chem.*, **266**, 9610–16.

Kyprianou, N., Alexander, R. B. and Isaacs, J. T. (1991). Activation of programmed cell death by recombinant human tumor necrosis factor plus topoisomerase II-targeted drugs in L929 tumor cells. *J. Natl. Cancer Inst.*, **83**, 346–50.

Lee, M. S., Wang, J. C. and Beran, M. (1992). Two independent amsacrine-resistant human myeloid leukemia cell lines share an identical point mutation in the 170 kDa form of human topoisomerase II. *J. Mol. Biol.*, **223**, 837–43.

Lee, M. P., Brown, S. D., Chen, A. and Hsieh, T.-S. (1993). DNA topoisomerase I is essential in *Drosophila melanogaster*. *Proc. Natl. Acad. Sci. USA*, **90**, 6656–60.

Lefevre, D., Riou, J. F., Ahomadegbe, J. C. et al. (1991). Study of molecular markers of resistance to m-AMSA in a human breast cancer cell line. Decrease of topoisomerase II and increase of both topoisomerase I and acidic glutathione S transferase. *Biochem. Pharmacol.*, **41**, 1967–79.

Leteurtre, F., Kohlhagen, G., Fesen, M. R. et al. (1994). Effects of DNA methylation on topoisomerase I and II cleavage activities. *J. Biol. Chem.*, **269**, 7893–900.

Lima, C. D., Wang, J. C. and Mondragon, A. (1994). Three-dimensional structure of the 67K N-terminal fragment of *E. coli* DNA topoisomerase I. *Nature*, **367**, 138–46.

Liu, L. F. (1989). DNA topoisomerase poisons as antitumor drugs. *Annu. Rev. Biochem.*, **58**, 351–75.

Liu, S. Y., Hwang, B. D., Liu, Z. C. and Cheng, Y. C. (1989). Interaction of several nucleoside triphosphate analogues and 10-hydroxycamptothecin with human DNA topoisomerases. *Cancer Res.*, **49**, 1366–70.

Long, B. H., Wang, L., Lorico, A. et al. (1991). Mechanisms of resistance to etoposide and teniposide in acquired resistant human colon and lung carcinoma cell lines. *Cancer Res.*, **51**, 5275–84.

Markovits, J., Pommier, Y., Kerrigan, D. et al. (1987). Topoisomerase II-mediated DNA breaks and cytotoxicity in relation to cell proliferation and the cell cycle in NIH 3T3 fibroblasts and L1210 leukemia cells. *Cancer Res.*, **47**, 2050.

Markovits, J., Junqua, S., Goldwasser, F. et al. (1995). Genistein resistance in human leukaemic CCRF-CEM cells: selection of a diploid cell line with reduced DNA topoisomerase IIβ isoform. *Biochem. Pharmacol.*, **50**, 177–86.

Mattern, M. R., Hofmann, G. A., Polsky, R. M. et al. (1993). *In vitro* and *in vivo* effects of clinically important camptothecin analogues on multidrug-resistant cells. *Oncol. Res.*, **5**, 467–74.

McLeod, H. L., Douglas, F., Oates, M. et al. (1994). Topoisomerase I and II activity in human breast, cervix, lung and colon cancer. *Int. J. Cancer*, **59**, 607–11.

McPherson, J. P., Brown, G. A. and Goldenberg, G. J. (1993). Characterization of a DNA topoisomerase IIα gene rearrangement in adriamycin-resistant P388 leukemia: expression of a fusion messenger RNA transcript encoding topoisomerase IIα and the retinoic acid receptor α locus. *Cancer Res.*, **53**, 5885–9.

Mirski, S. E. L. and Cole, S. P. C. (1995). Cytoplasmic localization of a mutant M_r 160 000 topoisomerase IIα is associated with the loss of putative bipartite nuclear localization signals in a drug-resistant human lung cancer cell line. *Cancer Res.*, **55**, 2129–34.

Negri, C., Chiesa, R., Cerino, A. et al. (1992). Monoclonal antibodies to human DNA topoisomerase I and the two forms of DNA topoisomerase I and IIα. *Exp. Cell Res.*, **206**, 128–33.

Niimi, S., Nakagawa, K., Sugimoto, Y. et al. (1992). Mechanism of cross-resistance to a camptothecin analogue (CPT-11) in a human ovarian cancer cell line selected by cisplatin. *Cancer Res.*, **52**, 328–33.

Nitiss, J. L., Liu, Y.-X., Harbury, P. et al. (1992). Amsacrine and etoposide hypersensitivity of yeast cells overexpressing DNA topoisomerase II. *Cancer Res.*, **52**, 4467–72.

Osheroff, N. (1989). Biochemical basis for the interactions of type I and type II topoisomerases with DNA. *Pharmacol. Ther.*, **41**, 223–41.

Osheroff, N., Corbett, A. H. and Robinson, M. J. (1994). Mechanism of action of topoisomerase II-targeted antineoplastic drugs. In *Advances in Pharmacology*, Volume 29B (ed. L. F. Liu), pp. 105–26. Academic Press.

Patel, S. and Fisher, L. M. (1993). Novel selection and genetic characterization of an etoposide-resistant human leukemic CCRF-CEM cell line. *Br. J. Cancer*, **67**, 456–63.

Perego, P., Capranico, G., Supino, R. and Zunino, F. (1994). Topoisomerase I gene expression and cell sensitivity to camptothecin in human cell lines of different tumor types. *Anti-Cancer Drugs*, **5**, 645–9.

Petrov, P., Drake, F. H., Loranger, A. et al. (1993). Localization of DNA topoisomerase II in Chinese hamster fibroblasts by confocal and electron microscopy. *Exp. Cell Res.*, **204**, 73–81.

Pommier, Y., Capranico, G., Orr, A. and Kohn, K. W. (1991). Local base sequence preferences for DNA cleavage by mammalian topoisomerase II in the presence of amsacrine or teniposide. *Nucl. Acids Res.*, **19**, 5973–80.

Potmesil, M. (1994). Camptothecins: from bench research to hospital wards. *Cancer Res.*, **54**, 1431–9.

Potmesil, M., Hsiang, Y., Liu, L. F. et al. (1988). Resistance of human leukemic and normal lymphocytes to drug-induced DNA cleavage and low levels of DNA topoisomerase II. *Cancer Res.*, **48**, 3537–43.

Pratesi, G., Capranico, G., Binaschi, M. et al. (1990). Relationships among tumor responsiveness, cell sensitivity, doxorubicin cellular pharmacokinetics and drug-induced DNA alterations in two human small-cell lung cancer xenografts. *Int. J. Cancer*, **46**, 669–74.

Prosperi, E., Sala, E., Negri, C. et al. (1992). Topoisomerase IIα and β in human tumor cells grown *in vitro* and *in vivo*. *Anticancer Res.*, **12**, 2093–100.

Ramachandran, C., Mead, D., Wellham, L. et al. (1995). Expression of drug resistance-associated mdr-1, GSTπ, and topoisomerase II genes during cell cycle traverse. *Biochem. Pharmacol.*, **49**, 545–52.

Riou, J.-F., Helissey, P., Grondard, L. and Giorgi-Renault, S. (1991). Inhibition of eukaryotic DNA topoisomerase I and II activities by indoloquinolinedione derivatives. *Mol. Pharmacol.*, **40**, 699–706.

Ritke, M. Y., Allan, W. P., Fattman, C. et al. (1994). Reduced phosphorylation of topoisomerase II in etoposide-resistant human leukemia K562 cells. *Mol. Pharmacol.*, **46**, 58–66.

Roca, J. and Wang, J. C. (1994). DNA transport by a type II DNA topoisomerase: evidence in favor of a two-gate mechanism. *Cell*, **77**, 609–16.

Roca, J., Berger, J. M., Harrison, S. C. and Wang, J. C. (1996). DNA transport by a type II topoisomerase: direct evidence for a two-gate mechanism. *Proc. Natl. Acad. Sci. USA*, **93**, 4057–62.

Ross, W., Rowe, T., Glisson, B. et al. (1984). Role of topoisomerase II in mediating epipodophyllotoxin-induced DNA cleavage. *Cancer Res.*, **44**, 5857–60.

Rubin, E., Pantazis, P., Bharti, A. et al. (1994). Identification of a mutant human topoisomerase I with intact catalytic activity and resistance to 9-nitro-camptothecin. *J. Biol. Chem.*, **269**, 2433–9.

Ryan, A. J., Squires, S., Strutt, H. L. and Johnson, R. T. (1991). Camptothecin cytotoxicity in mammalian cells is associated with the induction of persistent double strand breaks in replicating DNA. *Nucleic Acids Res.*, **19**, 3295–300.

Saijo, M., Ui, M. and Enomoto, T. (1992). Growth state and cell cycle dependent phosphorylation of DNA topoisomerase II in Swiss 3T3 cells. *Biochemistry*, **31**, 359–63.

Schneider, E., Horton, J. K., Yang, C.-H. et al. (1994). Multidrug resistance-associated protein gene overexpression and reduced drug sensitivity of topoisomerase II in human breast carcinoma MCF7 cell line selected for etoposide resistance. *Cancer Res.*, **54**, 152–8.

Schultz, P., Olland, S., Oudet, P. and Hancock, R. (1996). Structure and conformational changes of DNA topoisomerase II visualized by electron microscopy. *Proc. Natl. Acad. Sci. USA*, **93**, 5936–40.

Shibuya, M. L., Ueno, A. M., Vannais, D. B. et al. (1994). Megabase pair deletions in mutant mammalian cells following exposure to amsacrine, an inhibitor of DNA topoisomerase II. *Cancer Res.*, **54**, 1092–7.

Slesarev, A., Stetter, K. O., Lake, J. A. et al. (1993). DNA topoisomerase V is a relative of eukaryotic topoisomerase I from a hyperthermophilic prokaryote. *Nature*, **364**, 735–7.

Slichenmeyer, W. J., Rowinsky, E. K., Donehower, R. C. and Kaufmann, S. H. (1993). The current status of camptothecin analogues as antitumor agents. *J. Natl. Cancer Inst.*, **85**, 271–91.

Smith, K., Houlbrook, S., Greenall, M. et al. (1993). Topo IIα coamplification with erbB2 in human primary breast cancer and breast cancer cell lines: relationship to m-AMSA and mitoxantrone sensitivity. *Oncogene*, **8**, 933–8.

Smith, P. J., Morgan, S. A., Fox, M. E. and Watson, J. V. (1990). Mitoxantrone-DNA binding and the induction of topoisomerase II associated DNA damage in multi-drug resistant small cell lung cancer cells. *Biochem. Pharmacol.*, **40**, 2069–78.

Staron, K., Kowalska-Loth, B., Zabek, J. et al. (1995). Topoisomerase I is differently phosphorylated in two sublines of L5178Y mouse lymphoma cells. *Biochim. Biophys. Acta*, **1260**, 35–42.

Sugimoto, Y., Tsukahara, S., Oh-hara, T. et al. (1990a). Decreased expression of DNA topoisomerase I in camptothecin-resistant tumor cell lines as determined by a monoclonal antibody. *Cancer Res.*, **50**, 6925–30.

Sugimoto, Y., Tsukahara, S., Oh-hara, T. et al. (1990b). Elevated expression of DNA topoisomerase II in camptothecin-resistant human tumor cell lines. *Cancer Res.*, **50**, 7962–5.

Sullivan, D. M., Latham, M. D., Rowe, T. C. and Ross, W. E. (1989). Purification and characterization of an altered topoisomerase II from a drug-resistant Chinese hamster ovary cell line. *Biochemistry*, **28**, 5680–7.

Swaffar, D. S., Ireland, C. M. and Barrows, L. R. (1994). A rapid mechanism-based screen to detect potential anti-cancer agents. *Anti-cancer Drugs*, **5**, 15–23.

Swedlow, J. R., Sedat, J. W. and Agard, D. A. (1993). Multiple chromosomal populations of topoisomerase II detected *in vivo* by time-lapse, three-dimensional wide-field microscopy. *Cell*, **73**, 97–108.

Takano, H., Kohno, K., Ono, M. et al. (1991). Increased phosphorylation of DNA topoisomerase II in etoposide-resistant mutants of human cancer KB cells. *Cancer Res.*, **51**, 3951–7.

Takeda, S., Shimazoe, T., Sato, K. et al. (1992). Differential expression of DNA topoisomerase I gene between CPT-11 acquired and native-resistant human pancreatic tumor cell lines: detected by RNA/PCR-based quantitation assay. *Biochem. Biophys. Res. Comm.*, **184**, 618–25.

Tamura, H., Kohchi, C., Yamada, R. et al. (1991). Molecular cloning of a cDNA of a camptothecin-resistant human DNA topoisomerase I and identification of mutation sites. *Nucl. Acids Res.*, **19**, 69–75.

Tan, K. B., Mattern, M. R., Boyce, R. A. and Schein, P. S. (1987). Elevated DNA topoisomerase II activity in nitrogen mustard-resistant human cells. *Proc. Natl. Acad. Sci. USA*, **84**, 7668–71.

Tan, K. B., Mattern, M. R., Eng, W. K. et al. (1989). Nonproductive rearrangement of DNA topoisomerase I and II genes: correlation with resistance to topoisomerase inhibitors. *J. Natl. Cancer Inst.*, **81**, 1732–5.

Tan, K. B., Dorman, T. E., Falls, K. M. et al. (1992). Topoisomerase IIα and topoisomerase IIβ genes: characterization and mapping to human chromosomes 17 and 3, respectively. *Cancer Res.*, **52**, 231–4.

Tanizawa, A., Bertrand, R., Kohlhagen, G. et al. (1993). Cloning of Chinese hamster DNA topoisomerase I cDNA and identification of a single point mutation responsible for camptothecin resistance. *J. Biol. Chem.*, **268**, 25463–8.

Tanizawa, A., Kohn, K. W., Kohlhagen, G. et al. (1995). Differential stabilization of eukaryotic DNA topoisomerase I cleavable complexes by camptothecin derivatives. *Biochemistry*, **34**, 7200–6.

Towatari, M., Ito, Y., Morishita, Y. et al. (1990). Enhanced expression of DNA topoisomerase II by recombinant human granulocyte colony-stimulating factor in human leukemia cells. *Cancer Res.*, **50**, 7198–202.

Tsai-Pflugfelder, M., Liu, L. F., Liu, A. A. et al. (1988). Cloning and sequencing of cDNA encoding human DNA topoisomerase II and localization of the gene to chromosome region 17q21–22. *Proc. Natl. Acad. Sci. USA*, **85**, 7177–81.

Tsao, Y.-P., Russo, A., Nyamuswa, G. et al. (1993). Interaction between replication forks and topoisomerase I–DNA cleavable complexes: studies in a cell-free SV40 DNA replication system. *Cancer Res.*, **53**, 5908–14.

Volm, M. and Mattern, J. (1992). Expression of topoisomerase II, catalase, metallothionen and thymidylate-synthase in human squamous cell lung carcinomas and their correlation with doxorubicin resistance and with patients' smoking habits. *Carcinogenesis*, **13**, 1947–50.

Wall, M. E., Wani, M. C., Cooke, C. E. et al. (1966). The isolation and structure of camptothecin, a novel alkaloidal leukemia and tumor inhibitor from *Camptotheca acuminata*. *J. Am. Chem. Soc.*, **88**, 3888–90.

Wang, J. C. (1985). DNA topoisomerases. *Annu. Rev. Biochem.*, **54**, 665–97.

Wang, J. C. (1987). Recent studies of DNA topoisomerases. *Biochim. Biophys. Acta*, **909**, 1–9.

Wang, J. C. (1991). DNA topoisomerases: why so many? *J. Biol. Chem.*, **266**, 6659–62.

Wang, J. C. (1994). DNA topoisomerases as targets of therapeutics: an overview. In *Advances in Pharmacology*, vol. 29A (ed. L. F. Liu), pp. 1–19. Academic Press.

Wang, J. C. and Giaever, G. N. (1988). Action at a distance along a DNA. *Science*, **240**, 300–4.

Wasserman, R. A. and Wang, J. C. (1994). Analysis of yeast DNA topoisomerase II mutants resistant to the antitumor drug amsacrine. *Cancer Res.*, **54**, 1795–800.

Watt, P. M. and Hickson, I. D. (1994). Structure and function of type II DNA topoisomerases. *Biochem. J.*, **303**, 681–95.

Webb, C. D., Latham, M. D., Lock, R. B. and Sullivan, D. M. (1991). Attenuated topoisomerase II content directly correlates with a low level of drug resistance in a Chinese hamster ovary cell line. *Cancer Res.*, **51**, 6543–9.

Wells, N. J., Addison, C. M., Fry, A. M. et al. (1994). Serine 1524 is a major site of phosphorylation of human topoisomerase IIα protein *in vivo* and is a substrate for casein kinase II *in vitro*. *J. Biol. Chem.*, **269**, 29746–51.

Woessner, R. D., Chung, T. D. Y., Hofmann, G. A. et al. (1990). Differences between normal and ras-transformed NIH-3T3 cells in expression of the 170 kD and 180 kD forms of topoisomerase II. *Cancer Res.*, **50**, 2901–8.

Woessner, R. D., Mattern, M. R., Mirabelli, C. K. et al. (1991). Proliferation- and cell cycle-dependent differences in expression of the 170 kilodalton and 180 kilodalton forms of topoisomerase II in NIH-3T3 cells. *Cell Growth Differ.*, **2**, 209–14.

Woessner, R. D., Eng, W.-K., Hofmann, G. A. et al. (1992). Camptothecin hyper-resistant P388 cells: drug-dependent reduction in topoisomerase I content. *Oncology Res.*, **4**, 481–8.

Yang, L., Rowe, T. C., Nelson, E. M. and Liu, L. F. (1985). *In vivo* mapping of DNA topoisomerase II-specific cleavage sites on SV40 chromatin. *Cell*, **41**, 127–32.

Zee, A. G. J. van der, Hollema, H., de Jong, S. et al. (1991). P-glycoprotein expression and DNA topoisomerase I and II activity in benign tumors of the ovary and in malignant tumors of the ovary, before and after platinum/ cyclophosphamide chemotherapy. *Cancer Res.*, **51**, 5915–20.

Zee, A. G. J. van der, de Vries, E. G. E., Hollema, H. et al. (1994). Molecular analysis of the topoisomerase IIα gene and its expression in human ovarian cancer. *Ann. Oncol.*, **5**, 75–81.

Zini, N., Martelli, A. M., Sabatelli, P. et al. (1992). The 180 kDa isoform of topoisomerase II is localized in the nucleolus and belongs to the structural elements of the nucleolar remnant. *Exp. Cell Res.*, **200**, 460–6.

Zini, N., Santi, S., Ognibene, A. et al. (1994). Discrete localization of different DNA topoisomerases in HeLa and K562 cell nuclei and subnuclear fractions. *Exp. Cell Res.*, **210**, 336–48.

Zwelling, L. A., Estey, E., Silberman, L. et al. (1987). Effect of cell proliferation and chromatin conformation on intercalator-induced, protein-associated DNA cleavage in human brain tumor cells and human fibroblasts. *Cancer Res.*, **47**, 251.

Zwelling, L. A., Hinds, M., Chan, D. et al. (1989). Characterization of an amsacrine-resistant line of leukemia cells. *J. Biol. Chem.*, **264**, 16411–20.

Zwelling, L. A., Hinds, M., Chan, D. et al. (1990). Phorbol ester effect on topoisomerase II activity and gene expression in HL-60 human leukemia cells with different proclivities toward monocytoid differentiation. *Cancer Res.*, **50**, 7116–22.

5

Genes that modulate apoptosis: major determinants of drug resistance

JOHN A. HICKMAN

Apoptosis and drug resistance: introduction

There is rapidly expanding literature to show that anticancer drugs kill certain cell types by inducing apoptosis. Since there are gene products and signalling pathways that inhibit apoptosis, and others that promote it, it should not be surprising that modulation of their activity can bring about drug resistance. What makes these genes particularly attractive to those interested in mechanisms of drug resistance is a prediction that they would impose a pleotropic drug resistance, independent of particular mechanisms of damage; put simply, this is resistance to death. Pleotropic resistance of this type describes the reality of much of drug resistance observed in the clinic. This chapter reviews the influence of some of the genes that determine whether drug-induced perturbations can induce cell death.

Why *do* cells die after treatment with antitumor drugs and why, more often, do they not? New perceptions of mechanisms of drug resistance

Asking the question, 'why do tumor cells die after treatment with antitumor drugs?' obviously might provide some insights to the counter question of why, more often, they do not and are drug resistant. Until recently, there have been surprisingly few attempts to answer the question of why, in molecular terms, the cell dies after drugs or irradiation. This may be because it was considered that the imposition of cellular damage (such as DNA strand breaks) or the perturbation of cellular metabolism (such as a fall in thymidine pools) would bring about a passive decline in cell viability. Targeting a specific gene, for example, with a sequence-specific alkylating agent may prevent transcription of that gene product and disable the cell such that, in thermodynamic terms, it runs 'downhill'. Such a view has its roots in the pioneering work of Paul Ehrlich, the father of chemotherapy, who propounded the idea that the selectivity (albeit between unicellular pathogens and metazoan host cells) of chemotherapeutic agents was critically dependent upon the selective expression of a drug 'target' to which the toxophile must bind tightly. Drug resistance would naturally follow if the target was absent, overexpressed or mutated, or if insufficient drug was able to bind to the target, or if 'damage' was repaired.

These valid and coherent explanations of drug resistance form the basis of much of this monograph. But in a metazoan organism, such as man, cellular damage and debilitating perturbations to the metabolism of an individual cell set in train a series of conserved responses that are made in the context of the whole organism. Whilst these inducible responses include biochemical changes at the level of the perturbation (e.g. a post-translational increase in thymidylate synthase after inhibitors of the enzyme, or increases in DNA repair activity) others, critically, address the fate of the cell. In the social context of a multicellular organism, damaged cells present a problem to the host. A passive loss of viability results in the spilling of cellular contents and an associated inflammatory response; damage to the genome of cells may produce a passive decline in viability but if it does not, then in the context of proliferating cells the inheritance of mutations and chromosomal aberrations may allow aberrant growth and differentiation of millions of progeny away from the strict social controls necessary for homeostasis. It is now considered that the conserved and genetically programmed mode of cell death that is utilized in embryonic development, to sculpt the organs, is retained thereafter as a mechanism that can be activated to delete cells that might provoke inflammation and/or dysplasias. Morphologically, this type of cell death is described as apoptosis (reviewed by Dexter, Raff and Wyllie, 1995).

The induction of apoptosis by antitumor drugs suggests that a cellular decision to die (or not) is also a major arbiter of chemosensitivity

The observation that anticancer drugs induce the morphological features of a programed cell death, or apoptosis, is not entirely new. Experiments both in vivo (Ijiri and Potten, 1983) and in vitro (Searle et al., 1975) had shown that the conserved nuclear change of chromatin condensation and margination at the nuclear periphery, and the formation of apoptotic fragments, which are engulfed by neighbouring cells, were associated with the death of normal and tumor cells treated with different types of cytotoxins or irradiation (reviewed by Hickman, 1992; Dive and Wyllie, 1993; Hickman et al., 1994; Stewart, 1994). This phenomenon remained only a phenomenon until genes were identified that modulate, positively or negatively, the ability of a cell to undertake this adaptive form of cell death. The importance of these genes to the question of why tumors are resistant to therapy must depend upon the answer to the question of whether all cells die by apoptosis after treatment with cytotoxic drugs? For example, it has been claimed that in colonic tumor cell lines cell death is not by apoptosis (Slichenmyer et al., 1993) although normal colonic epithelia (Merritt et al., 1995) and colon carcinomas in vivo clearly show classical features of apoptosis (Bedi et al., 1995). The irradiation of fibroblasts in vitro renders them nonclonogenic but they are 'viable' in that they retain membrane and metabolic integrity. These cells are often described as reproductively cell dead (reviewed by Hendry and Scott, 1987); their long-term fate is uncertain, but they do not undergo a rapid death with features of apoptosis. However, primary rodent fibroblasts can be induced to undergo classical apoptosis with cytotoxic drugs and transfection of these cells with a suppressor of apoptosis, bcl-2, inhibits drug-induced apoptosis (Fanidi, Harrington and Evan, 1992). Perhaps the best criteria of whether a particular cell type undergoes an apoptotic cell death, even if it is a kinetically slow process, is to investigate whether transfection of suppressors or promoters of apoptosis influence survival.

With the caveat that not all cells may engage apoptosis, largely based on concerns arising from the behaviour of long-established cell lines, the observation that susceptible cells are stimulated to engage apoptosis, independent of the type of drug mechanism that induces cellular perturbation or damage, permits a new view of the molecular basis of selectivity and of resistance (Dive and Hickman, 1991; Fisher, 1994).

Drug target interactions are only the first stage in a programed cell death and are not the sole determinants of sensitivity and resistance

It has been proposed that the apoptotic machinery, responsible for the execution of the cell, is constitutively expressed in all cells and that cell death is a default position that is held in abeyance by contact with other cells or by trophic factors (Raff, 1992). This view may be tempered by an increasing understanding that the propensity of different cell types to undergo apoptosis is phenotypically determined by the differential expression of genes that encode 'sensors' of damage, such as *p53*, endogenous suppressors of apoptosis such as members of the *bcl*-2 family, components of the survival signalling pathways (as distinct from those for proliferation) such as *bcr-abl*, v-*abl*, *ras* and the IGF-1 receptor. In addition, activation of the *fas* ligand and receptor pathway of signalling for cell death may be an important component of the balance between survival and death in some tissues (Nagata, 1995). A review of the mechanisms of action of these gene products in modulating apoptosis is beyond the scope of this chapter, but each of them has been shown to play a pivotal role in the coupling of a damage signal (Figure 5.1) to the execution of a cell. The differentially expressed repertoire of these gene products suggests that a hierarchy may exist for the ease of engagement of apoptosis. This essentially suggests that some cells are *inherently* more resistant to cytotoxic drugs than others. For example, there is a hierarchy of cell death in the gastrointestinal tract with the stem cells of the small intestine undergoing apoptosis after irradiation more readily than those of the colon (Potten, 1992). Some of the molecular correlates of this hierarchy have now been established with differential expressions of both *p53* and *bcl*-2 playing key roles (Merritt et al., 1995). Thus, the small intestine is rarely the site of carcinomas (95% are in the colon and rectum), presumably because damaged stem cells are readily deleted by apoptosis. The greater survival potential of colonic stem cells, on the other hand, is permissive for carcinogenesis of an inherently death-resistant cell type: these cells are not readily deleted after DNA damage (Merritt et al., 1995). This may then explain why drugs, such as the thymidylate synthase inhibitors, are toxic to the small intestine and are only palliative in the treatment of carcinomas of the colon (Figure 5.2). It may also provide a framework for understanding not only cancer incidence – hematopoetic tumors may be rare because damaged cells readily undergo apoptosis – but also chemosensitivity and drug resistance: the carcinomas are relatively common because they are derived from cells that are able to sustain damage and, almost *ipso facto*, they will be resistant to cytotoxic drugs, especially when compared to the bone marrow.

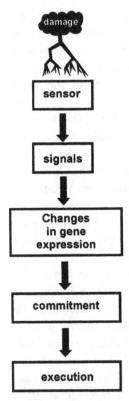

Figure 5.1. The concept of the sensing of drug-induced perturbations being coupled to a cascade of events leading to an irreversible cellular suicide by the process of apoptosis. Attenuation of any of hypothetical steps outlined would impose drug resistance.

'Sensing' DNA damage: the apparently paradoxical roles of *p53* in determining drug sensitivity and resistance

The majority of antitumor drugs used in the clinic damage DNA, either directly, as in the case of the alkylating agents and cisplatin; through the activity of enzymes such as the topoisomerases; or indirectly by induction of metabolic imbalance after the reduction of pools of deoxyribonucleotides (e.g. 5-FU-induced strand breaks). The tumor suppressor *p53*, the so-called 'guardian of the genome' (Lane, 1992), has recently been suggested to localize to single-stranded regions of DNA and to the termini of nonspecific DNA templates (Bayle, Elenbaas and Levine, 1995). Together with the possible recruitment of other factors to damage sites (polyADPribose polymerase, repair proteins), *p53* may then

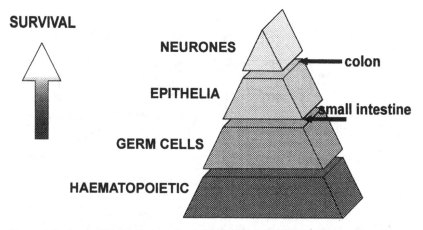

Figure 5.2. A possible hierarchy of cellular survival in different tissues, based upon their relative sensitivities to whole-body radiation. In this model tumor incidence reflects the difficulty of cell deletion and drug resistance the hierarchy of survival: epithelial tumors are therefore common and intrinsically more resistant to therapy, whereas hematopoietic tissue gives rise to few tumors but is intrinsically sensitive to cytotoxins, causing problems of host toxicity.

become activated as a transcriptional regulator after post-translational stabilization (Nelson and Kastan, 1994). The pattern of transcriptional regulation that ensues is critical in determining, according to cellular background, the outcome of a *p53*-dependent DNA damage response. There are at least three scenarios: repair with survival, repair but subsequent death, or failure to repair and death. The molecular events that surround the attraction of repair proteins, *p53*, the DNA-dependent kinase, the stoichiometry of their interactions and how this might 'quantitate' damage prior to cellular 'decisions' for repair and/or the activation of survival or death pathways is an exciting new area of investigation.

p53 has a somewhat paradoxical role in this decision-making: it can activate death by apoptosis (Yonish-Rouach et al., 1991) or initiate a cell cycle checkpoint that will promote repair of lesions that may be more lethal during DNA replication in S-phase (Kuerbitz et al., 1992). As a transcriptional activator it can increase the transcription of *waf*-1, to produce an inhibitor of cell cycle progression at G_1 (El-Diery et al., 1993) (Figure 5.3). *WAF*-1 is associated with the cyclin-dependent kinases required for G_1 to S phase progression so that functional *p53* in a tumor (>50% of human tumors have been estimated to be mutant or null for *p53*), might promote survival, making *p53*-defective tumors

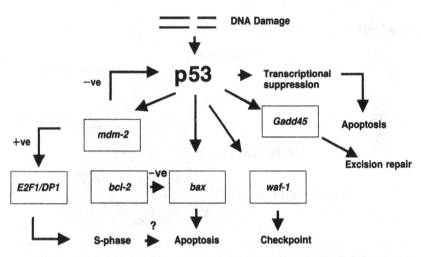

Figure 5.3. Some of the events that may follow the formation of DNA strand breaks and their 'sensing' by *p53*. The 'choice' of death or survival (via a checkpoint that provides time for repair) may be determined by the stoichiometry of activation of these and other players.

more sensitive to DNA damage. But, as Figure 5.3 shows (and only a few of the players are shown) this depends upon what *other* genes *p53* is activating or suppressing. *p53* has been shown to activate the transcription of the accelerator of cell death *bax* (see below) (Miyashita and Reed, 1995). *p53* stabilization may also lead to an increased synthesis of *mdm-2*, a suppressor of *p53* transcriptional activity (Momand et al., 1992). Interestingly (Figure 5.3), activation of *mdm-2* promotes S-phase stimulatory E2F1 transcriptional activity (Martin et al., 1995). The traverse of DNA-damaged cells into S-phase may then initiate apoptosis as replication forks collide with DNA damage. The other key players in the 'decision' of whether a DNA-damaged cell should survive, repair and/or die are the members of the *bcl-2* family, including *bax* (Figure 5.3). These are discussed further below. Whether the promotion of transcriptional activity of *p53* is important for the promotion of cell death in all cell types was not supported by studies of Caelles, Helmberg and Karin (1994), who showed that DNA damage-induced, *p53*-dependent apoptosis did not require new RNA or protein synthesis. Indeed, it was shown that Bcl-2 (Figure 5.3) can relieve the *p53* transcriptional repression and so inhibit cell death (Shen and Shenk, 1994).

Loss of functional *p53* may promote pleotropic drug resistance to DNA-damaging agents

The importance of *p53* in promoting DNA damage-induced apoptosis was demonstrated by studies of immature thymocytes in vitro or intestinal epithelia in vivo from homozygously *p53* null animals, generated by recombinant gene knockout procedures (Clarke et al., 1993; Lowe et al., 1993a, Merritt et al., 1994). Cells that had been γ-irradiated did not undergo apoptosis in comparison to those that were homozygously *p53* positive. *p53* null thymocytes also failed to undergo apoptosis after treatment with the topoisomerase II inhibitor etoposide but, importantly, did undergo normal levels of apoptosis after treatment with the non-DNA-damaging corticosteroid dexamethasone, suggesting that the non-DNA damage-induced pathway was discrete and *p53* independent.

Lowe et al. (1993b, 1994) showed that in fibroblasts, sensitized to undergo apoptosis by the expression of the adenovirus gene E1A, treatment with 5-FU, etoposide or adriamycin was significantly less cytotoxic against a *p53* null (−/−) background, 24 h to 72 h after treatment. However, Kastan and colleagues (Slichenmeyer et al., 1993) irradiated normal and *p53* null murine fibroblasts (which were therefore isogenic) and determined that there was no difference in survival as measured by a clonogenic assay. However, the authors claimed that one possible difference between their result and those obtained using thymocytes (Clarke et al., 1993; Lowe et al., 1993a) was that fibroblasts did not undergo apoptosis; this contentious question has been discussed above. Irradiation of proliferating lymphoid cells from *p53* null cells did not prevent apoptosis unless the cells were transfected with *bcl*-2 (see below) suggesting, again, that *p53*-independent modes of cell death may be initiated in some cell types (Strasser et al., 1994). Perhaps the most significant point made in this study was that *bcl*-2 acts 'downstream' of *p53* and that strategies to restore *p53* to cells with a null phenotype or *p53* mutations may not be effective if *bcl*-2 is expressed (see Figure 5.3).

In a study of Burkitt's lymphoma and lymphoid cell lines the mutation of *p53* made cells significantly resistant to γ-irradiation, etoposide, cisplatin and nitrogen mustard as measured by viability (Trypan Blue exclusion) at 72 h after treatment. Whether this reflects a delay in the kinetics of cell death rather than true changes in sensitivity is unclear (Fan et al., 1994). The potential of a *p53* wild-type tumor to sustain DNA damage but to enter the G_1 checkpoint, and therefore to be resistant to DNA damaging agents, was subverted in experiments by O'Connor and colleagues by transfection of the papillomavirus type 16 *E6* gene, the product of which stimulates the proteolysis of the p53 protein (Fan et al., 1994). The human breast carcinoma cell line MCF-7 is *p53* wild type but is resistant to cisplatin. Expression of *E6* induced sensitivity, not only because of the release from a G_1 checkpoint but also because *p53* up-regulates Gadd45, a protein that stimulates excision repair (Figure 5.3). Down-regulation of *p53* therefore reduced excision repair as well as allowing cisplatin-damaged cells to enter S-phase. Cisplatin-induced DNA damage was insufficient to induce apoptosis in non-proliferating immature mouse thymocytes, a cell type that is exquisitely sensitive to irradiation and to etoposide (Evans, Tilby and Dive, 1994). However, if the small population of *dividing* thymocytes was examined these were sensitive to cisplatin. This suggests that the *quality* of DNA damage is an important aspect of the signalling for the initiation of apoptosis. Presumably the intrastrand cross-links induced by cisplatin, and the distortion they induce in DNA, are not 'sensed' until replication forks collide with them, perhaps generating strand breaks. Similar conclusions were reached by Fan et al. (1994) when studying the induction of a *p53* G_1 by γ-irradiation, etoposide, cisplatin and nitrogen mustard: the former two agents induced a strong G_1 checkpoint compared to the latter two, presumably because *p53* only detects strand breaks.

The significance of the mutation of *p53* and of allelic loss in the progress of human neoplasias as an indicator of a poor prognosis is unquestionable. Whether the loss of *p53* function alone is responsible for pleotropic drug resistance to DNA-damaging drugs observed in many advanced cancers is doubtful. As multistage carcinogenicity progresses it is likely that the survival potential of the cancer cell is increased by a variety of oncogenic events. Only as this occurred would the progressing tumor be able to survive the increasing genetic instability associated with malignancy. A glance at Figure 5.3 immediately warns that even in the presence of wild-type *p53* drug sensitivity is not assured; the background in which *p53* functions is critical. Restoration of *p53* may indeed hold promise but its position in the hierarchy (upstream of *bcl*-2) should not be forgotten (nicely discussed with respect to chemotherapy by Strasser et al., 1994). Nor should it be forgotten that *p53* null cell lines such as the HL-60 myeloid leukemia are exquisitely sensitive to DNA-damaging agents, such as etoposide. There are as yet undiscovered *p53*-independent mechanisms of 'sensing' DNA damage, and a hunt for these will yield further insights into resistance mechanisms where a DNA damage signal becomes uncoupled from an appropriate response. A likely candidate pathway involves the activation of the transcription factor interferon regulatory factor (IRF-1), which is necessary for DNA damage-induced cell death in mitogen-activated T lymphocytes (Tamura et al., 1995).

The bcl-2 *gene suppresses apoptosis and provides pleotropic drug resistance*

One of the most exciting and insightful discoveries of the apoptosis field was that the product of the gene *bcl-2* suppresses cell death but has no effect on cell proliferation (Vaux, Cory and Adams, 1988; Hockenbery et al., 1990). Confirmation of the importance of *bcl-2* beyond its role as a gene involved in hematopoietic cell survival, and its translocation in follicular lymphomas [t(14:18)], was the finding that it was highly evolutionarily conserved, with a homologous sequence to the *ced-9* gene, which acts as suppressor of cell death in the worm *Caenorhabditis elegans* (Vaux, Haecker and Strasser, 1994).

The current dogma of how the 26 kDa Bcl-2 protein might promote cell survival is summarized in Figure 5.3. Bcl-2 is the archetypic member of a family of proteins that undergo homo- and heterodimerizations to each other via binding through conserved BH1 and BH2 domains (Yin, Oltval and Korsmeyer, 1994; Fong et al., 1994). The isolation of the Bcl-2 homologue Bax, as a protein that immunoprecipitated with Bcl-2 (Oltvai, Milliman and Korsmeyer, 1993), and the finding that its expression accelerated apoptosis suggested a model whereby Bax–Bax homodimers promote apoptosis whilst Bcl-2–Bax heterodimerization inhibits apoptosis by limiting Bax–Bax homodimerization (reviewed by Korsmeyer et al., 1993; Núñez et al., 1994; Reed, 1997). How Bax–Bax homodimers accelerate apoptosis is unclear. Knowledge of the family of *bcl-2*-like genes has been expanding with recent discoveries of sequence-related promoters of apoptosis (*bad*, *bak*, *bcl-X$_S$*) and inhibitors of apoptosis (*bcl-X$_L$*) (Boise et al., 1993; Chittenden et al., 1995; Farrow et al., 1995; Kiefer et al., 1995; Yang et al., 1995). The structural requirements for homo- and heterodimerization and the degree of redundancy in binding were determined by the yeast two-hybrid system (Sato et al., 1994). This model of change in the patterns of homo- and heterodimerizations was made all the more attractive when it was shown that *p53* was a direct transcriptional activator of the human *bax* gene (Miyashita and Reed, 1995) and that both wild-type and mutant *p53* might down-regulate the expression of *bcl-2* (Miyashita et al., 1994). However, in recent studies, including our own, activation of p53 by genotoxic damage (see Figure 5.3) does not result in modulation of the cellular protein *levels* of either Bcl-2 or Bax (Canman et al., 1995; Chresta, Masters and Hickman, 1995). In addition, recent evidence suggests that bcl-2 and bcl-X may function differently, providing different efficacies of protection according to cell type (Gottschalk et al., 1994).

Although the precise dynamics of the expression of the *bcl*-2 family members is under debate, there can be no question that the altered expression of these genes has a significant effect on cell survival after treatment with *all* classes of antitumor drugs (Table 5.1). It could be claimed that the overexpression of *bcl*-2 imparts real multidrug resistance, since it crosses the entire spectrum of the pharmacopoeia. It is quite extraordinary that cells treated with agents that induce considerable amounts of DNA damage maintain viability for considerable periods and may then go on to form colonies (see Table 5.1). In many of these studies a reduction in apoptotic cell number or a maintenance of cell viability has been measured in short-term assays and it is difficult to assume that these cells (the 'undead') may repair the damage to maintain their proliferative potential. Nevertheless, the maintenance of viability, the DNA damage in place, allows time for repair and, possibly, the fixation of mutations and chromosomal damage induced by the drugs. This is an extremely dangerous scenario, particularly if that tumor has a mutant p53 phenotype since this may promote genetic instability.

The over-expression of the death-promoting bcl-X_S protein in *bcl*-2-expressing MCF-7 human breast carcinoma cells sensitized them to the cytotoxicity of both etoposide and taxol (Sumantran et al., 1995). Strategies like this, to deliver apoptotic accelerators such as *bax* and *bcl*-X_S or inhibitors of *bcl*-2 or *bcl*-X_L, by expression of mimics that prevent them from binding to *bcl*-2, would seem to be an important route to take for the circumvention of this type of drug resistance. Consideration of Figures 5.1 and 5.3 places *bcl*-2 at the gateway to the execution phase of apoptosis. The question of 'who binds to whom', and of the stoichiometry of binding of partners is going to be increasingly important both in the design of drug strategies and also in prognosis. The expression pattern of *bcl*-2 is widespread in human tumors, and includes breast, lung and colon carcinomas, androgen-receptor negative prostate cancer, lymphomas, leukemias, neuroblastomas and gliomas (reviewed by Pezella and Gatter, 1995). In breast cancer a considerable number of studies suggest, paradoxically, that *bcl*-2 expression is a feature of a good prognosis, predicting efficacy of adjuvant treatments in node-positive disease (e.g. Gasparini et al., 1995). However, none of these studies have measured the expression or status of Bax, and it is possible that Bax levels rather than those of Bcl-2 are a predictor of response. Given the idea that the stoichiometry binding is of critical importance, measurement of a single parameter is obviously limiting. In addition, it is possible that the expression of *bcl*-2 in some tumors may represent an early stage of tumor survival and development, with more powerful survival modulators coming into play during tumor progression. Possible candidates are discussed in the next section.

Survival signals: inhibitors of drug-induced apoptosis

The survival of a cell in a multicellular organism is strongly dependent upon signals provided by other cells (Raff, 1992). These are provided either by cell–cell contacts, cell–matrix contact or by trophic factors. The prototypical survival factor is nerve growth factor which, in post-mitotic cells, is necessary for the continued survival of neurones (Levi-Montalcini, 1987). The delivery of discrete signals for survival, independent of those for proliferation, by so-called growth factors and by cytokines, was somewhat unexpected in a context wider than the neurotrophic factors (Harrington, Fanidi and Evan, 1994). Thus, the apoptosis-inducing ability of artificially elevating c-*myc* expression in primary rat fibroblasts was inhibited by insulin-like growth factor I (IGF1) (Harrington et al., 1994) and removal of cytokines such as IL-3 from a factor-dependent hematopoietic cell line induced not only a cessation in proliferation but also apoptosis (Williams et al., 1990). How these survival signals impinge on the engagement of apoptosis is unclear and their relative importance in the hierarchy of providing survival (whether they are 'upstream' or 'downstream' of *bcl*-2 for example, see Figure 5.3) is also unknown. The effects of a discrete survival-signalling pathway on drug sensitivity have been investigated using a temperature-sensitive mutant of the v-*abl* oncogene as a mimic of the *bcr-abl* onco-gene (Chapman, Whetton and Dive, 1994). An IL-3 dependent murine mast cell line (IC2.9) underwent apoptosis when IL-3 was withdrawn at the non-permissive temperature for the expression of v-*abl* (39°C) but maintained viability, without proliferation, in the absence of IL-3 but with v-*abl* active (32°F). Treatment with melphalan at the non-permissive temperature provided a complete protection against the onset of apoptosis over 120 h, at which time 100% of the cells not expressing active v-*abl* were dead. This complete maintenance of survival was more

Table 5.1. *The effect of over-expression of bcl-2 on the sensitivity of various cells to the major classes of antitumor drugs*

Drug	Cell type	Delay in apoptosis* or increase in clonogenicity	Reference
Nitrogen mustard	Murine lymphoid FL5.12	Delay to apoptosis	Walton et al., 1993
Camptothecin, CPT-11	Murine lymphoid FL5.12	Delay to apoptosis	Walton et al., 1993
	Murine leukemia L1210	Delay to apoptosis	Kondo et al., 1994
Etoposide	Murine bone marrow BAF3	Delay to apoptosis	Collins et al., 1992
	Human neuroblastoma NBL	Delay to apoptosis	Dole et al., 1994
	Murine S49.1 and WEHI17.2 T lymphoid	Delay to apoptosis	Miyashita and Reed, 1992
	Murine bone marrow	Delay to apoptosis	Kondo et al., 1994
	Murine B cell lymphoma CH31	Increase in clonogenicity	Kamesaki et al., 1993
Cisplatin	Murine bone marrow BAF3	Delay to apoptosis	Collins et al., 1992
	Human neuroblastoma NBL	Delay to apoptosis	Dole et al., 1994
Adriamycin	Murine M1 leukemia	Delay to apoptosis	Lotem and Sachs, 1993
	Murine bone marrow	Delay to apoptosis	Kondo et al., 1994
Gamma irradiation	p53-/- murine T lymphoma cells	Increase in clonogenicity	Strasser et al., 1994
	Murine bone marrow BAF3	Delay to apoptosis	Collins, et al., 1992
	Human lymphoid MUTU-BL	Delay to apoptosis	Fisher et al., 1993
Fluorodeoxyuridine (and other thymidylate synthase inhibitors)			
2-Chloro-2'-deoxy adenosine	Human pre-B cells (697)	Delay to apoptosis	Gao et al., 1995
Methotrexate	Murine M1 leukemia	Delay to apoptosis	Lotem and Sachs, 1993
	Human pre-B cells (697)	Increase in clonogenicity	Miyashita and Reed, 1993
Cytosine arabinoside	Murine M1 leukemia	Delay to apoptosis	Lotem and Sachs, 1993
	Murine S49.1 and WEHI17.2 T lymphoid	Delay to apoptosis	Miyashita and Reed, 1992

Table 5.1 (Cont.)

Dexamethasone	Human pre-B cells (697)	Delay to apoptosis	Alnemri et al., 1992
	Murine S49.1 and WEHI17.2 T lymphoid	Delay to apoptosis	Miyashita and Reed, 1992
	Human pre-B cells (697)	Increase in clonogenicity	Miyashita and Reed, 1992
Vincristine	Murine S49.1 and WEHI17.2 T lymphoid	Delay to apoptosis	Miyashita and Reed, 1992
	Human pre-B cells (697)	Increase in clonogenicity	Miyashita and Reed, 1993
4-Hydroxy-cyclophosphamide	Human pre-B cells (697)	Delay to apoptosis	Miyashita and Reed, 1993

*In many experiments changes in survival were measured in short-term viability assays and cannot preclude the possibility that death is delayed rather than inhibited. Other experiments have discounted this possibility by showing drug resistance as an increase in clonogenic potential when bcl-2 was overexpressed.

profound than any of the patterns of suppression of apoptosis observed in the presence of elevated levels of *bcl*-2 (Table 5.1). The authors could find no change in the cellular levels of Bcl-2 nor in its phosphorylated state. Analysis of the DNA damage showed that the 'undead' cells had a full complement of DNA cross-links (Chapman et al., 1995). Expression of v-*abl* elevated diacylglycerol levels and was associated with the specific translocation of protein kinase isoform βII to the nucleus, although how this might inhibit the engagement of apoptosis remains speculative (Evans et al., 1995). Importantly, however, Chapman et al. (1995) inhibited protein kinase C activity with the relatively specific agent calphostin C and completely restored the drug sensitivity to v-*abl* expressing cells. They suggest that whilst it is unlikely that calphostin C may be used in the clinic a treatment regime of a standard chemotherapeutic drug together with an inhibitor of a survival-signalling pathway might constitute an important strategy to re-establish drug sensitivity. The translocation of the c-*abl* oncogene to form the *bcr-abl* fusion (Philadelphia chromosome of chronic myelogenous leukemia) also provides a significant survival advantage to drug-treated cells and it is possible that the progression of CML is brought about by the survival of drug-treated cells (McGohan et al., 1994). Analysis of the signalling pathways activated by *bcr-abl* that inhibit apoptosis suggests that multiple pathways are used to activate RAS although other pathways are also important in its transformation of myeloid or lymphoid cells (Cortez, Kadlec and Pendergast, 1995).

The involvement of *ras* in survival signalling was suggested by the earliest study of the effects of oncogenes on apoptosis (Wyllie et al., 1987), where it was suggested that levels of spontaneous apoptosis were suppressed by c-H-*ras*. Expression of c-H-*ras* in rat rhabdomyoscarcoma cells provided a survival advantage after treatment with doxorubicin and, most importantly, gave a 3- to 5-fold increase in clonogenicity in soft agar (Nooter et al., 1995). The drug resistance of the c-H-*ras* transfectants was not due to any change in the cell cycle of the cells nor to intracellular drug accumulation. Since mutational activation of *ras* is a frequent event in human cancers, its involvement in the suppression of drug-induced cell death merits further attention.

Finally, Baserga and colleagues (Sell, Baserga and Rubin, 1995) have shown that the overexpression of receptors for insulin-like growth factor 1 provided significant protection against the cytotoxicity of etoposide. Transfected BALB/c3T3 cells were significantly protected from loss of viability over a 72 h period when up to 40 μM of etoposide was used, an effect that again could not be related to changes in proliferation. Since many oncogenes play subvertive roles in signalling pathways it will be interesting to determine how many of them provide not only signals for aberrant proliferation but also may promote survival. It is interesting that a mutation of a Grb-2 protein, coupling epidermal growth factor (EGF) receptors to downstream signalling pathways, promoted apoptosis (Fath et al., 1994) suggesting that the EGF receptor may have a survival signalling role.

Are pro- and anti-apoptotic genes the final arbiters of drug activity? Concluding remarks

The idea that since antitumor drugs initiate apoptosis then gene products that prevent apoptosis from being engaged will make tumors pleotropically resistant is simple and attractive. The 'decision' of a cell as to whether it should engage apoptosis after drug-induced perturbation is unlikely to result from the activation of a simple linear cascade of biochemistry. Rather, reiterative loops, involving the 'quantitation' of damage and an assessment of the survival status of the cell *vis à vis* position and status (e.g. its differentiated state, and therefore whether it has proliferative potential) will be set in motion. Some of these complex pathways of 'decision making' are shown in Figure 5.3, a simplistic view of just a few of the players set in motion in a *p53*-dependent cell death. Therefore, if a single gene and its product, predicted to be an arbiter of the apoptotic pathway, does not appear *on its own* to be a marker of a poor prognosis or to provide significant clonogenic survival advantage (and drug resistance) we should not be surprised. Cellular context is all-important. The hierarchical position of the players reviewed here and of those yet to emerge will hopefully be clarified in future years. Some of these should then present themselves as targets for modulation to remove the major impediment to drug therapy of disseminated tumors, pleotropic drug resistance, or resistance to death.

Acknowledgment

The author wishes to thank Carol Miles for secretarial assistance and the Zeneca Pharmaceutical and the Cancer Research Campaign for support.

194 J. A. Hickman

References

Alnemri, E. S., Fernandes, T. F., Haldar, S. et al. (1992). Involvement of bcl-2 in glucocorticoid-induced apoptosis of human pre-B-leukemias. *Cancer Res.*, 52, 491–5.

Bayle, J. H., Elenbaas, B. and Levine, A. J. (1995). The carboxyl-terminal domain of the p53 protein regulates sequence-specific DNA binding through its nonspecific nucleic acid-binding activity. *Proc. Natl. Acad. Sci. USA*, 92, 5729–33.

Bedi, A., Pasricha, P. J., Akhtar, A. J. et al. (1995). Inhibition of apoptosis during development of colorectal cancer. *Cancer Res.*, 55, 1811–16.

Boise, L. H., González-Garcia, M., Postema, C. E. et al. (1993). bcl-x, a bcl-2-related gene that functions as a dominant regulator of apoptotic cell death. *Cell*, 74, 597–608.

Caelles, C., Helmberg, A. and Karin, M. (1994). p53-Dependent apoptosis in the absence of transcriptional activation of p53-target genes. *Nature*, 370, 220–3.

Canman, C. E., Gilmer, T. M., Coutts, S. B. and Kastan, M. B. (1995). Growth factor modulation of p53-mediated growth arrest versus apoptosis. *Genes Devel.*, 9, 600–11.

Chapman, R. S., Whetton, A. D. and Dive, C. (1994). The suppression of drug-induced apoptosis by activation of v-ABL protein tyrosine kinase. *Cancer Res.*, 54, 5131–7.

Chapman, R. S., Whetton, A. D., Chresta, C. M. and Dive, C. (1995). Characterization of drug resistance mediated via the suppression of apoptosis by Abelson protein tyrosine kinase. *Mol. Pharmacol.*, 481, 334–43.

Chittenden, T., Harrington, E. A., O'Connor, R. et al. (1995). Induction of apoptosis by the Bcl-2 homologue Bak. *Nature*, 374, 733–6.

Chresta, C. M., Masters, J. R. W. and Hickman, J. A. (1996). Hypersensitivity of human testicular tumors to etoposide-induced apoptosis is associated with functional p53 and a high Bax to Bcl-2 ratio. *Cancer Res.*, 56, 1834–41.

Clarke, A. R., Purdie, C. A., Harrison, D. J. et al. (1993). Thymocyte apoptosis induced by p53-dependent and independent pathways. *Nature*, 362, 849–52.

Collins, M. K. L., Marvel, J., Malde, P. and Lopez-Rivas, A. (1992). Interleukin 3 protects murine bone marrow cells from apoptosis induced by DNA damaging agents. *J. Exp. Med.*, 176, 1043–51.

Cortez, D., Kadlec, L. and Pendergast, A. M. (1995). Structural and signaling requirements for BCR-ABL-mediated transformation and inhibition of apoptosis. *Mol. Cell. Biol.*, 15, 5531–41.

Dexter, T. M., Raff, M. C. and Wyllie, A. H. (eds) (1995). *The Role of Apoptosis in Development, Tissue Homeostasis and Malignancy*. Chapman & Hall, London.

Dive, C. and Hickman, J. A. (1991). Drug–target interactions: only the first step in the commitment to a programmed cell death. *Br. J. Cancer*, 64, 192–6.

Dive, C. and Wyllie, A. H. (1993). Apoptosis and cancer chemotherapy. In *Cancer Chemotherapy* (ed. J. A. Hickman and T. R. Tritton), pp. 21–56. Blackwell Scientific Publications, Oxford.

Dole, M., Nuñez, G., Merchant, A. K. et al. (1994). Bcl-2 inhibits chemotherapy-induced apoptosis in neurblastoma. *Cancer Res.*, 54, 3253–9.

El-Diery, W. S., Tokino, T., Veculesco, V. E. et al. (1993). WAF-1, a potential mediator of p53 tumor suppression. *Cell*, 75, 817–25.

Evans, D. L., Tilby, M. and Dive, C. (1994). Differential sensitivity to the induction of apoptosis by cisplatin in proliferating and quiescent immature rat thymocytes is independent of the levels of drug accumulation and DNA adduct formation. *Cancer Res.*, **54**, 1596–603.

Evans, C. A., Lord, J. M., Owen-Lynch, P. J. et al. (1995). Suppression of apoptosis by v-Abl protein tyrosine kinase is associated with nuclear translocation and activation of protein kinase C in an interleukin-3-dependent haematopoietic cell line. *J. Cell Sci.*, **108**, 2591–8.

Fan, S., El-Deiry, W. S., Bae, I. et al. (1994). p53 gene mutations are associated with decreased sensitivity of human lymphoma cells to DNA damaging agents. *Cancer Res.*, **54**, 5824–30.

Fanidi, A., Harrington, E. A. and Evan, G. I. (1992). Cooperative interaction between c-myc and bcl-2 proto-oncogenes. *Nature*, **359**, 554–6.

Fath, I., Schweighoffer, F., Rey, I. et al. (1994). Cloning of a Grb2 isoform with apoptotic properties. *Science*, **264**, 971–4.

Farrow, S. N., White, J. H. M., Martinou, I. et al. (1995). Cloning of a bcl-2 homologue by intervention with adenovirus E1B 19K. *Nature*, **374**, 731–3.

Fisher, D. E. (1994). Apoptosis in cancer therapy: crossing the threshold. *Cell*, **78**, 539–42.

Fisher, T. C., Milner, A. E., Gregory, C. D. et al. (1993). Bcl-2 modulation of apoptosis induced by anticancer drugs: resistance to thymidylate stress is independent of classical resistance pathways. *Cancer Res.*, **53**, 3321–6.

Fong, L., Wang, H.-G. and Reed, J. C. (1994). Interactions among members of the Bcl-2 protein family analyzed with a yeast two-hybrid system. *Proc. Natl. Acad. Sci. USA*, **91**, 9238–42.

Gao, X., Knudsen, T. B., Ibrahim, M. M. and Haldar, S. (1995). Bcl-2 relieves deoxyadenylate stress and suppresses apoptosis in pre-B leukemia cells. *Death and Differentiation*, **2**, 69–78.

Gasparini, G., Barbereschi, M., Dogliono, C. et al. (1995). Expression of *bcl-2* protein predicts efficacy of adjuvant treatments in operable node-positive breast cancer. *Clin. Cancer Res.*, **1**, 189–98.

Gottschalk, A. R., Boise, L. H., Thompson, C. B. and Quitáns, J. (1994). Identification of immunosuppressant-induced apoptosis in a murine B-cell line and its prevention by bcl-x but not bcl-2. *Proc. Natl. Acad. Sci. USA*, **91**, 7350–4.

Harrington, E. A., Bennett, M. R., Fanidi, A. and Evan, G. I. (1994a). C-Myc-induced apoptosis in fibroblasts is inhibited by specific cytokines. *EMBO J.*, **13**, 3286–95.

Harrington, E. A., Fanidi, A. and Evan, G. I. (1994b). Oncogenes and cell death. *Curr. Opin. Genet. Dev.*, **4**, 120–9.

Hendry, J. H. and Scott, D. (1987). Loss of reproductive integrity of irradiated cells, and its importance in tissues. In *Perspectives on Mammalian Cell Death* (ed. C. S. Potten), pp. 160–83. Oxford University Press, Oxford.

Hickman, J. A. (1992). Apoptosis induced by anticancer drugs. *Cancer Metast. Rev.*, **11**, 121–39.

Hickman, J. A., Potten, C. S., Merritt, A. J. and Fisher, T. C. (1994). Apoptosis and cancer chemotherapy. In *The Role of Apoptosis in Development, Tissue Homeostasis and Malignancy* (ed. T. M. Dexter, M. C. Raff and A. H. Wyllie), pp. 83–9. Chapman & Hall, London.

Hockenbery, D., Nuñez, G., Milliman, C. et al. (1990). Bcl-2 is an inner mitochondrial membrane protein that blocks programmed cell death. *Nature*, **348**, 334–6.

Ijiri, K. and Potten, C. S. (1983). Response of intestinal cells of differing topographical and hierarchical status to ten cytotoxic drugs and five sources of radiation. *Br. J. Cancer*, **47**, 175–85.

Kamesaki, S., Kamesaki, H., Jorgensen, T. J. et al. (1993). bcl-2 protein inhibits etoposide-induced apoptosis through its effects on events subsequent to topoisomerase ii-induced DNA strand breaks and their repair. *Cancer Res.*, **53**, 4251–6.

Kiefer, M. C., Brauer, M. J., Powers, V. C. et al. (1995). Modulation of apoptosis by the widely distributed Bcl-2 homologue Bak. *Nature*, **374**, 736–9.

Kondo, S., Yin, D., Morimura, T. and Takeuichi, J. (1994a). bcl-2 gene prevents induction of apoptosis in L1210 murine leukemia cells by SN-38, a metabolite of the campthothecin derivative CPT-11. *Int. J. Oncol.*, **4**, 649–54.

Kondo, S., Yin, D., Takeuchi, J. et al. (1994b). bcl-2 enables rescue from *in vitro* myelosuppression (bone marrow cell death) induced by chemotherapy. *Br. J. Cancer*, **70**, 421–6.

Korsmeyer, S. J., Shutter, J. R., Veis, D. J. et al. (1993). Bcl-2/Bax: a rheostat that regulates an anti-oxidant pathway and cell death. *Seminars Cancer Biol.*, **4**, 327–32.

Kuerbitz, S. J., Plunkett, B. S., Walsh, W. V. and Kastan, M. B. (1992). Wild-type p53 is a cell cycle checkpoint determinant following irradiation. *Proc. Natl. Acad. Sci. USA*, **89**, 7491–5.

Lane, D. P. (1992). p53, guardian of the genome. *Nature*, **358**, 15–16.

Levi-Montalcini, R. (1987). The nerve growth factor: thirty five years later. *EMBO J.*, **6**, 1145–54.

Lotem, J. and Sachs, L. (1993). Regulation by bcl-2, c-myc, and p53 of susceptibility to induction of apoptosis by heat shock and cancer chemotherapy compounds in differentiation-competent and -defective myeloid leukemic cells. *Cell Growth Differ.*, **4**, 41–7.

Lowe, S. W., Ruley, H. E., Jacks, T. and Housman, D. E. (1993a). p53-Dependent apoptosis modulates the cytotoxicity of anticancer agents. *Cell*, **74**, 957–67.

Lowe, S. W., Schmitt, E. M., Smith, S. W. et al. (1993b). p53 is required for radiation-induced apoptosis in mouse thymocytes. *Nature*, **362**, 847–53.

Lowe, S. W., Bodis, S., McClatchey, L. R. et al. (1994). p53 Status and the efficacy of cancer therapy in vivo. *Science*, **266**, 807–10.

Martin, K., Trouche, D., Hagemeier, C. et al. (1995). Stimulation of E2F1/DP1 transcriptional activity by MDM2 oncoprotein. *Nature*, **375**, 691–8.

McGohan, A., Bissonnette, R. P., Schmitt, M. et al. (1994). *BCR-ABL* maintains resistance of chronic myeloid leukemia (CML) through inhibition of apoptosis. *Blood*, **83**, 1179–87.

Merritt, A. J., Potten, C. S., Kemp, C. J. et al. (1994). The role of p53 in spontaneous and radiation-induced apoptosis in gastrointestinal tract of normal and p53-dependent mice. *Cancer Res.*, **54**, 614–17.

Merritt, A. J., Potten, C. S., Watson, A. J. M. et al. (1995). Differential expression of bcl-2 in intestinal epithelia. *J. Cell Sci.*, **108**, 2261–71.

Miyashita, T. and Reed, J. C. (1992). bcl-2 gene transfer increases relative resistance of S49.1 and WEHI7.2 lymphoid cells to cell death and DNA fragmentation induced by glucocorticoids and multiple chemotherapeutic drugs. *Cancer Res.*, **52**, 5407–11.

Miyashita, T. and Reed, J. C. (1993). Bcl-2 oncoprotein blocks chemotherapy-induced apoptosis in a human leukemia cell line. *Blood*, **81**, 151–7.

Miyashita, T. and Reed, J. C. (1995). Tumor suppressor p53 is a direct transcriptional activator of the human bax gene. *Cell*, **80**, 293–9.

Miyashita, T., Maysayoshi, H., Hanada, M. and Reed, J. C. (1994). Identification of a p53-dependent negative response element in the *bcl-2* gene. *Cancer Res.*, **54**, 3131–5.

Momand, J., Zambetti, G. P., Olson, D. C. et al. (1992). The *mdm-2* oncogene product forms a complex with the p53 protein and inhibits p53-mediated transactivation. *Cell*, **69**, 1237–45.

Nagata, S. (1997). Apoptosis by death factor. *Cell*, **88**, 355–65.

Nelson, W. G. and Kastan, M. B. (1994). DNA strand breaks: the DNA template alterations that trigger p53-dependent DNA damage response pathways. *Mol. Cell. Biol.*, **14**, 1815–23.

Nooter, K., Boersma, A. W. M., Oostrum, R. G. et al. (1995). Constitutive expression of the c-H-*ras* oncogene inhibits doxorubicin-induced apoptosis and promotes cell survival in a rhabdomyoscarcoma cell line. *Br. J. Cancer*, **71**, 556–61.

Núñez, G., Merino, R., Grillot, D. and González-García, M. (1994). Bcl-2 and Bcl-x: regulatory switches for lymphoid death and survival. *Immunology*, **12**, 592–8.

Oltvai, Z. N., Milliman, C. L. and Korsmeyer, S. J. (1993). Bcl-2 heterodimerizes in vivo with a conserved homolog, bax, that accelerates programmed cell death. *Cell*, **74**, 609–19.

Pezzella, F. and Gatter, K. (1995). What is the value of bcl-2 detection for histopathologists? *Histopathology*, **26**, 89–93.

Potten, C. S. (1992). The significance of spontaneous and induced apoptosis in the gastrointestinal tract of mice. *Cancer Metast. Rev.*, **11**, 179–95.

Raff, M. C. (1992). Social controls on cell survival and cell death. *Nature*, **356**, 397–400.

Reed, J. C. (1997). Double identity for proteins of the Bcl-2 family. *Nature*, **387**, 773–6.

Sato, T., Hanada, M., Bodrug, S. et al. (1994). Interactions among members of the Bcl-2 protein family analyzed with a yeast two-hybrid system. *Proc. Natl. Acad. Sci. USA*, **91**, 9238–42.

Searle, J., Lawson, T. A., Abbott, P. J. et al. (1975). An electron-microscope study of the mode of cell death induced by cancer-chemotherapeutic agents in populations of proliferating normal and neoplastic cells. *J. Pathol.*, **116**, 129–38.

Sell, C., Baserga, R. and Rubin, R. (1995). Insulin-like growth factor I (IGF-I) and the IGF-I receptor prevent etoposide-induced apoptosis. *Cancer Res.*, **55**, 303–6.

Shen, Y. and Shenk, T. (1994). Relief of p53-mediated transcriptional repression by the adenovirus E1B 19-kDa protein or the cellular Bcl-2 protein. *Proc. Natl. Acad. Sci. USA*, **91**, 8940–4.

Slichenmyer, W. J., Nelson, W. G., Slebos, R. J. and Kastan, M. B. (1993). Loss of a p53-associated G1 checkpoint does not decrease cell survival following DNA damage. *Cancer Res.*, **53**, 4164–8.

Stewart, B. W (1994). Mechanisms of apoptosis: integration of genetic, biochemical, and cellular indicators. *J. Natl. Cancer Inst.*, **86**, 1286–96.

Strasser, A., Harris, A. W., Jacks, T. and Cory, S. (1994). DNA damage can induce apoptosis in proliferating lymphoid cells via p53-independent mechanisms inhibitable by Bcl-2. *Cell*, **79**, 329–39.

Sumantran, V. N., Ealovega, M. W., Nũnez, G. et al. (1995). Overexpression of Bcl-x_s sensitizes MCF-7 cells to chemotherapy-induced apoptosis. *Cancer Res.*, **55**, 2507–10.

Tamura, T., Ishihara, M., Lamphier, M. S. et al. (1995). An IRF-1-dependent pathway of DNA damage-induced apoptosis in mitogen-activated T lymphocytes. *Nature*, **376**, 596–9.

Vaux, D. L., Cory, S. and Adams, J. M. (1988). *Bcl-2* gene promotes haemopoietic cell survival and cooperates with *c-myc* to immortalize pre-B cells. *Nature*, **335**, 440–2.

Vaux, D. L., Haecker, G. and Strasser, A. (1994). An evolutionary perspective on apoptosis. *Cell*, **76**, 777–9.

Walton, M. I., Whysong, D., O'Connor, P. M. et al. (1993). Constitutive expression of human bcl-2 modulates nitrogen mustard and campthothecin induced apoptosis. *Cancer Res.*, **53**, 1853–61.

Williams, G. T., Smith, C. A., Spooncer, E. et al. (1990). Haemopoietic colony stimulating factors promote cell survival by suppressing apoptosis. *Nature*, **343**, 76–82.

Wyllie, A. H., Rose, K. A., Morris, R. G. et al. (1987). Rodent fibroblast tumours expressing human *myc* and *ras* genes: growth, metastasis and endogenous oncogene expression. *Br. J. Cancer*, **56**, 251–9.

Yang, E., Zha, J., Jockel, J. et al. (1995). Bad, a heterodimeric partner for Bcl-x$_L$ and Bcl-2 displaces Bax and promotes cell death. *Cell*, **80**, 285–91.

Yin, X.-M., Oltval, Z. N. and Korsmeyer, S. J. (1994). BH1 and BH2 domains of Bcl-2 are required for inhibition of apoptosis and heterodimerization with Bax. *Nature*, **369**, 321–3.

Yonish-Rouach, E., Resnitzky, D., Lotem, J. et al. (1991). Wild-type p53 induces apoptosis of myeloid leukaemic cells that is inhibited by interleukin-6. *Nature*, **352**, 345–7.

6

Clinical implications of drug resistance

HENK M. W. VERHEUL and HERBERT M. PINEDO

Introduction

Drug resistance is the single most important stumbling block in the fight against metastatic cancer. In fact, 90% of the advanced cancers that can be eradicated by chemotherapy are rare tumor types, which altogether account for only 10% of all malignant tumor types. Tumor types that are responsive for chemotherapy can be categorized into three groups, according to whether chemotherapy produces cure, survival gain, or no survival gain (see also Table 6.1):

1. Tumor types in which a large fraction of patients can be cured. Here we should differentiate between those patients with advanced disease and those treated in an adjuvant setting for microscopic disease. Classical examples of the former include female choriocarcinoma, testicular carcinoma, and Hodgkin's disease. The best examples of microscopic disease that is curable with adjuvant chemotherapy are childhood embryonal rhabdomyosarcoma and breast and colon cancer in adults.
2. Advanced cancers that respond to systemic therapy resulting in an overall survival benefit. The best example of this category is advanced breast cancer.
3. Cancer types in which a small fraction of patients respond but an overall survival benefit is not achieved. Most representative of this category is colorectal cancer, where only responding patients show a survival benefit. This effect in responders is not translated into an overall survival advantage.

Nearly 50% of all patients with cancer suffer from malignancies that are intrinsically resistant to chemotherapy. The majority of the remaining half of patients develop drug resistance during the course of their treatment. However, it is still unclear whether drug resistance is the result

200 H. M. W. Verheul & H. M. Pinedo

Table 6.1. *Outcomes of chemotherapy in advanced diseases (De Vita, 1989)*

Cures:
Choriocarcinoma
Acute lymphocytic leukemia in children
Hodgkin's disease
Diffuse histiocytic lymphoma
Nodular mixed lymphoma
Testicular cancer
Ovarian cancer
Acute myelogenous leukemia
Wilms' tumor
Embryonal rhabdomyosarcoma
Burkitt's lymphoma

No cures, but improved survival:
Breast carcinoma
Chronic myelogenous leukemia
Chronic lymphocytic leukemia
Nodular poorly differentiated lymphocytic lymphoma
Small cell carcinoma of the lung
Soft tissues sarcomas
Gastric carcinoma
Malignant insulinoma
Endometrial carcinoma
Adrenal cortical carcinoma
Medulloblastoma
Neuroblastoma
Polycythemia vera
Prostatic cancer
Glioblastoma
Bladder carcinoma
Osteosarcoma
Ewing sarcoma

No cures, no improvement in survival:
Non small cell lung cancer
Carcinoma of the penis
Carcinoma of the cervix
Colon carcinoma
Head and neck carcinoma
Renal cell carcinoma
Malignant carcinoid tumors
Malignant melanoma
Thyroid carcinoma
Rectal carcinoma
Hepatocellular carcinoma

of the outgrowth of pre-existent resistant tumor cells, whether resistant cells develop as a result of exposure to suboptimal drug concentrations, or whether resistance stems from a combination of both of these.

In clinical practice, the main parameter used to establish whether a solid tumor is resistant to therapy is the tumor mass. A patient is classified as cured if the tumor is no longer detectable and the disease does not reappear during long-term follow-up. In addition, for a number of tumor types, follow-up of blood levels of tumor markers may be of great help in determining the type of response and the prognosis. In general, the faster a complete remission is achieved, the greater the chance that an individual patient is cured. Moreover, a high percentage of complete remissions in a particular tumor type is associated with a greater chance of achieving cures. Ultimately, however, only long-term follow-up will disclose whether an individual patient has been cured.

Clinical aspects of resistance related to the tumor

In the clinic the oncologist is faced with two types of resistance. A tumor which is a priori resistant contains more resistant cells than sensitive cells. If the growth of the resistant population outpaces the elimination of the sensitive cells, the final outcome will be interpreted as primary resistance by the clinician.

In theory all cells of a given tumor may be resistant from the time of diagnosis. In such patients, tumor growth continues from the time of initiation of treatment. At the other end of the scale the oncologist encounters patients with metastases that totally disappear, an observation frequently made in patients with testicular cancers. Between the two extremes is so-called acquired clinical resistance, when relapse follows initial clinical remission.

Theoretically there are two types of acquired clinical resistance. The first type is caused by the continuing growth of pre-existent resistant (mutant) clones. The ratio of the mass of the resistant cells (which depends on their doubling time) to the mass of the eradicated sensitive cells will ultimately determine the quality and duration of remission following chemotherapy. If there are a limited number of resistant cells with a long doubling time, a long duration of remission will be observed. If, however, the proportion of sensitive cells is low relative to the number of resistant cells and the doubling time of the resistant cells is short, then tumor response will be minor or none (see Figure 6.1). Sometimes chemotherapy induces massive cell kill with infiltration

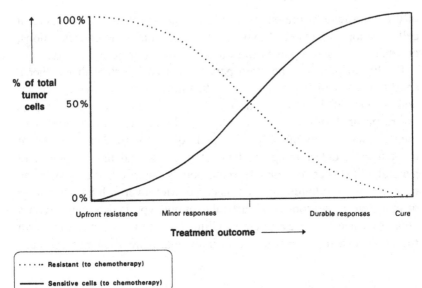

Figure 6.1. The clinical response to chemotherapy is determined by the proportion of sensitive compared to resistant tumor cells.

by mononuclear cells, resulting in an outflow of cytokines or a production of epithelial growth factors, which may promote interstitial changes such as fibrosis. Occasionally, under those circumstances, metastases may even maintain their original size. This result may be misinterpreted as resistance to drugs. With time, however, the fibrotic areas tend to shrink. The classical example of such shrinkage is seen in metastases from testicular cancer. Also, in testicular cancers and neuroblastomas, chemotherapy may induce differentiation into 'benign' lesions. However, it has recently been shown that such 'benign' lesions retain potential malignancy.

Positron emission tomography (PET scanning) offers the possibility of distinguishing between a malignant tumor focus and a benign lesion. This imaging technique may also differentiate malignant areas from benign areas within a particular lesion. Thus, PET scanning may become an important tool for defining the effect of chemotherapy on large solid tumor masses. Also, with the use of such techniques as magnetic resonance imaging (MRI), it is becoming clear that certain tumors, such as soft tissue sarcomas, may consist of large areas of fluid, which accumulate in cyst-like spaces and contain a wide variety of cytokines. Such tumor fluid can be misinterpreted as necrosis on CT images (see

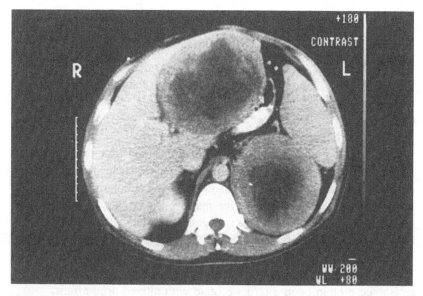

Figure 6.2. CT scan of a patient with a soft tissue sarcoma. This CT scan shows two pockets of fluid in a patient with a metastasized leiomyosarcoma, which might be easily misinterpreted as necrosis.

Figure 6.2). It is as yet unclear whether an attempt should be made to drain such fluid prior to the initiation of chemotherapy. The persistence of large areas of tumor fluid may render the response assessment difficult. These observations represent important advantages of the newer imaging techniques and should certainly prove helpful in better defining the response to treatment.

Causes of resistance at the cellular level

Theoretical considerations related to the tumor cell and tumor kinetics

Genetic considerations

Several theories regarding resistance have been put forward. One of the most widely accepted hypotheses is that of Goldie and Coldman, which is essentially based on the assumption that 'resistant cells are mutant cells'. Non-random mutations are associated with the capacity of tumor cells to resist the assault by a cytotoxic agent (Goldie and Coldman, 1984).

The mutation rate of somatic cells appears to be of the order of 10^{-6}–10^{-8} per DNA base pair per division and if the mutation is not fatal it will be carried along. This means that a tumor of more than 10^8 cells will contain at least one mutated cell that is resistant (Goldie and Coldman, 1979). This theory supports the concept that resistance is usually already present at diagnosis.

An alternative possibility is that a potentially sensitive tumor cell can develop into a resistant cell. Although acquired resistance following drug exposure has, in fact, been demonstrated during cellular proliferation in vitro, this phenomenon has never really been proven to exist in the clinic. Indeed, it is most likely that genetic mutations may be induced by chemotherapy itself. If the dose of the drug is too low for cell killing while the exposure time is sufficiently long, the chance of inducing mutations increases. Mutations may result in overexpression of a drug resistance protein or in a target protein with altered drug affinity.

The importance of growth fraction

A given drug kills a constant fraction of tumor cells rather than a constant number of cells (Skipper et al., 1964). The growth fraction of a tumor decreases with increasing tumor size, but also decreases in micrometastases. At 37% of the hypothesized maximal size of the tumor, the growth fraction will be optimal and the tumor will be therefore very sensitive to chemotherapy (Norton and Simon, 1977).

Anticancer drugs affect mainly proliferating cells, and larger tumors generally appear to be more resistant than smaller ones. However, when a clinical complete remission is achieved the remaining micrometastases may paradoxically be more resistant than the primary tumor to chemotherapy. Although no tumor cells can be detected in such cases, the intensiveness of the treatment regimen might make the difference between cure versus regrowth of the remaining tumor cells. Therefore, patients with no detectable tumor will benefit from full dose chemotherapy (in the adjuvant setting) or even from high dose chemotherapy (late-intensification after complete remission to standard-dose chemotherapy).

Resistance related to apoptosis

In recent years increased interest has been focused on studying the pathways of cell death. Although in normal tissues there is a balance between dying and dividing cells, in tumors cellular proliferation exceeds cell death. Chemotherapy may correct this imbalance in favour of cell death.

The apoptotic pathway, or programed cell death, is still not completely understood, although a great deal of knowledge has been gained. Several genes, including *bcl*-2 and *p53*, are involved in this mechanism (Dole et al., 1994; Fisher, 1994). In breast cancer and other tumor types, an inverse relationship has been found between the expression of the *p53* and *bcl*-2 genes (Silvestrini et al., 1994). Apoptosis seems to be dependent on normal *p53* function and can be blocked by overexpression of *bcl*-2. It appears that the cells of the more sensitive tumors (as mentioned in Table 6.1) may undergo apoptosis, whereas the cells of the incurable tumors are less capable of doing so. Changes responsible for the loss of programed cell death may be responsible not only for tumor development but also for drug resistance (Kastan, Canman and Leonard, 1995).

Biochemical mechanisms of cellular resistance

Experimental studies have identified a number of mechanisms of resistance, including transport deficiencies and biochemical changes at the cellular level. Decreased drug uptake has been reported to be a cause of resistance to several drugs. For example, the alteration or inactivation of 5-methyl-tetrahydrofolate, the transport system for methotrexate, results in decreased influx into the cell (Bertino et al., 1989). Another phenomenon, increased drug extrusion, is the result of increased synthesis of a protein that can pump out drugs, the classical example being the P-glycoprotein (Pgp, see below).

In addition, anticancer drugs can be inactivated intracellularly, as for example in the degradation of 5-fluorouracil to its inactive metabolite 5-fluorodihydrouracil (F-DHU). Dihydrouracil dehydrogenase, the enzyme responsible for this degradation, has been detected in most tissues, but in relatively low levels in tumor cells (Pinedo and Peters, 1988). The inactivation of alkylating agents and anthracyclines, on the other hand, is mainly attributable to glutathione. Another mechanism of cellular drug resistance is decreased conversion of a prodrug to its active metabolite. An example is the decreased conversion of the anticancer drug arabinoside cytosine (Ara-C) to its active metabolite Ara-CTP by the converting enzyme deoxycytidine. Yet another example of decreased drug activation is caused by low intracellular levels of carboxyesterase, which catalyses the conversion of the topoisomerase I inhibitor CPT-11 to its active metabolite SN-38 (Vendrik et al., 1992).

Gene amplification may be responsible for a proportional decrease in the formation of drug target complexes. This decreased formation can be due to decreased or increased target enzyme production, production of an altered enzyme with less affinity for the drug, or an increased level of normal substrate (Borst and Pinedo, 1995). Finally, increased repair of DNA damage has been reported as a weakly established mechanism of resistance for alkylating agents and platinum analogs (Harris, 1985). Direct evidence of this phenomenon in clinically resistant cancer is difficult to prove, however. Probably, those cancer cells become more like normal cells, which are thought to be resistant to chemotherapy because of their DNA repair mechanisms. Meenakshi et al. (1995) reported that in the L1210 cells, T lymphocytes, and human ovarian cancer cells, resistance to low levels of cisplastin was attributable to increased DNA repair. They found several genes, *ERCC1*, *ERCC3* and *ERCC6*, to be involved in this process. mRNA levels for these genes in malignant tissues were noted to be significantly higher in patients who did not respond to cisplatin treatment than in those who did respond.

Classical multidrug resistance

Classical multidrug resistance (MDR) is associated with overexpression of Pgp, a surface glycoprotein with a molecular weight of 170 kDa. Pgp is known as an efflux transport protein, which reduces the cellular accumulation of drugs, resulting in drug resistance. The relationship between the degree of expression of this glycoprotein at the cell membrane and the degree of resistance was reported in 1976 by Juliano and Ling. This membrane protein, like others, can be detected by immunocytochemistry. Three monoclonal antibodies (MoAbs) commonly used for detection of Pgp are C219 and JSB (cytoplasmic) and MRK16 (external epitopes). A sister of the Pgp gene, which is recognized by the MoAb C219, has been very recently detected, although its role is not yet understood (Childs et al., 1995). Pgp is responsible for the resistance of a cell to several drugs, including vinca alkaloids, epipodophyllotoxins, doxorubicin and paclitaxel. To date, however, Pgp has never been proven to account for clinical resistance, despite reports of good correlations between Pgp expression and tumor relapse or resistance. Chan et al. (1990) have shown that children with soft tissue sarcomas and neuroblastomas that expressed Pgp had a higher recurrence rate than those whose tumors were Pgp negative. In a study of 79 patients with acute lymphocytic leukemia, Tiirikainen et al. (1993) concluded that Pgp expression at the time of diagnosis correlated with a low remission rate.

Non-P-glycoprotein mediated MDR

Non-P-glycoprotein mediated MDR has been reported in association with the multidrug resistance-associated protein (MRP), which is localized mainly on the cell membrane. Cole et al. (1992) have cloned the gene that encodes for MRP. In addition, although MRP is expressed in many normal tissues, its role there has yet to be defined. The function of MRP cannot be modified by Pgp resistance modifiers and the contribution of this protein to drug resistance is still unclear.

The function of the MRP pump, unlike that of the Pgp pump, is strongly dependent on Glutathione (GSH). Jedlitschky et al. (1994) have reported that the MRP pump mediates ATP-dependent glutathione S-conjugates transport and that lower levels of intracellular GSH inhibit the ability of the MRP pump to eject positively charged groups. According to these researchers, while the MRP pump is responsible for the efflux of negatively charged intracellular groups, positively charged groups must be conjugated to GSH before they are pumped out of the cell by MRP. Although Feller et al. (1995) could not confirm such a relationship they likewise reported that a decrease of intracellular GSH leads to inactivation of the MRP pump.

The first clinical analyses in tumor tissues have recently been reported. Burger et al. (1994) found high expression of MRP in 15 of 21 patients with chronic lymphatic leukemia but in only 3 of 16 patients with acute myelocytic leukemia (AML). This expression was not related to prior chemotherapy although the investigators did not attempt to correlate their findings with treatment results. Kuss et al. (1994) reported that disease-free survival was longer in patients with AML who had reduced expression of the MRP gene than in those with higher levels of expression.

Lung resistance-related protein (LRP)

Another gene that might be responsible for drug resistance has recently been found. This gene encodes for the lung-resistant-related protein (*LRP56*). The *LRP56* gene is overexpressed in tumor cells that have been treated with anthracyclines in vitro (Scheper et al., 1993). Izquierdo et al. (1995) demonstrated that a poor response to treatment and reduced overall survival correlated with enhanced LRP expression in metastatic ovarian cancer. This phenomenon has also been suggested for AML (List et al., 1993).

The precise role of LRP in the process of drug resistance is still unclear. However, the location of the LRP gene on chromosome 16, near the MRP gene, combined with the correlation between LRP gene expression and therapeutic outcome, suggest that LRP may play an important part in drug resistance (Scheffer et al., 1995).

Glutathione-related resistance

Glutathione (GSH) and glutathione-S-transferase (GST) cause drug resistance by an unknown mechanism. The concentration of both GSH and GST are elevated in resistant cells. Kramer et al. (1988) and Dusre et al. (1989) have reported that GSH depletion leads to a partial reversal of resistance to alkylating agents. The maximum increase in the resistance to tumor cells treated with alkylating agents is about 20-fold (Frei et al., 1988). In a phase I study with thiotepa and ethacrynic acid, O'Dwyer et al. (1991) have shown an inhibition of GSH transferase in the peripheral mononuclear cells. No clinical data thus far have been reported, however.

Topoisomerase I inhibitors

A reduction in metabolic activation has been implicated in the development of resistance to the topoisomerase I inhibitor irinotecan (CPT-11). A reduced level of carboxyesterase, the enzyme needed for conversion of CPT-11, leads to a decreased concentration of SN-38, the active metabolite of the topoisomerase I inhibitor. In addition, decreased activity of the target enzyme DNA topoisomerase I and/or a mutation in the gene that encodes for this enzyme, seems to contribute to resistance to camptothecin (Gupta et al., 1988; Tamura et al., 1991).

Topoisomerase I inhibitors have a reduced effect on non-proliferative cells as found in the multilayered postconfluent cultures of colon and ovarian human tumor cell lines (Pizao et al., 1994). mRNA expression of topoisomerase I in peripheral mononuclear (PMN) cells and colon mucosa has been reported by O'Dwyer et al. (1994). These studies have shown great variability of expression in the PMN cells, as compared to the colon mucosa. In phase I and II studies of the topoisomerase I inhibitors, samples of different tissues from patients will need to be examined for topoisomerase protein levels in order to determine whether these predict treatment outcome.

Topoisomerase II inhibitors

Certain drugs such as doxorubicin, VP-16, m-AMSA and others, are topoisomerase II inhibitors.

Resistance based on alterations in topoisomerase II has been termed atypical MDR. Cells may develop resistance to topoisomerase II inhibitors when target enzyme levels decrease or when the gene encoding for the enzyme is mutated, which may lead to an altered enzyme with reduced affinity for the drugs. Studies performed by Tan et al. (1989) and Deffie et al. (1989) have indeed shown a mutation in the topoisomerase II gene in cases of atypical MDR.

Increased phosphorylation seems to contribute to the resistance of human cancer KB cells to etoposide, a phenomenon that is also accompanied by low intracellular levels of topoisomerase II (Takano et al., 1991). However, no clinical study has yet shown a clear correlation between topoisomerase II levels and treatment outcome.

Thymidylate synthase and 5-fluorouracil

Altered specificity of dihydrofolate reductase (DHFR) and thymidylate synthase (TS), the target enzymes for 5-fluorouracil (5-FU) and other new inhibitors such as Tomudex, leads to decreased formation of drug–target complexes. Excess production of TS inhibits the action of 5-FU (Peters et al., 1994a). In clinical samples Spears et al. (1988) and Swain et al. (1989) have shown a correlation between the degree of TS inhibition and the tumor response to 5-FU. The main causes of resistance to 5-FU are an increased intracellular level of TS and a decreased level of the tetrahydrofolate cofactor needed for the binding of 5-FU to TS to form the tertiary complex. Peters et. al. (1994b) have recently documented the predictive correlation between residual and total TS activity and the response to 5-FU treatment in colorectal cancers. In addition, Johnston et al. (1993) have demonstrated that TS levels and TS gene expression predict the response to 5-FU.

Causes of resistance related to the tumor microenvironment

In addition to the genetic basis of cellular drug resistance and other factors such as growth fraction, and the anatomical and physiological conditions, the tumor microenvironment also appears to contribute to the sensitivity or resistance of solid tumors to drugs. Indeed, the drug has to traverse several hurdles before it reaches the cancer cell. Critical determinants include the degree to which the tumor is vascularized. In general, the distance between the capillaries and the malignant cells will be shorter in well-vascularized tumors than in poorly vascularized tissues. More specific local conditions come into play, including factors facilitating the exit from the vessel into the surrounding matrix, the interstitium, factors influencing migration of the molecules through the matrix, and, finally, factors existing at the level of the target cell membrane. In this respect, little is known about the differences between the conditions in primary tumors and those in metastases.

Obviously these barriers are not present in hematologic malignancies such as leukemia, where leukemic blood cells live in circumstances comparable to those in suspension culture. Under the latter conditions the anticancer drug only has to take the last hurdle, as there is no matrix to be crossed. Conditions closely resembling those in leukemia exist in cases of intrathecal and intraperitoneal chemotherapy, although multiple layers of tumor cells may exist on the cavity wall. Conditions in other hematological malignancies, such as lymphoma and myeloma, resemble those in leukemia to some extent. Indeed, these tumors are better vascularized than solid tumors. Also, in lymphoma and myeloma, drug transport is facilitated by a matrix that is loose compared to the matrix in solid tumors.

Jain (1989, 1994) has demonstrated that in several solid tumor types there is a high pressure gradient extending from the centre of the lesion toward the edge of the tumor. This phenomenon may impede the access of drugs to the center of the tumor. Failure of the drug to reach the tumor may also be due to pharmacological sanctuaries, such as the brain and testis. Shirai et al. (1994) have shown a possible role for Pgp in the endothelial cells of the brain barrier. In cultures of brain capillary endothelial cells, inhibition of the uptake of cyclosporin A has been found following incubation with verapamil. In the clinic, brain meta-stases may progress during chemotherapy, while no tumor relapse occurs in other organs. For many years it has been assumed that this is caused by the blood–brain barrier.

Other potential factors contributing to the resistance of solid tumors to drugs are the hypoxia and the decrease in local pH resulting from poor vascularization. Hypoxia and low pH have been demonstrated to contribute to resistance in cultured cells of solid tumors (Tannock and Roth, 1989), but clinical studies are urgently needed to establish the precise role of this phenomenon.

Screening for drug resistance

Preclinical in vitro models

The molecular basis of drug sensitivity and drug resistance is still poorly understood, while drug development has been mainly empirically based. Attempts to comprehend the mechanism of action of anticancer drugs have been made in the laboratory, although more recently clinical studies have been undertaken to overcome drug resistance through a variety of approaches aimed at modulating drug action. Many of these approaches have failed to add significantly to the success of cancer chemotherapy. Advances are to be expected from the development of drugs with new targets.

Drug screening has been based on in vitro systems and in vivo models. Most in vitro studies have been performed in monolayer cultures, in which the cell surface is readily exposed to the drug. Efforts have been made to develop models that more closely resemble the in vivo con-ditions of solid tumors.

Hamburger and Salmon (1977) reported an in vitro model of a bioas-say of human tumor stem cells. The tumor cells were incubated on a soft agar layer in a special medium at 37°C for 3 days and thereafter treated with different agents. This model should have been able to predict the sensitivity of different human tumor cells to anticancer drugs but, with time, it became apparent that the cloning of the human tumor cells in this model was too difficult for practical use. In 1992 Pizao et al. developed a V-bottom shaped system with multilayered postconfluent tumor cell cultures. This system might appear to predict for sensitivity and resistance of solid tumors to drugs. The biology of the system is definitely more similar to the biology of human solid tumors than are the circumstances in suspension cultures. Kobayashi et al. (1993) reported an in vitro multicellular tumor spheroid culture system in which the cells showed a drug resistance spectrum similar to that observed in vivo.

Preclinical studies

In vivo studies stand closer to reality. Preclinical investigations with murine models have made a major contribution to experimental chemo-therapy (Goldie, Coldman and Gudauskas, 1982) and have helped lay the foundation for clinical chemotherapy. However, experiments have now taught us that the murine solid tumor screening panels used to date have frequently yielded false-positive results. With time it has become apparent that it is essential to perform animal studies using human tumor xenografts in nude (immune deficient) mice. The validity of xenografts has been demonstrated by comparing the clinical response to chemo-therapy with the response of the same tumor type implanted in the xenograft (Winograd et al., 1987). Fidler (1990) have elegantly shown the importance of the site of inoculation of the tumor and they advocate implantation of the tumor cells in the organ of origin in order to obtain more representative results.

Tumors with documented resistance in individual patients have occasionally been studied in xenografts, resulting in good correlations. However, the xenograft system has still never been proven to have any clinical significance for the treatment of an individual patient. Nonethe-less, because of its high correlation with clinical results, this model remains ideal for testing new drugs and new combinations of drugs (Fiebig, 1988). In addition, the xenograft represents an excellent model for delineating the optimal drug dosage, schedule, and route of adminis-tration.

Despite all the advantages of the xenograft model over the murine tumor model, false-positive results (epi-doxorubicin in colon cancer; Pezzoni and Giuliani, 1988) and false-negative results (methotrexate in head and neck cancer; Braakhuis and Snow, 1988) have been reported. Perhaps the best correlation has been reported by Boven (1988) for platinum analogues in ovarian cancer xenografts.

Clinical studies

Clinical trials aiming at understanding and overcoming drug resistance should be widely encouraged. In order for new schedules to be investigated on a rational basis they must be supported by good laboratory research. Attempts should be made to use clinical samples to investigate the effect of the drugs at the tumor cell level. First and foremost, we need to know whether all the tumor cells are being reached, including those in the centre of solid tumors.

With the introduction of hematopoietic growth factors, bone marrow transplantation and peripheral stem cell transplantation, attempts are being made to achieve higher extracellular levels of the drugs in solid tumors. In many of these latter studies drugs have been selected on the basis of the achievable doses, supported by the general philosophy that 'more is better'. This is an unrealistic approach. The starting point should be the selection of drugs on the basis of their established efficacy in the particular tumor type to be studied. In an attempt to expose the tumor cells to the highest possible drug concentrations, routes of local drug administration have been introduced, such as intraperitoneal, intrathecal and intraarterial chemotherapy (see page 217).

In addition the search for new ways to predict drug resistance is gaining ground. Several genes responsible for the genetic changes underlying various types of drug resistance have been identified and cloned. The human *MDR* gene is perhaps most representative. This gene is expressed in response to cellular damage by cytotoxic drugs, even if the tumor cells are only briefly exposed to the drugs (Chaudhary and Roninson, 1993). It is still unknown whether this observation has any clinical significance.

An interesting clinical phenomenon that we have observed in some patients is an acceleration in the growth of metastases following removal of the primary tumor. It is tempting to relate this phenomenon to a recent preclinical observation that a decrease in anti-angiogenic factors may be responsible. According to this hypothesis the primary tumor is responsible for the production of angiogenesis inhibitors or for the production of an enzyme that catalyzes the synthesis of these inhibitors. This possibility has been recently substantiated by the findings of O'Reilly et al. (1994), who demonstrated a potent angiogenesis inhibitor possibly produced by the primary tumor in the Lewis lung carcinoma model. After removal of the primary tumor these investigators observed an outburst of metastases that was clearly related to neovascularization of these deposits. The angiogenesis-inhibiting protein, which they called angiostatin, is a 38 kDa split product of plasminogen.

Clinical implications

Detection of drug resistant tumor cells

There is an urgent need for assays that can predict clinical drug resistance. In this section a number of recent developments will be briefly reviewed.

Resistance proteins

The classical example of a drug resistance assay is the assay for Pgp in clinical samples. In a number of clinical studies the level of Pgp has been shown to correlate with resistance to natural compounds, such as anthracyclines. In acute leukaemia Pgp expression at diagnosis has been associated with a low remission rate following the first cycle of induction therapy (Tiirikainen et al., 1993). In a second study in patients with Pgp-positive acute nonlymphoblastic leukemia, Pgp expression predicted a lower complete remission rate and a shorter duration of survival (Campos et al., 1992). The expression of the *MDR1* gene was established by a semiquantitative slot blot procedure and with immunocytochemistry. The *MDR1* gene is highly expressed in many clinically resistant tumors and is an adverse prognostic factor in some cancers (Fisher and Sikic, 1995).

However, a study by Pirker et al. (1991) has clearly shown that there is no absolute correlation between clinical response and the absence of Pgp/*MDR1*. Presumably there are more resistance-related proteins, including the recently described MRP, which complicates the interpretation of single assays. One may anticipate the discovery of more efflux proteins in the future. Therefore, the development of functional assays should be encouraged. Schuurhuis et al. (1995) have demonstrated a correlation between the clinical response in AML and the functional MDR phenotype. Although reduced accumulation was observed with phenotype overexpression of both Pgp/*MDR1* and MRP, accumulation was occasionally low in samples that were negative for both proteins. Sampling of fresh leukemia cells from de novo or relapsed patients revealed reduced drug accumulation in cells from patients who failed to achieve a complete response to daunomycin or mitoxantrone in combination with Ara-C. These findings support the hypothesis that functional assays are more reliable than assays that only test for the presence of drug-resistance proteins.

Alterations in key enzymes can affect the mechanisms of action of a number of drugs. The concentration of TS in malignant cells in clinical biopsies of metastatic colorectal cancer has been shown to predict for response to 5-FU (Peters et al., 1994b). In the future, the TS concentration may be used as the determinant of whether 5-FU chemotherapy should be started or not. Only those patients with colon cancers that are expected to be sensitive to 5-FU should be treated with 5-FU. Furthermore, it is a well recognized phenomenon that exposure to 5-FU will enhance TS in tumor cells and this, in turn, is related to the development of resistance. This increase may be prevented by interferon-alpha, which could account for the higher response rate observed with the combination of the two agents. One might also wonder whether increases in cellular TS levels caused by 5-FU will result in enhanced tumor growth. Johnston et al. (1993) have clearly shown that the TS level in tumor samples from newly operated patients is predictive of ultimate survival.

The tumor suppressor gene p53

This appears to play a significant role in tumorigenesis. Several studies have found that p53 mutation correlates with a high risk of tumor aggressivity and recurrence (Ito et al., 1994). *p53* mutations have been demonstrated in most tumor types including the colon, lung, oesophagus, breast, liver, brain, reticuloendothelial tissues, and hematopoietic tissues. For example, Peyrat et al. (1995) have shown that *p53*, as detected by immunochemistry, is an important prognostic factor in patients undergoing surgery for locoregional breast cancer. This phenomenon will certainly have clinical implications. The combination of Pgp expression and nuclear *p53* accumulation in locally advanced breast carcinoma cells at diagnosis seems to predict for shorter survival (Linn et al., 1996).

Tumor angiogenesis

Quantitative pathologic studies using microvessel counting have shown that highly vascular early breast cancers have a poor prognosis (Craft and Harris, 1994). Since these first reports, almost all of the many studies performed have indicated that angiogenesis is an independent prognostic factor (reviewed by Gasparini and Harris, 1995). Further studies are needed to investigate whether the microvessel assay is an important indicator in other tumor types as well. In an animal model the onset of angiogenesis has been demonstrated to coincide with the appearance of tumor cells within the efferent tumor circulation and with metastasis (Liotta et al., 1974).

Positron emission tomography

A noninvasive method of detecting drug-resistant tumor cells would be of great help in determining whether further treatment is warranted in an individual patient (see Figure 6.3). Positron emission tomography provides an elegant noninvasive means of detecting viable cells following chemotherapy. This technique makes use of the increased rates of glycolytic activity in malignant tumor cells by applying 18-fluorodeoxyglucose to detect malignant cells. In a comparison of PET scans with the pathology of the resected lymph nodes in 80 patients with testicular cancers, Mechev and Sakolo (1994) found a high predictive value for the PET scan with 83% sensitivity and 90.9% specificity. Lewis et al. (1994) reported that the detection of small metastases by PET scanning prior to scheduled surgery led to changes in treatment planning in 41% of lung cancer patients. This technique proved to be more sensitive than conventional imaging techniques.

Imaginary resistance and local chemotherapy

The possibility of imaginary resistance should also be taken into consideration. Patients are often treated with suboptimal doses of chemotherapy and this is the best example of 'resistance' that can be easily resolved. Imaginary resistance can also be caused by sequestration of the tumor, resulting in less drug or even no drug reaching the malignant cells. There are several ways of coping with this type of resistance and these will be discussed below.

Intrathecal chemotherapy

Intrathecal administration of a drug bypasses the blood–brain barrier and may be indicated for treating leptomeningeal carcinomatosis. The underlying basis of this barrier is probably a special sort of plasma membrane glycoprotein, such as Pgp (Shirai et al., 1994). MDR experi-

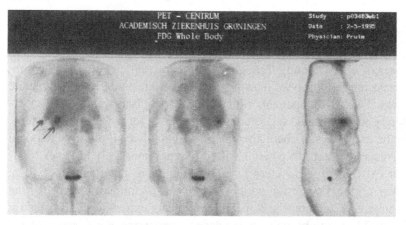

Figure 6.3. PET scan showing liver metastases. Clearly visible on this PET scan are two hot spots in the liver of a patient with metastatic colorectal carcinoma, who had been treated with intra-arterial chemotherapy that was complicated by a thrombotic accident. After the thrombotic accident the right liver lobe shrunk and the left lobe became hypertrophic. One year after the accident the carcinoembryonic antigen (CEA) level rose in this patient, but neither the CT scan nor the MRI could detect the expected liver metastases. At last the PET scan showed the two liver metastases and the patient's metastases were resected.

ments in knock-out mice have elegantly shown the role of Pgp at the blood–brain level. Schinkel et al. (1994) have demonstrated that disruption of this protein results in higher brain drug concentrations following administration of vinblastine.

Intraperitoneal chemotherapy

Preclinical studies (Los et al., 1993) have shown the great advantage of intraperitoneal administration of cisplatin over the intravenous route. It has been known for several years that this approach may be very effective in metastatic ovarian carcinoma, with response rates as high as 80%. Systemic toxicity is mild and is mainly attributable to cisplatin (Markman, 1991). A recent randomized trial comparing intraperitoneally and intravenously administered cisplatin has shown that the intraperitoneal route affords a significant survival benefit in patients with minimal disease following debulking surgery (Alberts et al., 1995). Other agents for which this route has proven useful include 5-FU, mitoxantrone and mitomycin. However, mitoxantrone and doxorubicin may cause severe toxic effects, including abdominal pain and bowel obstruction, following intraperitoneal administration.

Isolated perfusion therapy

In 1958, Creech and Krementz reported the administration of very high doses of chemotherapy through an extracorporeal circuit. They demonstrated the feasibility of isolating the limbs, intestines, liver, pelvis and lungs. Twenty-four patients with malignant neoplasia were treated accordingly and the results suggested good palliation for far-advanced lesions. In the early days of chemotherapy Stehlin and Lee (1960) used regional perfusion to treat 116 patients with different tumor types in the extremities. At that time no clear response rates were reported. Since then, many regional perfusion studies have been performed, mainly for the treatment of sarcomas and melanomas in the extremities. The greatest benefit has been observed when poorly vascularized tumors were treated with drugs showing a rapid total body clearance. The advantages of this approach are based mainly on the high doses that can be locally administered and, essentially, on a lack of systemic side-effects. By perfusing melphalan in patients with advanced melanoma of the limbs, Klaase et al. (1994) achieved a 54% complete remission rate, with a median duration of 9 months. Local intra-arterial cisplatin therapy provides comparable results (Guchelaar et al., 1992; Thompson and Gianouts 1992). More recently, dramatic tumor shrinkage has been observed with the perfusion of TNF-α. However, because tumors usually recur following regional perfusion, this approach should be considered a palliative treatment or a way of preventing mutilating surgery (see Figure 6.4).

Intraarterial infusion

With this approach, tumor exposure to the drug is enhanced, but systemic exposure is similar to that with the intravenous route (Curley et al., 1992). Intra-arterial infusion is being applied in tumors of the extremities, the bladder (hypogastric artery) and the liver (hepatic artery). It goes without saying that drugs infused intra-arterially into the extremities and the bladder should not require activation at other sites in the body.

Thanks to hepatic drug extraction, higher concentrations can be achieved when a drug is administered via the hepatic artery, although this depends on the extraction factor (see Table 6.2). The method is especially applicable for hepatic metastases from colorectal cancer but is also used for hepatic metastases from other tumor types, including breast cancer. Hohn *et al.* (1989) have reported that intra-arterial chemo-

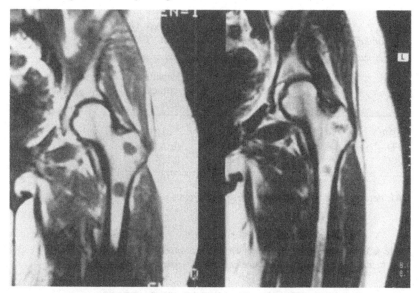

Figure 6.4. MRI of palliative isolated arterial perfusion. This MRI shows clearly a very dangerous metastasis (left) in the left hip of a patient with a metastatic breast carcinoma. After isolated arterial chemotherapy the patient experienced an almost complete local remission and was no longer in danger of fracture.

therapy produced durable responses in patients with unresectable liver metastases from gastrointestinal cancers. In patients with liver metastases from colorectal cancer, systemic 5-FU chemotherapy achieves response rates of only 10–20%, whereas intra-arterial 5-FU chemotherapy yields significantly higher response rates of 42–62%. However, these improved response rates do not translate into a significant prolongation of overall survival (Takats et al., 1994).

Dose and schedule

In order to achieve the optimal treatment dose and schedule, the drug's mechanism of action, pharmacologic properties, toxicity, and possible interactions with other drugs need to be taken into account (Cassidy, 1994). Higher drug doses will usually increase the response rate. Focan et al. (1993) compared an intensified and a non-intensified schedule of epirubicin in patients with locally advanced breast cancer and recurrent metastatic breast cancer. The response rate was 27% higher in the group that received the intensified schedule (69% versus 41%). Blomqvist et

Table 6.2. *Pharmacokinetic characteristics of drugs commonly used for hepatic arterial administration (Takats et al., 1994)*

Drug	Estimated increase in hepatic exposure by HAI over peripheral infusion	Hepatic extraction ratio
FUDR	× 100–400	0.95
5-FU	× 50–100	0.30–0.40
Mit C	× 3–5	0.10–0.20

HAI, hepatic arterial infusion; Mit C, mitomycin C

Table 6.3. *Potential for increasing single dose intensity based on a hematopoietic supportive care regimen (Petros and Peters, 1993)*

Low dose					High dose
None	CSF	CSF + PBPC	ABMT	ABMT + CSF	ABMT + CSF + PBPC

CSF, colony stimulating factors; PBPC, peripheral stem cell transplantation; ABMT, allogenic bone marrow transplantation.

al. (1993) compared a weekly schedule of 5-FU plus epirubicin plus cyclophosphamide (FEC) chemotherapy with a monthly schedule providing the same total dose. The monthly schedule caused more toxicity, but also yielded a higher response rate (47% versus 30%).

In most studies, however, higher response rates have not translated into survival benefits. Hematological growth factors, bone marrow transplantation, and peripheral stem cell transplantation have been of great help in minimizing hematologic toxicity and thereby permitting the administration of higher doses and more intensive cycles of chemotherapy. It remains to be seen, however, whether the megadoses that are being combined with hematopoietic support will result in a higher cure rate in chemosensitive tumors. Petros and Peters (1993) tried to order hematopoietic supportive care regimens based on the idea of the relevance of dose intensity (see Table 6.3).

Modulation of drug resistance

Reverters of drug resistance

The reversal of Pgp-mediated multidrug resistance has attracted major attention in recent years. Agents that have been investigated clinically as potential reverters of this type of resistance and reviewed by Fisher and Sikic (1995) include verapamil (Milroy, 1993), cyclosporin (Bartlett et al., 1994), progesterone (Christen et al., 1993), RU 486 (Gruol et al., 1994), BIBW22BS (Jansen et al., 1994) and PSC 833 (Giaccone et al., unpublished). The calcium channel blocker verapamil, which has a high affinity for Pgp, has been the reference drug for such studies (Plumb et al., 1990). In a pilot study by Dalton et al. (1989), patients with myeloma who were resistant to vincristine plus adriamycin plus dexamethasone (VAD) chemotherapy went into a second remission when verapamil was added to VAD. However, the serious cardiac side effects caused by verapamil precluded an increase in its dosage.

Similarly cyclosporin A, a relatively potent inhibitor of Pgp with immunomodulating properties, cannot be investigated clinically at an optimal dose because of its very severe side effects, including nausea and vomiting, myelosuppression, and hyperbilirubinemia. Bartlett et al. (1994) have reported a large increase in the area under the curve (AUC) of doxorubicin and its metabolite doxorubicinol without increased toxicity, when a maximum of 60% of the conventional doxorubicin dose was given in combination with cyclosporin A. PSC 833, a cyclosporin A analogue, is a new modulator with reduced side effects and is currently being evaluated in phase I studies. To date, no clinical study has shown an important effect of resistance reverters, except for a modest effect in AML.

Mülder et al. (1996) have tested the effect of human plasma on daunorubicin accumulation in two MDR-resistant cell lines, SW1573/2R160 and GLC4/ADR, that express Pgp and MRP, respectively. These investigators found a dose–response relationship between the amount of plasma and daunorubicin accumulation. Plasma cortisol was found to be responsible for 35% of this effect. It is therefore most likely that MDR-reverting agents will provide only minor additive effects on top of the plasma effect. Before starting therapy with a reverting agent, it is mandatory to measure the reverting effect of the patient's own plasma. Only in this way can the real contribution of the reverter be assessed.

Enhancers of 5-FU cytotoxicity

Resistance can also be overcome by increasing the binding of the cyto-toxic agent to its target. The classical example is that of leucovorin (LV), which improves the binding of FdUMP to TS, particularly in cells which are deficient in folates.

In advanced colorectal cancer the combination of 5-FU and LV has been reported to result in higher response rates, but no survival benefit as compared to single-agent 5-FU. Both the combination of 5-FU and LV and the combination of 5-FU, LV and methotrexate have been shown to yield similar response rates (Glimelius, 1993). Wadler et al. (1989) have reported promising results with 5-FU and α-interferon, but without any survival benefit thus far. Similar to the report from the Italian Group for the Study of Digestive Tract Cancer, the addition of α-interferon to the combination of 5-FU and LV did not result in a better treatment outcome in 56 patients (Labianca et al., 1994). Cunningham et al. (1995) have concluded that chemotherapy given by hepatic arterial infusion afforded no clear survival benefit as compared to systemic infusion of 5-FU with or without α-interferon. On the contrary, they pointed out that intra-arterial therapy was associated not only with more local complications but also with a higher death rate.

Modulation of tumor GSH levels

Elevated concentrations of GST have been reported in resistant ovarian cancer cells, although the reason for this elevation is not yet known. Of interest, buthionine sulfoxamine (BSO) appears to modulate resistance in these cells by causing an excessive reduction in GSH concentration, which leads to a stress situation in the cell (Muggia and Los, 1993). The mechanism of action of BSO is not fully understood but it has been proven effective in ovarian cancers. In one study four of nine patients with refractory ovarian cancers showed a partial response. Tumor biopsies revealed that BSO reduced GSH levels to 20% of baseline concentrations (O'Dwyer et al., 1994). These findings need to be confirmed on a larger scale.

Alternative approaches to enhancing the antitumor effect

The use of drug combinations and alternating non-cross-resistant chemo-therapeutic agents is based on Goldie and Coldman's mathematical model (1984). In tumors with increased GST activity, combinations of cytotoxic drugs have been successful in achieving enhanced tumor cell kill.

Treatment of stage IV Hodgkin's disease with an alternating schedule of non-cross-resistant chemotherapy regimens consisting of MOPP (mechlorethamine, procarbazine and prednisone) followed by ABVD (doxorubicin, bleomycin, vinblastine and decarbazine) has resulted in a significantly better outcome as compared to the MOPP regimen alone (Bonadonna et al., 1986). However, alternating schedules have not always proven to be more successful than sequential schedules. More recently, Bonadonna et al. (1995) reported the results of a randomized study performed over a period of 10 years, which included 405 patients treated for resectable breast cancer with more than three positive axillary lymph nodes. They compared an alternating schedule with a sequential schedule of non-cross-resistant adjuvant chemotherapy, using single-agent doxorubicin and the combination of cyclophosphamide, methotrexate, and 5-fluorouracil (CMF). The patients who were treated with four cycles of doxorubicin followed by eight courses of CMF had a median relapse-free survival of 86 months, as compared with 47 months for the patients who received the alternating schedule of two cycles of CMF followed by one dose of doxorubicin, four times. This finding does not fully support the mathematical model of Goldie and Coldman.

Another interesting alternative approach to enhancing tumor activity is the administration of liposome-encapsulated drugs. In animals with tumor implants of the J6456 lymphoma, Gabizon (1992) studied the effect of anthracyclines encapsulated in long circulating liposomes. A major pharmacokinetic drawback is that liposomes are taken up by the reticuloendothelial system, but this uptake can be dramatically decreased by coating with PEG (polyethylene glycol)-derived phospholipids. The PEG liposomes are capable of delivering the cytotoxic agent to the tumor, resulting in an antitumor effect superior to that of free doxorubicin in animals. In addition, this method of drug delivery decreases the side-effects of the drug. Gabizon et al. (1994) have reported an accumulation of Doxil (a doxorubicin liposome formation containing PEG) in malignant pleural effusions in 16 patients between three and seven days after intravenous injection.

New drugs

New cytotoxic agents will be indispensable in helping to solve the problems of drug resistance. The recent discovery of effective agents with new cellular targets opens up untapped possibilities in the fight against cancer resistance. Noteworthy examples include the topoisomerase I inhibitors and the taxanes.

The topoisomerase I inhibitors, exemplified by CPT-11 and topotecan, act by stabilizing DNA complexes in the cleavable form. These drugs have recently proven to have clinical efficacy in non-small cell lung cancer, small cell lung cancer, uterine cancer, ovarian cancer, colorectal cancer, and non-Hodgkin's lymphoma. Abigerges et al. (1995) have reported eight responses in a phase I study of CPT-11 in 64 previously treated patients. Complete remissions were observed in one patient with cervical cancer and one patient with head and neck cancer and partial responses were seen in six patients with metastatic colorectal carcinoma. Topotecan seems to be less active, with only minor responses being reported among 87 patients with non-small cell lung cancer, ovarian cancer, and renal cell carcinoma (von Hoff et al., 1994).

Taxanes enhance the formation of polymerized microtubules and subsequentially prevent them from depolymerization. Phase II studies have shown these agents to be active in ovarian cancer (Francis et al., 1994) and breast cancer (Spielman, 1994) with proven resistance to conventional agents and in previously untreated urothelium cancer (Roth et al., 1994).

Conclusions and perspectives

In great contrast to the promise of preclinical results, only moderate success has been achieved in the clinical modulation of drug resistance. Many in vitro and in vivo studies have been performed with the aim of developing ways of modulating or bypassing drug resistance. Although these studies have resulted in a better understanding of the mechanisms of drug resistance, they have also raised many new questions.

One major disappointment has been that the unravelling of the works of the Pgp-efflux pump has thus far not resulted in a clinical solution to the problem of classical MDR, despite the clinical use of such modulating agents as verapamil and cyclosporin. The problem of imaginary resistance needs further attention. Investigators should concentrate their efforts on increasing the intratumoral concentrations of antineoplastic agents. Perhaps the best example is isolated perfusion therapy, a classic approach that has become the focus of renewed interest. New possibilities for the application of higher dosages by using hematopoietic growth factors with or without stem cell transplantations need to be evaluated in randomized clinical studies. At present, too many scattered studies with limited numbers of patients are presently being performed. Whatever the approach being investigated, it remains crucial to develop methods for predicting clinical drug resistance in individual patients. Such methods would clearly benefit cancer patients, both by increasing the effectiveness of treatment and by reducing toxicity. We urgently need clinical investigations to explain why preclinical findings are not being successfully translated to the clinic.

References

Abigerges, D., Chabot, G. G., Armand, J. P. et al. (1995). Phase I and pharmacologic studies of the camptothecin analog irinotecan administered every 3 weeks in cancer patients. *J. Clin. Oncol.*, **13**, 210–21.

Alberts, D. S., Liu, P. Y., Hannigan, E. V. et al. (1995). Phase II study of intraperitoneal cisplatin (CDDP)/intravenous (IV) cyclophosphamide (CPA) vs IV CDDP/CPA in patients with optimal disease stage III ovarian cancer: A SWOG-GOG-ECOG intergroup study (Int 0051). *Proc. ASCO*, **14**, 760.

Bartlett, N. L., Lum, B. L., Fisher, G. A. et al. (1994). Phase I trial of doxorubicin with cyclosporine as a modulator of multidrug resistance. *J. Clin. Oncol.*, **12**, 835–42.

Bertino, J. R. and Romanini, A. (1989). Resistance to methotrexate in experimental models and in patients. In *Chemistry and Biology of Pteridines* (ed. H. Curtsind et al.), pp. 1089–99. Germany.

Blomqvist, C., Elomao, I., Rissanen, P. et al. (1993). Influence of treatment schedule on toxicity and efficacy of cyclophosphamide, epirubicin, and fluorouracil in metastatic breast cancer: a randomized trial comparing weekly and every-4-week administration. *J. Clin. Oncol.*, **3**, 467–73.

Bonadonna, G., Zambetti, M., Valgussa, P. et al. (1995). Sequential or alternating doxorubicin and CMF regimens in breast cancer with more than three positive nodes. *J. Am. Med. Assoc.*, **273**, 542–7.

Borst, P. and Pinedo, H. M. (1995). Drug resistance. In *Oxford Textbook of Oncology* (ed. M. Peckham et al.), pp. 586–601.

Boven, E. (1988). Screening of analogs in human ovarian cancer xenografts. In *Human Tumour Xenografts in Anticancer Drug Development* (ed. B. Winograd et al.), pp. 71–3. Springer Verlag, Berlin, Heidelberg, New York.

Braakhuis, B. J. M. and Snow, G. B. (1988). Activity of conventional drugs in head and neck cancer xenografts. In *Human Tumour Xenografts in Anticancer Drug Development* (ed. B. Winograd et al.), pp. 37–9.

Burger, H., Nooter, K., Zaman, G. J. (1994). Expression of the multidrug resistance-associated protein (MRP) in acute and chronic leukemias. *Leukaemia*, **6**, 990–7.

Campos, L., Guyotat, D., Archimbaud, E. et al. (1992). Clinical significance of multidrug resistance P-glycoprotein expression on acute nonlymphoblastic leukaemia cells at diagnosis. *Blood*, **79**, 473–6.

Cassidy, J. (1994). Chemotherapy administration: doses, infusions and choice of schedule. *Ann. Oncol.*, **5** (suppl.), S25–S30.

Chan, H. S. L., Thorner, P. S., Haddad, G. et al. (1990). Immunohistochemical detection of P-glycoprotein: prognostic correlation in soft tissue sarcoma of childhood. *J. Clin. Oncol.*, **8**, 689–704.

Chaudhary, P. M. and Roninson, I. B. (1993). Induction of multidrug resistance in human cells by transient exposure to different chemotherapeutic drugs. *J. Natl. Cancer. Inst.*, **85**, 632–9.

Childs, S., Yeh, R. L., Georges, E. and Ling, V. (1995). Identification of a sister gene to P-glycoprotein. *Cancer Res.*, **55**, 2029–34.

Christen, R. D., McClay, E. F., Plaxe, S. C. et al. (1993). Phase I/pharmacokinetic study of high-dose progesterone and doxorubicin. *J. Clin. Oncol.*, **11**, 2417–26.

Cole, S. P. C., Bhardwaj, G., Gerlach, J. H. et al. (1992). Overexpression of a novel transporter gene in a multidrug resistance human lung cancer cell line. *Science*, **258**, 1650–4.

Craft, P. S. and Harris, A. L. (1994). Clinical prognostic significance of tumour angiogenesis. *Ann. Oncol.*, **5**, 305–11.

Creech, O. and Krementz, E. T. (1958). Chemotherapy of cancer: regional perfusion utilizing an extracorporeal circuit. *Ann. Surgery*, **148**, 616–32.

Cunningham, D., Hill, M. E., Watson, M. and Norman, A. R. (1995). Survival after systematic therapy for metastatic colorectal cancer. *Lancet*, **345**, 328–9.

Curley, S. A., Byrd, D. R., Newman, R. A. et al. (1992). Reduction of systemic drug exposure after hepatic arterial infusion of doxorubicin with complete hepatic venous isolation and extracorporeal chemofiltration. *Surgery*, **114**, 579–85.

Dalton, W. S., Grogan, T. M., Meltzer, P. S. et al. (1989). Drug-resistance in multiple myeloma and non-Hodgkins lymphoma: detection of P-glycoprotein and potential circumvention by addition of verapamil to chemotherapy. *J. Clin. Oncol.*, **7**, 415–24.

Deffie, A. M., Batra, J. K. and Goldberg, G. J. (1989). Direct correlation between DNA topoisomerase II activity and cytotoxicity in adriamycin-sensitive and resistant P388 leukaemia cell lines. *Cancer Res.*, **49**, 58–62.

De Vita, V. T. (1989). The problem of resistance; keynote address. In *Drug Resistance: Mechanisms and Reversal* (ed. E. Mihich), pp. 7–33. John Liddeey C.C.

Dole, M., Nunez, G., Merchant, A. K. et al. (1994). Bcl-2 inhibits chemotherapy-induced apoptosis in neuroblastoma. *Cancer Res.*, **54**, 3253–9.

Dusre, L., Mimnaugh, E. G., Myers, C. E. and Sinha, B. K. (1989). Potentiation of doxorubicin cytotoxicity by buthionine sulfoximine in multidrug-resistant human breast tumour cells. *Cancer Res.*, **49**, 511–15.

Feller, N., Broxterman, H. J., Wahrer, D. C. and Pinedo, H. M. (1995). ATP-dependent efflux of calcein by the multidrug resistance protein (MRP): no inhibition by intracellular glutathione depletion. *FEBS Letters*, **368**, 385–8.

Fidler, I. J. (1990). Critical factors in the biology of human cancer metastasis: twenty-eight G. H. A. Clowes memorial award lecture. *Cancer Res.*, **50**, 6130–8.

Fiebig, H. H. (1988). Comparison of tumour response in nude mice and in patients.

Human Tumour Xenografts in Anticancer Drug Development (ed. B. Winograd et al.), pp. 25–30. Springer Verlag, Berlin, Heidelberg, New York.

Fisher, G. A. and Sikic, B. I. (1995). Clinical studies with modulators of multidrug resistance. In *Drug Resistance in Clinical Oncology and Hematology* (ed. B. I. Sikic), **9**, 363–82.

Fisher, D. E. (1994). Apoptosis in cancer therapy: crossing the threshold. *Cell*, **78**, 539–42.

Focan, C., Andrien, J. M., Closon, M. T. et al. (1993). Dose-response relationship of epirubicin-based first-line chemotherapy for advanced bresat cancer: a prospective randomized trial. *J. Clin. Oncol.*, **11**, 1253–63.

Francis, P., Schneider, J., Hann, L. et al. (1994). Phase II trial of docetaxel in patients with platinum-refractory advanced ovarian cancer. *J. Clin. Oncol.*, **12**, 2301–8.

Frei 3d, E. and Canellos, G. P. (1980). Dose: a critical factor in cancer chemotherapy. *Am. J. Med.*, **69**, 585–94.

Frei 3d, E., Teicher, B. A., Holden, S. A. et al. (1988). Resistance to alkylating agents: basic studies and therapeutic implications. In *Mechanisms of drug resistance in neoplastic cells* (ed. P. V. Woolley and K. D. Tew), pp. 69–86.

Gabizon, A. (1992). Selective tumour localization and improved therapeutic index of anthracyclines encapsulated in long-circulating liposomes. *Cancer Res.*, **52**, 891–6.

Gabizon, A., Catane, R., Uziely, B. et al. (1994). Prolonged circulation time and enhanced accumulation in malignant exudates of doxorubicin encapsulated in polyethylene-glycol coated liposomes. *Cancer Res.*, **54**, 987–92.

Gasparini, G. and Harris, A. L. (1995). Clinical importance of the determination of tumour angiogenesis in breast carcinoma: much more than a new prognostic tool. *J. Clin. Oncol.*, **13**, 765–82.

Glimelius, B. (1993). Biochemical modulation of 5-fluorouracil: A randomized comparison of sequential methotrexate, 5-fluorouracil and leucovorin versus sequential 5-fluorouracil and leucovorin in patients with advanced symptomatic colorectal cancer. *Ann. Oncol.*, **4**, 235–40.

Goldie, J. H. and Coldman, A. J. (1979). A mathematic model for relating the drug sensitivity of tumours to their spontaneous mutation rate. *Cancer Treat. Rep.*, **63**, 11–12.

Goldie, J. H. and Coldman, A. J. (1984). The genetic origin of drug resistance in neoplasms: implication for systemic therapy. *Cancer Res.*, **44**, 3643–53.

Goldie, J. H., Coldman, A. J. and Gudauskas, G. A. (1982). Rationale for the use of alternating non-cross-resistant chemotherapy. *Cancer Treat. Rep.*, **66**, 439–49.

Goldin, A. and Schabel, F. M. (1981). Clinical concepts derived from animal chemotherapy studies. *Cancer Treat. Rep.*, **65**, 11–19.

Gruol, D. J., Zee, M. C., Trotter, J. and Bourgeois, S. (1994). Reversal of multidrug resistance by RU 486. *Cancer Res.*, **54**, 3088–91.

Guchelaar, H. J., Hoekstra, H. J., de Vries, E. G. et al. (1992). Cisplatin and platinum pharmacokinetics during hyperthermic isolated limb perfusion for human tumours of the extremities. *Br. J. Cancer*, **65**, 898–902.

Gupta, R. S., Gupta, R., Eng, B. et al. (1988). Camptothecin-resistant mutants of Chinese hamster ovary cells containing a resistant form of topoisomerase I. *Cancer Res.*, **48**, 6404–10.

Hamburger, A. W. and Salmon, S. E. (1977). Primary bioassay of human tumour stem cells. *Science*, **197**, 461–3.

Harris, A. L. (1985). DNA repair: relationship to drug and radiation resistance, metastasis and growth factors. *Int. J. Radiat. Biol.*, **48**, 675–90.

Hohn, D., Stagg, R., Friedman, M. et al. (1989). A randomised trial of continuous intravenous versus hepatic intra-arterial floxidurine in patients with colorectal cancer metastatic to the liver: the Northern California Oncology Group Trial. *J. Clin. Oncol.*, **7**, 1646.

Ito, K., Watanabe, K., Nasim, S. et al. (1994). Prognostic significance of p53 overexpression in endometrial cancer. *Cancer Res.*, **54**, 4667–70.

Izquierdo, M. A., Zee, van der A. G. J., Vermorken, J. B. et al. (1995). Drug resistance-associated marker Lrp for prediction of response to chemotherapy and prognosis in advanced ovarian carcinoma. *J. Natl. Cancer Inst.*, **87**, 1230–7.

Jain, R. K. (1989). Delivery of novel therapeutic agents in tumours: physiological barriers and strategies. *J. Natl. Cancer Inst.*, **8**, 570–6.

Jain, R. K. (1994). Barriers to drug delivery in solid tumours. *Sci. American*, July, 42–9.

Jansen, W. J., Pinedo, H. M., Kuiper, C. M. et al. (1994). Biochemical modulation of 'classical' multidrug resistance by BIBW22BS, a potent derivate of dipyridamole. *Ann. Oncol.*, **5**, 733–9.

Jedlitschky, G., Leier, I., Buchholz, U. et al. (1994). ATP-dependent transport of glutathione S-conjugates by the multidrug resistance-associated protein. *Cancer Research*, **54**, 4833–6.

Johnston, P. G., Fisher, E. et al. (1993). Thymidylate synthase expression is an independent predictor of survival/disease free survival in patients with rectal cancer. *Proc. Am. Soc. Clin. Oncol.*, **12**, 202 (abstr. 599).

Juliano, R. L. and Ling, V. (1976). A surface glycoprotein modulating drug permeability in Chinese hamster ovary cells mutants. *Biochim. Biophys. Acta*, **455**, 152–6.

Kastan, M. B., Canman, C. E. and Leonard, C. J. (1995). P53, cell cycle control and apoptosis: implications for cancer. *Cancer Metast. Rev.*, **14**, 3–15.

Katagiri, A., Tomita, Y., Nishiyama, T. et al. (1993). Immunohistochemical detection of P-glycoprotein and GSTP1-1 in testis cancer. *Br. J. Cancer*, **68**, 125–9.

Klaase, J. M., Kroon, B. B., van Geel, A. N. et al. (1994). Prognostic factors for tumour response and limb recurrence-free interval in patients with advanced melanoma of the limbs treated with regional isolated perfusion with melphalan. *Surgery*, **115**, 39–45.

Kobayashi, J., Man, S., Graham, C. H. et al. (1993). Acquired multicellular-mediated resistance to alkylating agents in cancer. *Proc. Natl. Acad. Sci.*, **90**, 3294–8.

Kramer, R. A., Zakher, J. and Kim, G. (1988). Role of the glutathione redox cycle in acquired and de novo multidrug resistance. *Science*, **241**, 694–7.

Kuss, B. J., Deeley, R. G., Cole, S. P. et al. (1994). Deletion of gene for multidrug resistance in acute myeloid leukaemia with inversion in chromosome 16: prognostic implications. *Lancet*, **343**, 1531–4.

Labianca, R., Giaccone, G., Barni, S. et al. (1994). Double modulation of 5-fluorouracil in advanced colorectal cancer with low-dose interferon-α2b and folinic acid. The 'GISCAD' experience. *Eur. J. Cancer*, **30A**, 1611–16.

Lewis, P., Griffin, S., Marsden, P. et al. (1994). Whole-body F-fluorodeoxyglucose positron emission tomography in preoperative evaluation of lung cancer. *Lancet*, **344**, 1265–6.

Linn, S. C., Honkoop, A. H., Hoekman, K. et al. (1996). P53 and P-glycoprotein are often co-expressed and are associated with poor prognosis in breast cancer. *Brit. J. Cancer*, **74**, 63–8.

Liotta, L., Kleinerman, J. and Saidel, G. M. (1974). Quantitative relationship of intravascular tumour cells, tumour vessels, and pulmonary metastases following tumour implantation. *Cancer Res.*, **34**, 997–1004.

List, A. F., Spier, C. S. et al. (1993). Non-P-glycoprotein mediated multidrug resistance: identification of a novel drug resistance phenotype with prognostic relevance in acute myeloid leukemia. *Blood*, **82**, abstr. 443.

Lopez, R., Peters, G. J., Smitskamp-Wilms, E. et al. (1994). In vitro sequence-dependent synergistic effect suramin and camptothecin. *Eur. J. Cancer*, **11**, 1670–4.

Los, G., Tuyt, L., van Vugt, M. et al. (1993). Combination treatment of cis- and carboplatin in cancers restricted to the peritoneal cavity in the rat. *Cancer Chemother. Pharmacol.*, **32**(6), 425–33.

Markman, M. (1991). Intraperitoneal chemotherapy. *Semin. Oncol.*, **18**, 248–54.

Meenakshi, D., Vionnet, J. and Bostich Bruton, F. (1995). Nucleotide excision repair mediates clinical resistance to platinum compounds in human ovarian cancer. (Abstract) *Proc. Am. Assoc. Cancer Res.*, **36**, 1295.

Milroy, R. (1993). A randomised clinical study of verapamil in addition to combination chemotherapy in small cell lung cancer. *Br. J. Cancer*, **68**, 813–18.

Mross, K., Hamm, K. and Hossfeld, D. K. (1993). Effects of verapamil on the pharmacokinetics and metabolism of epirubicin. *Cancer Chemother. Pharmacol.*, **31**, 369–75.

Muggia, F. M. and Los, G. (1993). Platinum resistance: laboratory findings and clinical implications. *Stem Cells*, **11**, 182–93.

Mülder, H. S., Pinedo, H. M., Timmer, A. T. et al. (1996). Multidrug resistance-modifying components in human plasma with potential clinical significance. *J. Exp. Ther. Oncol.*, **1**(1), 13–22.

Norton, L. and Simon, R. (1977). Tumour size, sensitivity to therapy, and design of treatment schedules. *Cancer Treat. Rep.*, **7**, 1307–17.

O'Dwyer, P. J., La Creta, F., Nash, S. et al. (1991). Phase I study of thiotepa in combination with the glutathione transferase inhibitor ethacrynic acid. *Cancer Res.*, **51**, 6059–65.

O'Dwyer, P. J., LaCreta, F. P., Haas, N. B. et al. (1994). Clinical, pharmacokinetic and biological studies of topotecan. *Cancer Chemother. Pharmacol.*, **34**, S46–S52.

O'Reilly, M., Holmgren, L., Shing, Y. et al. (1994). Angiostatin: a novel angiogenesis inhibitor that mediates the suppression of metastases by a Lewis lung carcinoma. *Cell*, **79**, 315–28.

Peters, G. J., van der Wilt, C. L., van Groeningen, C. J. et al. (1994a). Thymidylate synthase inhibition after administration of fluorouracil with or without leucovorin in colon cancer patients: implications for treatment with fluorouracil. *J. Clin. Oncol.*, **12**, 2035–42.

Peters, G. J., Van der Wilt, C. L. and Van Groeningen, C. J. (1994b). Predictive value of thymidylate synthase and dihydropyrimidine dehydrogenase. *Eur. J. Cancer*, **10**, 1408–11.

Petros, W. P. and Peters, W. P. (1993). Haematopoietic colony-stimulating factors and dose intensity. *Semin. Oncol.*, **20**, 94–9.

Peyrat, J., Bonneterre, J., Lubin, R. et al. (1995). Prognostic significance of circulating P53 antibodies in patients undergoing surgery for locoregional breast cancer. *Lancet*, **345**, 621–2.

Pezzoni, G. and Giuliani, F. C. (1988). Predictability of clinical response of several human and murine tumour models to four anthracycline derivatives. *Human Tumour Xenografts in Anticancer Drug Development* (ed. B. Winograd et al.), pp. 75–8. Springer Verlag, Berlin, Heidelberg, New York.

Pinedo, H. M. and Peters, G. J. (1988). 5-Fluorouracil: biochemistry and pharmacology. *J. Clin. Oncol.*, **6**, 1653–64.

Pirker, R., Wallner, J., Geissler, K. et al. (1991). MDR1 gene expression and treatment outcome in acute myeloid leukaemia. *J. Natl. Cancer Inst.*, **83**, 708–12.

Pizao, P. E., Lyaruu, D. M., Peters, G. J. et al. (1992). Growth, morphology and chemosensitivity studies on postconfluent cells cultured in 'V'-bottomed microtiter plates. *Br. J. Cancer*, **66**, 660–5.

Pizao, P. E., Smitkamp-Wilms, E., van Arke-Otte, J. et al. (1994). Antiproliferative activity of the topoisomerase I inhibitors topotecan and camptothecin, on sub- and postfluent tumour cell cultures. *Biochem. Pharmacol.*, **48**, 1145–54.

Plumb, J. A., Milroy, R. and Kaye, S. B. (1990). The activity of verapamil as a resistance modifier in vitro in drug resistant human tumour cell lines is not stereospecific. *Biochem. Pharmacol.*, **39**, 787–92.

Roth, B. J., Dreicher, R., Einhorn, L. H. et al. (1994). Significant activity of paclitaxel in advanced transitional-cell carcinoma of the urothelium: a phase II trial of the Eastern Cooperative Oncology Group. *J. Clin. Oncol.*, **12**, 2264–70.

Schabel, F. M. Jr, Griswold, D. P. Jr., Corbett, T. H. and Laster, W. R. Jr (1983). Increasing therapeutic response rates to anticancer drugs by applying the basic principles of pharmacology. *Pharmacol. Ther.*, **20**, 283–305.

Schabel, F. M. Jr, Griswold, D. P. Jr, Corbett, T. H. and Laster, W. R. Jr (1984). Increasing the therapeutic response rates to anticancer drugs by applying the basic principles of pharmacology. *Cancer*, **54**, 1160–7.

Scheffer, G. L., Wijngaard, P. L., Flens, M. J. et al. (1995). The drug resistance related protein LRP is the human major vault protein. *Nature Medicine*, **6**, 578–82.

Scheithauer, W., Schenk, T. and Czejka, M. (1993). Pharmacokinetic interaction between epirubicin and the multidrug resistance reverting agent D-verapamil. *Br. J. Cancer*, **68**, 8–9.

Scheper, R. J., Broxterman, H. J., Scheffer, G. L. et al. (1993). Overexpression of a Mr (110 000) vesicular protein in non P-glycoprotein-mediated multidrug resistance. *Cancer Res.*, **53**, 1475–9.

Schinkel, A. H., Smit, J. J. M., van Tellingen, O. et al. (1994). Disruption of the mouse *mdr1a* P-glycoprotein gene leads to a deficiency in the blood–brain barrier and to increased sensitivity to drugs. *Cell*, **77**, 491–502.

Schuurhuis, G. J., Broxterman, H. J., Ossenkoppele, G. J. et al. (1995). Functional multidrug resistance phenotype associated with combined overexpression of Pgp/MDR1 and MRP together with cytosine–aravinoside sensitivity may predict clinical response in acute myeloid leukaemia. *Clin. Cancer Res.*, **1**, 81–93.

Shirai, A., Naito, M., Tatsuta, T. et al. (1994). Transport of cyclosporin A across the brain capillary endothelial cell monolayer by P-glycoprotein. *Biochim. Biophys. Acta*, **1222**, 400–4.

Silvestrini, R., Veneroni, S., Daidone, M. G. et al. (1994). The bcl-2 protein; a prognostic indicator strongly related to p53 protein in lymph node-negative breast cancer patients. *J. Natl. Cancer Inst.*, **86**, 499–504.

Skipper, H. E., Schabel, F. M. Jr and Wilcox, W. S. (1964). Experimental evaluation of potential anticancer agents. XIII On the criteria of kinetics associated with curability of experimental leukaemia. *Cancer Chemother. Rep.*, **35**, 1–111.

Spears, C. P., Gustavsson, B. G., Berne, M. et al. (1988). Mechanisms of innate resistance to thymidylate synthase inhibition after 5-fluorouracil. *Cancer Res.*, **48**, 5894–900.

Spielman, M. (1994). Taxol (paclitaxel) in patients with metastatic breast carcinoma who have failed prior chemotherapy: interim results of a multinational study. *Oncology*, **51**, (suppl 1), 25–8.

Stehlin, J. S. and Lee, R. (1960). Regional chemotherapy for cancer: experiences with 116 perfusions. *Ann. Surg.*, **151**, 605–19.

Swain, S. M., Lippman, M. E., Egan, E. F. et al. (1989). Fluorouracil and high-dose leucovorin in previously treated patients with metastatic breast cancer. *J. Clin. Oncol.*, **7**, 890–9.

Takano, H., Kohn, K., Ono, M. et al. (1991). Increased phosphorylation of DNA topoisomerase II in etoposide-resistant mutants of human cancer KB cells. *Cancer Res.*, **51**(15), 3951–7.

Takats, de P. G., Kerr, D. J., Poole, C. J. et al. (1994). Hepatic arterial chemotherapy for metastatic colorectal carcinoma. *Br. J. Cancer*, **69**, 372–8.

Tamura, H., Kohchi, C., Yamada, R. et al. (1991). Molecular cloning of a cDNA of a camptothecin-resistant human DNA topoisomerase I and identification of mutation sites. *Nucl. Acids Res.*, **19**(1), 69–75.

Tan, K. B., Mattern, M. R., Eng, W. K. et al. (1989). Nonproductive rearrangement of DNA topoisomerase I and II genes: correlation with resistance to topoisomerase inhibitors. *J. Natl. Cancer Inst.*, **81**, 1732–5.

Tannock, I. F. and Roth, D. (1989). Acid pH in tumours and its potential for therapeutic exploitation. *Cancer Res.*, **49**, 4373–84.

Thompson, J. F. and Gianouts, M. P. (1992). Isolated limb perfusion for melanoma: effectiveness and toxicity of cisplatin compared with that of melphalan and other drugs. *World J. Surg.*, **16**, 227–33.

Tiirikainen, M. I., Elonen, E., Ruutu, T. et al. (1993). Clinical significance of P-glycoprotein expression in acute leukaemia as analyzed by immunocytochemistry. *Eur. J. Haematol.*, **50**, 279–85.

Vendrik, C. P. J., Bergers, J. J., de Jong, W. H. and Steerenberg, P. A. (1992). Resistance to cytostatic drugs at the cellular level. *Cancer Chemother. Pharmacol.*, **29**, 413–29.

Von Hoff, D. D., Burris III, H. A. et al. (1994). Preclinical and phase I trials of topoisomerase I inhibitors. *Cancer Chemother. Pharmacol.*, **34**, S41–S45.

Wadler, S., Schwartz, E. L., Goldman, M. et al. (1989). Fluorouracil and recombinant alfa-2a-interferon: an active regimen against advanced colorectal carcinoma. *J. Clin. Oncol.*, **7**, 1769–75.

Winograd, B., Bouen, E., Lobbezou, M. W. and Pinedo, H. M. (1987). Human tumor xenografts in the nude mouse and their value as test models in anticancer drug development (review). *In Vivo*, **1**, 1–13.

7

The reversal of multidrug resistance

WILLIAM S. DALTON

Introduction

The use of cytotoxic drugs is a relatively recent advance in the treatment of cancer. Prior to the 20th century, essentially the only treatment for cancer was surgical removal of the tumor. Not until the discovery of the mustards in the 1940s did the use of chemicals become promising in the treatment of cancer (Marshall, 1964; DeVita, 1978). Over the past five decades new cytotoxic agents have been developed, either by isolating chemicals from natural products, such as the vinca alkaloids, or by synthesizing novel compounds, such as folic acid antagonists. In spite of the discovery of almost a hundred new compounds that are used in the clinic today, most cancers that have spread from the original site of origin are considered incurable. Many of these drugs are capable of inducing remissions in numerous types of cancers; however, these remissions are usually not permanent and the patient ultimately dies of drug-resistant disease. The development of drug-resistant cancers is considered to be the most significant obstacle to the cure of cancer today.

One of the most well-documented causes of drug resistance is the multidrug resistant phenotype (MDR) (Gerlach et al., 1986; Dalton and Miller, 1991). This phenotype is due to the overexpression of P-glycoprotein (Pgp) the protein encoded by the human *MDR1* gene (Gros et al., 1986; Ueda et al., 1987). The *MDR1* gene is a member of the ATP-binding cassette superfamily of genes. This superfamily of genes encodes for membrane transport proteins that are expressed in normal tissues throughout the body. The overexpression of this gene in cancer cells is believed to result in resistance to many diverse cytotoxic drugs, most of them natural products. Cancers that are derived from tissues that normally express Pgp, such as renal cancer, have a high incidence of Pgp at time of diagnosis. Other cancers, such as leukemias and myelomas, are believed to acquire this resistant mechanism after treatment with natural product agents including anthracyclines and vincristine. Cancer cells which overexpress Pgp accumulate less intracellular cytotoxic drug via the pumping action of Pgp. In order to overcome MDR, means of preventing the expression of MDR1/Pgp or inactivating the pumping action of Pgp must be developed.

A major development in the field was the finding of Tsuruo et al., showing that verapamil, a calcium channel blocker, can sensitize vincristine-resistant P388 leukemia cells to the cytotoxic actions of vincristine and vinblastine (Tsuruo et al., 1981, 1983). They also showed the MDR reversal effect of verapamil in mice bearing vincristine-resistant Ehrlich ascites tumors. Furthermore, Tsuruo and colleagues reported that agents such as the phenothiazines, enhance anticancer drug cytotoxicity by increasing their accumulation and retention in P388 leukemia MDR cells. Since these findings, a wide variety of agents have been identified to reverse the Pgp mediated MDR (Beck, 1991). This chapter will focus on the clinical studies performed to reverse MDR and consider potential outcomes and possible future clinical designs to overcome clinical drug resistance.

Detection of MDR1/P-glycoprotein in the clinic

Not all resistance to cytotoxic drugs is mediated by the overexpression of MDR1/Pgp. It is therefore necessary to target tumor types known to overexpress Pgp for studies to reverse MDR. Since the cloning of the *MDR1* gene, assays are now available to detect MDR1/Pgp in cancer cells (Goldstein et al., 1989; Dalton and Grogan, 1991; Chan et al., 1994). These assays use monoclonal antibodies for the detection of the Pgp protein and molecular probes for detection of the MDR mRNA. As with any assay, there are issues of target sensitivity and specificity that must be dealt with in the clinical situation. The detection of Pgp in clinical specimens is further complicated by the known expression of MDR1/Pgp in normal tissues (Thiebaut et al., 1987; Cordon-Cardo et al., 1990). Clinical assays must be able to distinguish Pgp expression in tumor cells versus normal cells. This is particularly relevant in hematopoietic cancer. MDR1 is expressed at high levels in the CD34 positive hematopoietic stem cell (Chaudhary and Roninson, 1991). Klimecki et al. have also demonstrated that certain normal peripheral blood cells, the CD56 positive and the CD8 positive lymphocytes, have high levels of functioning Pgp on the surface of their cells (Klimecki et al., 1994). Thus, any assay which uses bulk tissue homogenates for the detection of MDR1/Pgp, such as standard mRNA assays or immunoblot assays, may be measuring levels in normal cells. For this reason, assays that are able to discriminate normal cells from cancer cells are more reliable in determining the presence and significance of Pgp in drug-resistant cancer. Immunocytochemical assays using monoclonal antibodies best meet the necessary criteria for clinical detection of Pgp. RNA in situ hybridization is another possibility, but this assay is labor intensive and there may be problems with sensitivity. Flow cytometric assays that are capable of dual labeling (using tumor specific markers as well as markers for Pgp) may also meet the criteria of distinguishing Pgp expression in malignant cells versus normal cells. A recent international workshop on the clinical detection of MDR1/Pgp was held in Memphis, Tennessee and it was recommended that immunocytochemistry was the method of choice for solid tumors and that flow cytometric assays using monoclonal antibodies that recognize an external epitope (for example MRK16, IUC2, 4E3) were best suited for hematopoietic tumors (Beck et al., 1995). Confirmatory assays such as RT/PCR were also recommended to enhance the specificity of these assays.

Assays that demonstrate a functional Pgp molecule in tumor cells may also be necessary. Willman's group at the University of New Mexico have reported the detection of Pgp on the surface of leukemic cells that appears to be non-functional (Leith et al., 1995). Post-translational modification, such as phosphorylation, may be important in influencing the function of the Pgp molecule (Hamada et al., 1987). Three color flow cytometric assays using specific antibodies for Pgp and cell lineage, as well as a transport dye such as Rhodamine 123, may be able to address the issue of a functional Pgp molecule in malignant cells.

Reversing multidrug resistance

Preclinical studies

As mentioned above, Tsuruo et al. (1981) made the seminal observation that verapamil could reverse MDR by blocking the pumping action of Pgp. Since that time a number of agents have been discovered to over-come MDR by inhibiting Pgp function (Beck, 1991). Most of these agents can be classified as belonging to five general groups: (1) calcium

Table 7.1. *Chemosensitizing agents that inhibit P-glycoprotein function*

Type/Chemical class	Example
Calcium channel blockers	Phenyl alkylamines, e.g. verapamil
Calmodulin inhibitors	Phenothiazines
Immunosuppressants	Cyclosporins, FK506
Indole alkaloids	Reserpine
Steroids	Progesterone
Detergents	Tween 80
Antimalarials	Quinine
Anti-arrhythmics	Amiodarone

channel blockers, (2) immunosuppressive agents, (3) calmodulin inhibitors, (4) steroidal agents, and (5) miscellaneous (see Table 7.1). The exact mechanism by which these agents inhibit Pgp is not known, but they probably can be specified as competitive versus non-competitive inhibitors. Competitive inhibitors would be expected to bind Pgp at sites which are also involved in the binding of cytotoxic agents. These agents may themselves be substrates for Pgp and may be actively pumped out of the cell. Verapamil and cyclosporin A are classified as competitive inhibitors and the intracellular concentration of these agents is less in MDR positive cells (Yusa and Tsuruo, 1989; Ford and Hait, 1990). Progesterone, on the other hand, is known to bind Pgp but is not a substrate for Pgp (Ueda et al., 1992). One possible non-competitive mechanism would involve the binding of the inhibitor at sites distant to cytotoxic drug-binding sites, thereby altering the allosteric conformation of the protein. This alteration in Pgp structure could prevent the binding and efflux of cytotoxic drugs. Another possible mechanism of Pgp inhibition involves alterations in phosphorylation. Protein kinase C is believed to phosphorylate Pgp and some of the reversing agents known to reverse MDR also inhibit this enzyme (Aftab et al., 1991). Structure–function analysis of Pgp should help determine the means by which certain agents bind and inhibit Pgp function (Kajiji et al., 1994). This information should be helpful in designing more effective new agents, and may allow for a rationale approach to combining MDR reversing agents that have different mechanisms of inhibition.

In vivo animal models have been developed to evaluate chemosensitizing drugs to reverse Pgp function (Cress et al., 1988; Galski et al., 1989; Horton et al., 1989). The standard murine model involves inoculating

murine tumor cells into the peritoneum of mice and then injecting cytotoxic drugs with or without the chemosensitizer intraperitoneally. This
model has shown activity for a number of drugs known to reverse MDR
in vitro, but has been criticized as being a 'furry test-tube' and does not
truly test the in vivo capacity of chemosensitizers to reverse MDR.
To address this concern, murine models have been developed using
extraperitoneal tumors and injecting drugs at a site distant from the
tumor inoculum. These studies have demonstrated activity for some
chemosensitizers; however, they also illustrate that other critical factors,
besides inhibition of Pgp function in tumor cells, can contribute to
improve clinical effectiveness or toxicity (Horton et al., 1989). These
factors include pharmacokinetic interactions between the chemosensitizing drugs and the cytotoxic drugs. Chemosensitizing drugs can delay
the clearance of cytotoxic drugs thereby increasing the concentration of
the latter in both tumor and normal tissues. It is conceivable that by
inhibiting Pgp function in normal tissues, such as in the liver and kidney,
cytotoxic drug elimination is impeded and the duration of drug exposure
(as measured by the $C \times T$) is prolonged. This pharmacokinetic interaction might explain, at least in part, any increased clinical efficacy
and/or toxicity attributable to the additional use of a chemosensitizer.
These preclinical studies illustrated that future clinical studies would
need to consider this potential confounding variable when interpreting
results.

Clinical studies

The very first clinical studies investigating the potential use of chemosensitizing agents in combination with cytotoxic drugs used drugs that had
been developed for other uses, but had also demonstrated the ability to
reverse MDR in vitro. Table 7.2 lists some of the studies using the
'first generation' agents verapamil and cyclosporin A. The most promising results occurred in the treatment of hematopoietic malignancies
(Dalton and Sikic, 1994). Studies in hematopoietic cancers were the first
to demonstrate 'proof of concept' by measuring Pgp in cancer cells
and response to cytotoxics plus chemosensitizers. Myeloma and acute
leukemia were particularly suitable for study because of the ability to
measure Pgp on the surface of tumor cells and the effect of chemosensitizers on cytotoxic drug uptake into these cells. Dalton et al. (1989)
demonstrated that high dose infusion verapamil in combination with
vincristine/adriamycin/dexamethasone (VAD) could reverse MDR in

Table 7.2. *Clinical studies to reverse MDR1/Pgp using 'first generation' agents*

Agent	Study type	Reference
Racemic verapamil	1. Phase I: Vlb + Verap	Benson et al. (1985)
	2. Ovarian cancer: Dox + Verap	Ozols et al. (1987)
	3. Solid tumors: Dox + Verap	Presant et al. (1986)
	4. Pediatric leukemia: Vlb + VP-16 + Verap	Cairo, et al. (1989)
	5. Myeloma/NHL: VAD + Verap	Dalton et al. (1989)
	6. NHL/Hodgkin's: C-VAD + Verap	Miller et al. (1991)
	7. Myeloma: VAD + Vemp Salmon et al., (1991)	
Cyclosporin A	1. Phase I: VP-16 + CsA	Lum et al. (1992)
	2. Phase I: Vlb + CsA	Samuels et al. (1993)
	3. Phase I: Dox + CsA	Erlichman et al. (1993)
	4. Phase I: Dox + CsA	Bartlett et al. (1994)
	5. AML: AraC/Daun + CsA	List et al. (1993)
	6. AML: Mitox/VP-16 + CsA	Marie et al. (1993)
	7. Myeloma: VAD + CsA	Sonneveld et al. (1992)

AraC, cytosine arabinoside; CsA, cyclosporin A; Daun, daunomycin; Dox, doxorubicin; Mitox, mitoxantrone; Verap, verapamil.

a subset of patients with myeloma who had progressed on VAD alone. A follow-up study by Salmon et al. (1991) confirmed these initial results, but also demonstrated that the responses were short lived (approximately 6 months) and toxicity due to verapamil was high. It was concluded that high dose verapamil could transiently reverse MDR, but that the inherent cardiac toxicity of verapamil prevented the routine use of this drug for reversing resistance (Pennock et al., 1991). A recent randomized study in relapsing myeloma patients using low dose oral verapamil in combination with VAD showed no improvement in outcome compared to VAD alone (Dalton et al., 1995). Newer, more effective, and less toxic agents were needed to reverse MDR in the clinic.

Cyclosporin A is another 'first generation' agent which may be effective in reversing clinical MDR. Studies using high-dose infusion cyclosporin A as a chemosensitizer have shown promising results in patients with drug-resistant myeloma and acute myelogenous leukemia (AML). In three studies, the number of Pgp positive cells was reduced by the combination of cyclosporin A and chemotherapy (Sonneveld et al., 1992; List et al., 1993; Marie et al., 1993). These studies suggested that cyclosporin A is effective in eliminating Pgp positive cells in drug-resistant patients. Toxicity due to cyclosporin A was primarily hepatic with hyperbilirubinemia being predominant. Toxicities that could be attributed to the cytotoxic agents also appeared to increase when cyclosporin A was added, namely myelosuppression, nausea/vomiting, and neurotoxicity (Sonneveld et al., 1992; List et al., 1993; Weber, Dimopoulos and Alexanian, 1993). This increase in chemotherapeutic drug toxicity is probably due to the decreased clearance of the cytotoxic drugs caused by cyclosporin A (Lum et al., 1992; 1993; Samuels et al., 1993). While these results are preliminary, and confounding factors such as alteration in cytotoxic drug clearance need to be considered, it does appear that eliminating Pgp-positive cells from malignancies may be a possibility. As with verapamil, the studies with cyclosporin A demonstrate that more effective and less toxic chemosensitizing agents need to be developed in order to eliminate clinical MDR.

'Second generation' chemosensitizing agents have been developed to try and improve efficacy and reduce toxicity. These agents are basically derivatives of the 'first generation' agents. Dex-verapamil is a stereoisomer of racemic verapamil and has approximately 25% of the cardiac activity of the racemic mixture, but appears to be equally potent in reversing MDR (Gruber, Peterson and Reizenstein, 1988). Because the primary toxicity of racemic verapamil is cardiotoxicity, the reduced cardiac activity seen with dex-verapamil should enhance the therapeutic index. Clinical trials are now ongoing with this agent (Dalton et al., 1992; Wilson et al., 1993). Another 'second generation' agent is the cyclosporin derivative, PSC-833 (Boesch et al., 1991). This is a non-immunosuppressive drug that appears to have more intrinsic MDR reversing activity than cyclosporin A. Phase I/II clinical trials are currently being conducted and phase III randomized trials in myeloma and acute myelogenous leukemia are scheduled to begin in 1996.

Drug development for 'third generation' chemosensitizers is currently ongoing (Hyafil et al., 1993). These agents, unlike the 'first generation' agents, are specifically designed to inhibit P-glycoprotein in tumors. The characteristics of the 'ideal' third generation chemosensitizer would probably include the following: (1) high level of efficacy based on the ability to inhibit Pgp function at low doses – this would ensure the possibility that effective doses could be obtained at tumor sites; (2) no pharmacokinetic interactions with cytotoxic drugs – this would lessen the chance of increasing the toxicity of cytotoxic drugs by increasing cytotoxic drug exposure; and (3) preferential inhibition of tumor Pgp function compared to normal Pgp function – this would reduce the novel toxicities due to altered cytotoxic drug distribution. While it is unlikely that all these 'ideal' characteristics can be met, the design of drugs for the specific use of reversing clinical MDR should result in more effective, less toxic chemosensitizers for the clinic.

Design of future clinical trials must consider several critical factors. First, the tumor type treated must express Pgp at some time during the progression of disease. It is conceivable that in addition to reversing Pgp-mediated MDR, chemosensitizing agents may actually prevent the emergence of Pgp in tumors that eventually acquire this phenotype. Using chemosensitizers in 'up-front' chemotherapy may omit Pgp as a mechanism of resistance in certain tumors that are felt to acquire this phenotype by drug selection. In order to address this possibility, Pgp will need to be measured serially in patients enrolled in phase III trials. Second, the question of altered pharmacokinetics and delayed clearance of cytotoxic drugs due to the addition of the chemosensitizer must be addressed prior to performing phase III studies. Adjusting doses of cytotoxic drugs to achieve similar drug exposure (area under the curve, AUC) in both arms of a phase III trial is an ideal approach, but may not be feasible because of the patient-to-patient variability in drug disposition. This approach may be particularly problematic in patients with AML where a reduction in dose of the anthracycline may seriously undertreat a patient who may not have a significant alteration in pharmacokinetics. A more practical approach for dose modification may be to try and achieve dose equivalent toxicity with and without the chemosensitizer. Phase I trials would first determine a dose of chemosensitizer necessary to achieve a required drug concentration known to reverse MDR in preclinical studies. Doses of the cytotoxic drug in combination with the chemosensitizer would be initially low compared to usual standard doses (initial dose being dependent on the anticipated change in AUC) and gradually increased to the point where equal toxicity is seen compared to the cytotoxic drug alone. Once these doses are determined in Phase I/II trials, then Phase III trials can be conducted to determine efficacy.

There are at least three potential outcomes for Phase III trials examining the efficacy of chemosensitizers in reversing clinical MDR. In order to interpret these clinical outcomes adequately it will be important to determine the presence of Pgp in patient specimens at serial time points, before and after treatment. The three potential outcomes are as follows:

1. The use of chemosensitizers eliminates Pgp positive cells and improves overall survival.
2. Chemosensitizers are ineffective in eliminating Pgp positive cells and clinical outcome is not improved. This possibility would be demonstrated by finding Pgp positive cells at the time of tumor progression in patients who have received the combination of chemosensitizer plus cytotoxic drugs.
3. Chemosensitizers eliminate Pgp positive cells from tumors but clinical outcome is not improved. This possibility would be demonstrated by performing serial Pgp assays in patients before and after treatment with chemosensitizers plus cytotoxic drugs. If the treatment converts a Pgp positive tumor to a Pgp negative tumor, then the goal of eliminating Pgp as a mechanism of resistance has been achieved, but a non-Pgp mechanism of resistance has emerged at the time of relapse. In this case, it is likely that eliminating Pgp is necessary, but not sufficient to overcome clinical drug resistance.

In summary, numerous studies have shown that Pgp is present in drug-resistant tumors. Studies in hematopoietic malignancies, especially myeloma, AML and non-Hodgkin's lymphoma have further demonstrated that the presence of Pgp is a poor prognostic factor. Overcoming or preventing this mechanism of resistance may improve chemotherapeutic response and overall survival. Initial studies with 'first generation' chemosensitizers have produced promising results and encourages the development of more effective agents to be tried in the clinic. The development of second and third generation agents that are more effective and less toxic than the first generation agents should improve on the results from the initial studies performed to date. Future trials of these agents must consider several critical factors: (1) a working definition of clinical resistance must be determined prior to beginning the study so that patient populations may be compared; (2) accurate assays for Pgp detection in patients enrolled in trials must be performed in order to interpret clinical outcome; (3) the pharmacokinetic consequences of adding a chemosensitizer to cytotoxic drugs must be assessed; and (4) the existence of non-Pgp mechanisms that are not affected by available chemosensitizers must be evaluated in patient specimens to determine their clinical relevance. Performance of these clinical trials will advance our ability to improve clinical outcome of patients with drug-resistant malignancies.

References

Aftab, D. T., Ballas, L. M., Loomis, C. R. and Hait, W. N. (1991). Structure–activity relationships of phenothiazines and related drugs for inhibition of protein kinase C. *Mol. Pharmacol.*, **40**, 798–805.

Bartlett, N. L., Lum, B. L., Fisher, G. A. et al. (1994). Phase I trial of doxorubicin with cyclosporine as a modulator of multidrug resistance. *J. Clin. Oncol.*, **12**, 835–42.

Beck, W. T. (1991). Modulators of P-glycoprotein associated multidrug resistance. In *Molecular and Clinical Advances in Anticancer Drug Resistance* (ed. R. F. Ozols), pp. 151–70. Kluwer Academic Publishers, Philadelphia.

Beck, W. T., Grogan, T., Willman, C. et al. (1996). The St Jude workshop on methods to detect P-glycoprotein-associated multidrug resistance: Findings and consensus recommendations. *Cancer Res.*, **56**, 3010–20.

Benson, A. B., Trump, D. L., Koeller, J. M. et al. (1985). Phase I study of vinblastine and verapamil given by concurrent iv infusion. *Cancer Treat. Rep.*, **69**, 795–9.

Boesch, D., Muller, K., Pourtier-Manzanedo, A. and Loor, F. (1991). Restoration of daunomycin retention in multidrug-resistant P388 cells by submicromolar concentrations of SDZ PSC 833, a nonimmunosuppressive cyclosporin derivative. *Exp. Cell Res.*, **196**, 26–32.

Cairo, M. S., Siegel, S., Anas, N. and Sender, L. (1989). Clinical trial of continuous infusion verapamil, bolus vinblastine, and continuous infusion VP-16 in drug-resistant pediatric tumors. *Cancer Res.*, **49**, 1063–6.

Chan, J. S. L., Haddad, G., Zheng, L. et al. (1994). A sensitive multilayer immunofluorescent method for flow cytometric detection of P-glycoprotein in myeloma and tumor cells. *Lab. Invest.* (in press).

Chaudhary, P. M. and Roninson, I. B. (1991). Expression and activity of P-glycoprotein, a multidrug efflux pump, in human hematopoietic stem cells. *Cell*, **66**, 85–94.

Cordon-Cardo, C., O'Brien, J. P., Boccia, J. et al. (1990). Expression of the multidrug resistance gene product (P-glycoprotein) in human normal and tumor tissues. *J. Histochem. Cytochem.*, **38**, 1277–87.

Cress, A. E., Roberts, R. A., Bowden, G. T. and Dalton, W. S. (1988). Modification of keratin by the chemotherapeutic drug mitoxantrone. *Biochem. Pharmacol.*, **37**, 3043–6.

Dalton, W. S. and Grogan, T. M. (1991). Does P-glycoprotein predict response to chemotherapy, and if so, is there a reliable way to detect it? *J. Natl. Can. Inst.*, **83**(2), 80–1.

Dalton, W. S. and Miller, T. P. (1991). Multidrug resistance. In *Cancer: Principles and Practice of Oncology*, PPO Updates (ed. V. T. DeVita Jr, S. Hellman and S. A. Rosenbery), pp. 1–13. J. B. Lippincott, Philadelphia.

Dalton, W. S. and Sikic, I. S. (1994). Controversies in science: The multidrug-resistance gene (MDR 1) represents a potential target for reversing drug resistance in human malignancies. *J. NIH Res.*, **6**, 54–61.

Dalton, W. S., Grogan, T. M., Meltzer, P. S. et al. (1989). Drug-resistance in multiple myeloma and non-Hodgkin's lymphoma: detection of P-glycoprotein and potential circumvention by addition of verapamil to chemotherapy. *J. Clin. Oncol.*, **7**(4), 415–24.

Dalton, W. S., Birchfield, G., Miller, T. P. et al. (1992). Phase I trial of R-verapamil as a chemosensitizing agent. *Proc. Amer. Assoc. Can. Res.*, **33**, 234.

Dalton, W. S., Crowley, J. J., Salmon, S. S. et al. (1995). A phase III randomized
    study of oral verapamil as a chemosensitizer to reverse drug resistance in
    patients with refractory myeloma. A Southwest Oncology Group study.
    Cancer, 75(3), 815–20.
DeVita, V. T. Jr (1978). The evolution of therapeutic research in cancer. N. Engl.
    J. Med., 298, 907–10.
Erlichman, C., Moore, M., Thiessen, J. J. et al. (1993). Phase I pharmacokinetic
    study of cyclosporin A combined with doxorubicin. Cancer Res., 53(20),
    4837–42.
Ford, J. M. and Hait, W. N. (1990). Pharmacology of drugs that alter multidrug
    resistance in cancer. [Review]. Pharmacol. Rev., 42, 155–99.
Galski, H., Sullivan, M., Willingham, M. C. et al. (1989). Expression of a human
    multidrug resistance cDNA (MDR1) in the bone marrow of transgenic
    mice: resistance to daunomycin-induced leukopenia. Mol. Cell. Biol., 9,
    4357–63.
Gerlach, J. H., Kartner, N., Bell, D. R. and Ling, V. (1986). Multidrug resistance.
    Cancer Surv., 5, 25–46.
Goldstein, L. J., Galski, H., Fojo, A. et al. (1989). Expression of a multidrug
    resistance gene in human cancers. J. Natl. Can. Inst., 81(2), 116–24.
Gros, P., Neriah, Y. B., Croop, J. M. and Housman, D. E. (1986). Isolation and
    expression of a complementary DNA that confers multidrug resistance.
    Nature, 323, 728–31.
Gruber, A., Peterson, C. and Reizenstein, P. (1988). D-verapamil and L-verapamil
    are equally effective in increasing vincristine accumulation in leukemic cells in
    vitro. Int. J. Cancer, 41, 224–6.
Hamada, H., Hagiwara, K., Nakajima, T. and Tsuruo, T. (1987). Phosphorylation of
    the Mr 170 000 to 180 000 glycoprotein specific to multidrug-resistant tumor
    cells: effects of verapamil, trifluoperazine, and phorbol esters. Cancer Res.,
    47(11), 2860–5.
Horton, J. K., Thimmaiah, K. N., Houghton, J. A. et al. (1989). Modulation by
    verapamil of vincristine pharmacokinetics and toxicity in mice bearing human
    tumor xenografts. Biochem. Pharmacol., 38, 1727–36.
Hyafil, F., Vergely, C., Du Vignaud, P. and Grand-Perret, T. (1993). In vitro and in
    vivo reversal of multidrug resistance by GF 120918, an acridonecarboxamide
    derivative. Cancer Res., 53, 4595–602.
Kajiji, S., Dreslin, J. A., Grizzuti, K. and Gros, P. (1994). Structurally distinct
    MDR modulators show specific patterns of reversal against P-glycoproteins
    bearing unique mutations at serine939/941. Biochemistry, 33(17),
    5041–8.
Klimecki, W. T., Futscher, B. W., Grogan, T. M. and Dalton, W. S. (1994).
    P-glycoprotein expression and function in circulating blood cells from normal
    volunteers. Blood, 83(9), 2451–8.
Leith, C. P., Chen, I.-M., Kopecky, K. et al. (1995). Correlation of multidrug
    resistance protein expression with functional dye/drug efflux in acute myeloid
    leukemia by multiparameter flow cytometry: Identification of discordant
    MDR/efflux and MDR1/Efflux-cases. Blood, 86, 2329–42.
List, A. F., Spier, C., Greer, J. et al. (1993). Phase I/II trial of cyclosporine as a
    chemotherapy-resistance modifier in acute leukemia. J. Clin. Oncol., 11,
    1652–60.
Lum, B. L., Kaubisch, S., Yahanda, A. M. et al. (1992). Alteration of etoposide
    pharmacokinetics and pharmacodynamics by cyclosporine in a phase I trial to
    modulate multidrug resistance. J. Clin. Oncol., 10, 1635–42.

Lum, B. L., Fisher, G. A., Brophy, N. A. et al. (1993). Clinical trials of modulation of multidrug resistance. Pharmacokinetic and pharmacodynamic considerations. *Cancer*, **72**, 3502–14.

Marie, J. P., Bastie, J. N., Coloma, F. et al. (1993). Cyclosporin A as a modifier agent in the salvage treatment of acute leukemia (AL). *Leukemia*, **7**, 821–4.

Marshall, E. K. (1964). Historical perspectives in chemotherapy. In *Advances in Chemotherapy*, Vol. 1 (ed. A. Goldin and I. F. Hawking), pp. 1–8. Academic Press, New York.

Miller, T. P., Grogan, T. M., Dalton, W. S. et al. (1991). P-glycoprotein expression in malignant lymphoma and reversal of clinical drug resistance with chemotherapy plus high-dose verapamil. *J. Clin. Oncol.*, **9**(1), 17–24.

Ozols, R. F., Cunnion, R. E., Klecker, R. W. Jr et al. (1987). Verapamil and Adriamycin in the treatment of drug-resistant ovarian cancer patients. *J. Clin. Oncol.*, **5**, 641–7.

Pennock, G. D., Dalton, W. S., Roeske, W. R. et al. (1991). Systemic toxic effects associated with high-dose verapamil infusion and chemotherapy administration. *J. Natl. Can. Inst.*, **83**(2), 105–10.

Presant, C. A., Kennedy, P. S., Wiseman, C. et al. (1986). Verapamil reversal of clinical doxorubicin resistance in human cancer. A Wilshire Oncology Medical Group pilot phase I–II study. *Am. J. Clin. Oncol.*, **9**, 355–7.

Salmon, S. E., Dalton, W. S., Grogan, T. M. et al. (1991). Multidrug-resistant myeloma: laboratory and clinical effects of verapamil as a chemosensitizer. *Blood*, **78**(1), 44–50.

Samuels, B. L., Mick, R., Vogelzang, N. J. et al. (1993). Modulation of vinblastine resistance with cyclosporine: a phase I study. *Clin. Pharmacol. Ther.*, **54**, 421–9.

Sonneveld, P., Durie, B. G., Lokhorst, H. M. et al. (1992). Modulation of multidrug-resistant multiple myeloma by cyclosporin. The Leukaemia Group of the EORTC and the HOVON. *Lancet*, **340**, 266–9.

Thiebaut, F., Tsuruo, T., Hamada, H. et al. (1987). Cellular localization of the multidrug-resistance gene product P-glycoprotein in normal human tissues. *Proc. Natl. Acad. Sci.*, **84**, 7735–8.

Tsuruo, T., Iida, H., Tsukagoshi, S. and Sakurai, Y. (1981). Overcoming of vincristine resistance in P388 leukemia in vivo and in vitro through enhanced cytotoxicity of vincristine and vinblastine by verapamil. *Cancer Res.*, **41**, 1967–72.

Tsuruo, T., Iida, H., Nojiri, M. et al. (1983). Circumvention of vincristine and Adriamycin resistance in vitro and in vivo by calcium influx blockers. *Cancer Res.*, **43**, 2905–10.

Ueda, K., Clark, D. P., Chen, C. I. et al. (1987). The human multidrug resistance (mdr1) gene. cDNA cloning and transcription initiation. *J. Biol. Chem.*, **262**, 505–8.

Ueda, K., Okamura, N., Hirai, M. et al. (1992). Human P-glycoprotein transports cortisol, aldosterone, and dexamethasone, but not progesterone. *J. Biol. Chem.*, **267**, 24248–52.

Weber, D. M., Dimopoulos, M. A. and Alexanian, R. (1993). Increased neurotoxicity with VAD-cyclosporin in multiple myeloma. *Lancet*, **341**, 558–9.

Wilson, W. H., Bates, S. E., Foyo, A. et al. (1995). Controlled trial of dexverapamil, a modulator of drug resistance, in lymphomas refractory to EPOCH chemotherapy. *J. Clin. Oncol.*, **13**, 1995–2004.

Yusa, K. and Tsuruo, T. (1989). Reversal mechanism of multidrug resistance by verapamil: direct binding of verapamil to P-glycoprotein on specific sites and transport of verapamil outward across the plasma membrane of K562/ADM cells. *Cancer Res.*, **49**, 5002–6.

8

Effect of dose and schedule on chemotherapeutic drug resistance

DAVID FENNELLY, GEORGE RAPTIS, JOHN P. A. CROWN and LARRY NORTON

Introduction

Conventionally dosed chemotherapy regimens are capable of obtaining high rates of response in a wide variety of malignancies. For example, the majority of patients with previously untreated metastatic breast cancer will experience significant tumor shrinkage. This is encouraging because tumor volume regression usually diminishes the symptoms of cancer: if this benefit is not counterbalanced by drug toxicity, the patient's quality of life improves (Coates, Gebski and Bishop, 1987). Nevertheless, complete responses in breast cancer and other diseases are less frequent, and the remissions, when achieved, are rarely durable. The cellular mechanisms by which tumors escape eradication by chemotherapy are collectively termed drug resistance. Drug resistance is expressed in two forms: biochemical or absolute resistance, by which a cell cannot be killed with any dose level of drug; and relative resistance, by which the cell might require a higher level of drug to be killed. Absolute resistance cannot be overcome by any strategy that manipulates dose or schedule. Relative resistance, in distinction, is amenable to such manipulations, and is a topic of major practical importance in modern oncology. Manipulations of dose, and to some extent schedule, have long been demonstrated to be of value in the treatment of hematological malignancies. Lately, the value of induction and late intensification, a strategy hypothesized on theoretical grounds to be of potential value (Norton and Simon, 1977), has proven to be of benefit in the treatment of some forms of acute leukemia (Zittoun et al., 1995). The primary purpose of this chapter is to propose, illustrate, and discuss key concepts concerning dose, schedule, and their effect on drug resistance. To this end we will concentrate on several 'solid' tumors that are less responsive to chemotherapy than most hematological cancers: breast and ovarian carcinomas.

Drug resistance

The concept that failure to cure cancer with drugs is largely due to the existence of cells biochemically resistant to drug action is founded on theoretical as well as empirical considerations (De Vita, 1988). In 1943 Luria and Delbruck found that bacteria that had never before been exposed to bacteriophage spontaneously developed mutations that made them resistant to infection (Luria and Delbruck, 1943). A mutation occurring early in the history of a particular culture allows time for this clone to grow to become a large fraction of all of the bacteria present. Within a decade the same mathematical pattern was found to apply to the appearance of methotrexate resistance in L1210 cells (Law, 1952). Hence, biochemical drug resistance could be acquired spontaneously, and does not always require the presence of the drug. The initial application of this concept to clinical practice was based on the extrapolation that if at the time of first treatment a cancer could have already developed resistance to a drug, then treatment of that cancer with any single drug was likely to fail. By the same reasoning, combinations of drugs might work: it should be unlikely that any one cell could spontaneously become resistant to many drugs, particularly drugs with different biochemical sites of action (Frei et al., 1961). This was the basis for the development of combination chemotherapy, the mainstay of modern oncologic treatment (Burchenal et al., 1951).

More recently, the relevance of the Delbruck–Luria model to the treatment of human cancer has been re-examined (Goldie and Coldman, 1979, 1986; Goldie, 1987). Drs Goldie and Coldman have calculated that at a tenable rate of one mutation per million mitoses, the probability of finding no mutants to any one drug in a total population of 10^5 cells is about 90%. However, the probability of there being no resistant mutants in 10^7 cells is only 0.045%. Since even one drug-resistant mutant can prevent cure, they have predicted that the property of incurability should be acquired quickly as a tumor grows from 10^5 to 10^7 cells. Hence, there should be major advantage to the perioperative or even preoperative chemotherapy of primary breast cancer (Burchenal et al., 1951). This leads to the thought that as many effective drugs as possible should be applied as soon as possible. The object is to prevent cells that are already resistant to one drug from mutating to resistance to other drugs. If the toxicity to normal organs would preclude using many drugs at the same time at full dosage (DeVita, Young and Cannellos, 1975), then these authors have theorized that the strict alternation of two or more regimens would be the next best approach (Coldman and Goldie, 1982).

It is important to state that the Goldie–Coldman Hypothesis is an hypothesis, not an established fact. Many clinical data are inconsistent with its conclusions. In one trial, for example, patients with advanced breast cancer received cyclophosphamide, doxorubicin and 5-fluoro-uracil (CAF) with or without tamoxifen as their first treatment for advanced (metastatic) breast cancer (Kardinal et al., 1988). History of prior adjuvant chemotherapy did not affect the response rate, response duration, or overall survival. Similarly, patients with recurrent disease a year or more after adjuvant cyclophosphamide, methotrexate and 5-fluorouracil (CMF) respond as well to CMF as those who had been randomly allocated not to receive adjuvant CMF (Valagussa, Tancini and Bonadonna, 1986). Hence, contrary to the Goldie–Coldman Hypothesis, breast cancer cells not cured by adjuvant CMF are not universally resistant to CMF (Valagussa et al., 1988). Another debatable prediction of the Goldie–Coldman Hypothesis is that chemotherapy cannot be effective unless it is started as soon as possible after diagnosis (Goldie and Coldman, 1986). In contrast, a randomized trial in node-positive primary breast cancer found that 7 months of chemotherapy starting within 36 hours of surgery was no more effective than 6 months of chemotherapy starting within five weeks after surgery (Ludwig Breast Cancer Study Group, 1988). This study demonstrated that a short delay in initiating chemotherapy did not reduce the efficacy of the drugs. Similarly, the worldwide overview of all randomized trials found no pattern of improved results with early institution of chemotherapy or even with preoperative chemotherapy (Early Breast Cancer Trialists' Collaborative Group, 1992). In some studies, delayed therapy conveyed some advantages. The Cancer and Leukemia Group B treated node-positive patients with stage II breast cancer with either 8 months of CMF plus vincristine and prednisone (CMFVP) followed by 6 months of vinblastine, doxorubicin, thiotepa, and fluoxymesterone (VATH) or with an equivalent total duration (14 months) of CMFVP alone (Ainser et al., 1987). Patients receiving the VATH experienced better disease-free survival. Hence, absolute biochemical resistance to VATH did not develop rapidly in the cancer cells that failed to be eradicated by the CMFVP.

In distinction with the concept of absolute resistance, the effect of high-dose levels of chemotherapy in achieving higher response rates may be based on the observation that much drug resistance is relative rather than absolute (Goldie and Coldman, 1986). In diseases such as lymphoma, advanced breast cancer, and ovarian cancer some component of this resistance must be relative rather than absolute, since response rates are augmented with higher doses of drugs (Levin and Hryniuk, 1987; Tannock et al., 1988). Relative drug resistance depends upon the dose level employed, and the shape of the dose–response relationship (Kendal and Frost, 1986). In most animal experiments the killing of cancer cells is greater when the dose level is greater (Goldie, 1987). For this reason, it has long been hypothesized that clinical results could be improved by increasing dose intensity – the amount of drug given per unit of time – by increasing dose level. We will below add to this the concept that dose intensity could be profitably increased by shortening the time between chemotherapy administrations even if we keep dose level constant. Reducing inter-treatment time by decreasing dose levels, might, of course, be dangerous, depending upon the shape of the curve describing the dose–response relationship. However, simultaneously increasing dose level and shortening the time between treatments is theoretically the most efficacious approach. We will examine some clinical examples of the development of this concept, which might be labeled *dose-density* to distinguish it from dose intensity as a function of escalation of dose level alone.

Dose–response (without hematopoietic support)

Rising dose–response relationships have been documented for many chemotherapeutic agents in the laboratory and clinic. Skipper (1986a) and Schabel and later Teicher et al. (1988) found steep dose–response relationships for alkylating agents in in vitro tumor systems. Similarly, rising dose–response relationships are frequently encountered in the clinic. Higher doses of alkylating agents (Smith et al., 1983), cisplatin (Forastiere et al., 1982), cytosine arabinoside (Rudnick et al., 1979), doxorubicin (Jones et al., 1987), and methotrexate (Jaffe et al., 1978) have all been shown to produce high probabilities of response. When used as first chemotherapy for stage IV breast cancer, high-dose combination regimens have produced complete response rates of approximately 50% (Peters et al., 1988; Kaiser et al., 1990; Bezwoda, Seymour and Vorobiof, 1992a). Eddy, in his review of high-dose chemotherapy for metastatic breast cancer, reported that the complete response rates to high-dose regimens was more than 4-fold higher than that reported for lower doses (Eddy, 1992). Responses have also been documented in patients previously failing to respond to conventional doses of these agents. Early trials of high-dose chemotherapy with autologous bone marrow rescue included patients whose disease was refractory to conventionally dosed regimens. Complete response rates of 25% were reported in these series, suggesting that seemingly resistant cancer cells could be killed by brief exposure to very high dose levels (Eder et al., 1986). While most of these patients have relapsed with breast cancer, about 20% of those with chemotherapy-responsive disease have remained disease-free with follow-up in excess of 5 years (Jones et al., 1990; Kennedy et al., 1991; Dunphy and Spitzer, 1992; Williams et al., 1992).

These data, described in further detail below, have been the origin of considerable interest by clinicians and laboratory scientists in the qualitative and quantitative aspects of drug dose and cell kill. Much of this interest has been focused on the use of the alkylating agents: e.g. cyclophosphamide, BCNU, thiotepa, and melphalan. This is because steep dose–response relationships for alkylating agents have been discovered in in vitro tumor systems. For example, Frei et al. studied MCF 7 breast cancer cells (Frei et al., 1985). When data for radiation therapy are plotted graphically, a linear increase in dose results in a logarithmic increase in cell kill. Both thiotepa and melphalan exhibited rising dose–response curves, although they were curvilinear, rather than exponential, related to the proportion and degree of resistance in the original population.

Antimetabolites, in contrast, were seen to lose effect very rapidly after reaching cell-kill percentages of 90% to 99%. Part of this effect is related to the influence of dose on the emergence of biochemical drug resistance. For methotrexate and doxorubicin, high levels of resistance were produced with increasing selection pressure. For thiotepa and melphalan, drug concentration could be progressively increased to approximately 20-fold, after which any incremental increase in drug dose resulted in total cell death. These authors established a cell line that was stable at 20-fold resistance. After several months of unperturbed growth, resistance to alkylating agents in the colonies was found to vary between 3- and 15-fold (Frei et al., 1989). These data indicate that the lesser deviation from exponentiality for the alkylating agents is due to a relative 'resistance to resistance development'. Furthermore, the fact that a maximum of 3–15-fold resistance could be achieved suggests that the doses of drug that can be delivered in the clinical setting, as described below, might be capable of eradicating an entire population of tumor cells. With modern methods of hematological support, alkylating agents demonstrate significant potential for proportional dose escalation. Most alkylating agents have proportional dose escalation ratios of 4 to 10. Thiotepa is especially impressive in this regard, with a proportional dose escalation ratio of 30. This is perhaps the most attractive feature of alkylating agents in the setting of high-dose therapy.

The shape of the dose–response relationship in the clinical setting is of great practical importance. Even in the usual outpatient range, well below that requiring sophisticated hematopoietic support, there is evidence of a rising dose–response curve. Indeed, some data hint at a linear relationship. A randomized trial of post-operative adjuvant chemotherapy for node-positive breast cancer patients compared three plans of CAF (cyclophosphamide, doxorubicin, methotrexate) (Budman et al., 1997). Let X equal a certain total cumulative dose of chemotherapy: The three regimens gave either $2X$ over 4 months (arm I), $2X$ over 6 months (arm II), or X over four months (arm III). Arm I was superior to arm III in reducing the rate of recurrence, although no difference has as yet been reported between arm I and arm II. Should later analyses confirm these data, we would here have evidence of a strictly proportional dose–response relationship. The cumulative influence over 6 months of arm III is kX, where k is a constant. This cumulative influence is the sum of kX over the first 4 months plus zero for the two remaining months. The value kX is half of the influences of either arms II or III. Arm II yields $2kX$ over six months while arm I yields $2kX$ also, but as $2kX$ over the first 4 months, then zero for the other 2 months. A proportional dose–response relationship would predict that arm III should be inferior to both arms II and III, which it seems to be at present. A proportional dose–response relationship signifies that it would be possible to improve clinical results merely by increasing the dose level of the drugs employed (Frei and Canellos, 1980; DeVita, 1986). However, other data suggests that the dose–response relationship for some drugs is actually inferior to that predicted by strict proportionality. An example is a recent study of doxorubicin plus cyclophosphamide (AC) in the adjuvant setting that has yet to find an advantage to an escalation of the cyclophosphamide dose (Dimitrov et al., 1994). Reasons for the failure of alkylating agent dose-escalation to improve clinical results are discussed below.

For advanced ovarian cancer, the prognosis remains poor in spite of real advances in treatment. Reported 5 year survival rates are in the range of 15–20% (Silverberg, Boring and Squires, 1990). Like breast cancer, ovarian cancer is a tumor that demonstrates high response rates, occasional cures, but frequent relapses from therapy. One method of attempting to overcome this emerging drug resistance involves dose escalation. Levin and Hryniuk, in a classic retrospective analysis, explored the role of dose intensity in the treatment of this disease. Dose intensity is defined as amount of drug divided by the time of administration. These authors analyzed 33 trials of chemotherapy, both those applying cisplatin and those not containing cisplatin. They looked at doses received, relative dose intensity achieved (an average of the dose-intensities of the various components of a combination regimen), and overall response and survival. They demonstrated a statistically significant correlation between increasing dose intensity of cisplatin and both response rate and overall survival (Levin and Hryniuk, 1987). They defined the dose intensity of cisplatin as the amount of drug in mg/m^2 delivered per unit time in weeks. Analysis of the dose intensity of other drugs such as cyclophosphamide and adriamycin failed to reveal a significant correlation between increasing dose intensity and overall response. This retrospective analysis was based primarily on published trials involving mainly suboptimally debulked stage III and IV patients, with nearly 90% of patients having residual disease of greater than 2 cm in diameter. As pointed out by McGuire, outcome and average dose intensity are not highly correlated ($r2 = 0.17–0.23$) (McGuire, 1993).

Another important feature is the amount of dose escalation required to obtain a clinical effect. In Levin and Hryniuk's analysis the dose intensity achieved ranged from 30% to 110% of a standard. This is a relative range of only 3- to 4-fold. If it is true that the benefit of dose-intensive therapy lies in its ability to overcome relative drug resistance, then the in vitro models available would suggest that a greater than 5-fold increase would be desirable (Behrens et al., 1987). This may be the reason that no clear-cut dose–response relationship is universally acknowledged. At present data are available from a number of randomized trials that have not settled the issue of the value of dose intensity (Ehrlich et al., 1983; Ngan et al., 1989; Bella et al., 1992; Jones, Wiltshaw and Harper, 1992; Kaye et al., 1992; Colombo et al., 1993; Conte et al., 1993; McGuire et al., 1996). Kaye et al. (1992) reported

on a randomized study of two doses of cisplatin given with cyclophosphamide. Patients were randomized to receive six q 3 weekly cycles of
cyclophosphamide with either cisplatin 50 mg/m^2 or 100 mg/m^2. This
study was stopped early due to the emergence of a significant survival
advantage at 18 months of 73% for the higher dose arm versus 48% for
the low dose arm. The Gynecologic Oncology Group similarly performed a prospective randomized study concentrating on a population
with suboptimally debulked disease ($\geq$ 1 cm residual disease following
laparotomy). In this large study, which evaluated 460 patients, a trend
towards both progression-free and overall survival was seen for the
higher dose arm. A third study randomized patients to receive either
standard-dose or high-dose carboplatin, as based on a pharmacokinetic-
ally defined dose model. Frequencies of response were 58% versus 36%
in favor of the high-dose arm, a statistically significant result. Bella et
al. (1992) randomly assigned patients to receive 600 mg/m^2 either over a
9 week period or a 20 week period. Median survival was not significantly
different, but 4 year survival was 31% for the higher dose-density arm
versus 13% for the standard dose arm. Conte et al. (1993) reported on
the use of high-doses versus standard doses of cisplatin used in combination with cyclophosphamide and epidoxorubicin in patients with bulky
residual disease following laparotomy. Patients were randomized to
receive cisplatin 50 mg/m^2, epidoxorubicin 60 mg/m^2, and cyclophosphamide 600 mg/m^2, all on day one of each 28-day cycle (called P E C
50) versus a regimen consisting of epidoxorubicin and cyclophosphamide as above with cisplatin 50 mg/m^2 given on day one and two (P E C
100). All patients had residual disease $\geq$ 2 cm following laparotomy.
Overall response rates reported were 55.7% for P E C 50 versus 43.6%
for P E C 100. Median survival has not been reached. However, there is
already a trend in the direction of a survival improvement of 4 months
in the higher dose treatment arm. Further follow-up will be required to
determine if this trend translates to a clinically significant improvement in
survival. Ehrlich et al. (1983) randomized patients to cisplatin 100 mg/m^2
q 4 weekly for three cycles with adriamycin and cyclophosphamide
versus cisplatin 50 mg/m^2 q 3 weekly for six cycles with adriamycin
and cyclophosphamide. The pathological complete response rate for the
high-dose arm was 20% versus 47% for the standard-dose arm, with an
overall response rate of 88% for the high-dose arm versus 75% for the
standard arm. Although not reaching statistical significance there is a
trend towards improved survival of 27.5 versus 23.5 months in favor of
the high-dose arm. Of note is that over 30% of patients had $\geq$ 3 cm

residual disease following surgery. Colombo et al. (1993) reported on a randomized study of cisplatin 75 mg/m^2 q 3 weekly for six cycles versus a dose intense regimen of cisplatin 50 mg/m^2 per week for nine cycles. Patients by virtue of the trial design were to receive the same total dose of cisplatin with patients in the dose-intense arm receiving twice the dose intensity achieved in the standard arm. Overall response rates were 66% for the dose-intense arm versus 61% for the standard arm. Again a trend towards improved progression-free (21 vs. 18 months) and overall survival (36 vs. 33 months) was noted. Further follow-up will again be required to further evaluate this trend.

An overview of all these trials fails to answer the question of the true value of increased dose intensity (largely by increasing dose level) in the treatment of advanced ovarian cancer. However, some important points are clear. First, those studies that focused on patients with suboptimally debulked disease consistently reported negative results regarding statistically significant improvements in response rates and overall survival. Furthermore, studies focusing on patients with optimally debulked disease have reported positive end-points both in terms of response rate and overall survival. Secondly, in three of the studies cited the more dose-intensive treatment arm delivered fewer overall cycles of chemotherapy. Studies employing fewer treatment cycles have usually produced negative results, while none of the positive studies incorporated this treatment design. Positive trials demonstrated improvement in the pathologic complete response rate as opposed to the overall response rate (partial plus complete remission), and improvement in long-term survival as distinguished from median survival.

Based on Levin's initial work the focus of strategies to improve dose intensity have consistently focused on platinum delivery. It is accepted that by increasing dose of platinum delivered, responses can be obtained in tumors previously refractory to platinum therapy (Hreschyshyn, 1973; Barker et al., 1981; Bruckner et al., 1984). With the advent of carboplatin, a platinum analog with a more benign toxicity profile, investigators' attention turned to attempts to increase platinum dose intensity using carboplatin. Joddrell and colleagues analyzed in a retrospective fashion the relationship between total carboplatin exposure (AUC, or 'area under the curve' in mg/ml/min) and ultimate outcome. They calculated the exposure to platinum on the basis of creatinine clearance at the time of the first cycle of chemotherapy resulting in an AUC value. They were able to demonstrate that peak response was seen at an AUC of 6 mg/ml/min, and that increasing the dose of platinum resulted in increased toxicity without improvement in response rates. In their analysis, the first cycle AUCs only were used to predict ultimate outcome. It is likely that treatment delays and dose reductions in subsequent cycles resulted in some of the disparity between dose and response in this analysis. This factor serves to emphasize the importance of manipulations to allow not only increased doses of cytotoxic therapy but also timely retreatment.

One method of increasing the dose of platinum delivered is to combine cisplatinum with other platinum analogues. This is a feasible approach as both cisplatin and carboplatin have demonstrated similar efficacy in the treatment of advanced ovarian cancer, in addition to having non-overlapping toxicities, and this may allow full dosage of both platinum analogues to be administered with acceptable toxicity. A number of investigators have evaluated the role of this approach in ovarian cancer. Lund et al. initially reported on a phase II study combining carboplatin and cisplatin performed by the Copenhagen Ovarian Cancer Study Group. Using a dose of 300 mg/m^2 with cisplatin 100 mg/m^2 given q 4 weekly, they reported an overall pathologic response rate of 62%, with a pathologic complete response rate of 22% (Lund et al., 1989). In a subsequent study they reported on a regimen combining cisplatin and carboplatin with ifosfamide in 37 previously untreated patients. Carboplatin 200 mg/m^2 was given on day 1, cisplatin 50 mg/m^2 on days 2 and 3 with ifosfamide 1500 mg with mesna on days 1 to 3. Over 80% of patients in this study had residual disease ≥ 2 cm. The reported pathologic complete response rate in this study was an impressive 42%. Additionally it was reported that of the patients with a pathological CR 53% had initially had residual disease ≥ 5 cm (Lund et al., 1990). Piccart et al. (1990) evaluated, in a phase II study, the role of combined platinum therapy. They employed a carboplatin dosage of 300 mg/m^2 on day 1 followed by cisplatin 50 mg/m^2 on days 2 and 3. The overall reported response rate was 62% with a pathological complete response rate of 22%. The patient population in this study consisted largely of patients with bulky residual disease following laparotomy. The dose-limiting toxicity in this study was thrombocytopenia. The Belgian Study Group evaluated this combined platinum approach in previously untreated patients with advanced ovarian cancer. They performed a phase I/II trial in 30 patients with bulky residual ovarian carcinoma, using a carboplatin dose of 300 mg/m^2 on day 1 followed by cisplatin 100 mg/m^2 on day 2 with aggressive 48 hour hydration. Their reported pathological complete response rate of 22% was similar to that reported in the Danish study.

A number of other combined platinum studies in patients with ovarian cancer are now reported in the literature (Trump et al., 1987; Gill et al., 1991; Hardy et al., 1991; Dittrich et al., 1993; Waterhouse, Reynolds and Natale, 1993). The planned platinum dose intensity for these trials varies between 37.5 and 63 mg/m^2/week. It is clear that due to myelotoxicity frequent dose reductions were necessary, and thus the delivered platinum dose intensity was significantly lower.

Analysis of these and other studies demonstrate that in spite of this treatment schema, the dose intensity achieved is less than twice that achieved with standard therapy. Based on our knowledge of the relationship between dose intensity and response, and the relative drug resistance that emerges, this increase is unlikely to be clinically significant.

The use of intraperitoneal chemotherapy is potentially beneficial in the situation where tumor is confined to the peritoneal cavity, which is, after all, an extravascular space. Intraperitoneal chemotherapy has the theoretical advantage of achieving higher drug concentrations at the level of the tumor that can be achieved by intravenous therapy alone (Dedrick, 1978; Markman et al., 1985; Markman, 1991). The pharmacologic rationale is based on the difference between plasma and peritoneal clearance rates of antineoplastic agents and resultant differences in drug concentrations in these two compartments. Cisplatin, a drug with a high plasma clearance and a low peritoneal clearance, is an agent well suited to intraperitoneal administration. These pharmacokinetics result in increased drug delivery to the tumor, increased tumor exposure time, with decreased systemic toxicity. Additionally it is recognized that optimal responses to intraperitoneal therapy require minimal volume disease, usually less than one centimeter in diameter. Cisplatin delivered by the intraperitoneal route, whether administered as a single agent or in several cisplatin-based combination regimens, has demonstrated efficacy as salvage therapy in ovarian cancer patients with small-volume residual disease (largest tumor mass ≤ 0.5–1 cm in diameter) (Markman, 1991). In a recent review of our institution's experience with salvage cisplatin-based intraperitoneal therapy in patients with ovarian cancer, 42% (15/36) of patients who had previously responded to a systemic platinum regimen and who started the second-line program with small-volume residual disease achieved a surgically defined complete response (Markman et al., 1991b). In contrast, among 14 patients with small-volume disease who had previously failed to demonstrate a response to systemic platinum, the surgically defined complete response rate was only 7% ($P < 0.025$). In individuals whose largest mass was > 1 cm at the initiation of cisplatin-based intraperitoneal therapy, the surgical complete response rate was 10%, even if the patient had previously demonstrated an objective response to systemic platinum. This experience has more critically defined the patient population who may experience benefit from a platinum-based salvage intraperitoneal program. It also indicates that one cannot discount dose escalation as a means of overcoming drug resistance until one explores truly increased levels of drug exposure at the site of the cancer cells.

It is clear from the above discussion that the interpretation of data generated by dose-intense clinical regimens is complicated on several levels. The first concerns the issue of the efficacy of solitary exposures to drug (the so-called 'single cycle', which is actually a single course) in causing tumor volume regression. The second involves the matter of the degree of dose escalation. A third revolves around the distinction between dose intensity and dose density. These three issues are discussed sequentially below.

Multicycle regimens

The inability of high-dose chemotherapy to eradicate clones of highly resistant cancer cells, in spite of massive degrees of tumor volume regression, might account for the frequency with which relapse from complete remission is observed following this modality. However, an analysis of curative chemotherapy for other neoplastic diseases suggests another possibility. Successful treatment programs for chemotherapy-curable cancers have two features in common. The first is the availability of a regimen that produces frequent complete responses. The second is the feasibility of delivering a minimum number of courses of that regimen in full doses. These two requirements are logical extrapolations from animal studies (Skipper, 1967). Laboratory experiments have shown that multiple administrations of chemotherapy are usually more effective than a solitary treatment that delivers the same cumulative dosage (Goldie and Coldman, 1979). While there are no randomized clinical trials of single versus multiple courses of the same 'effective' chemotherapy in patients with curable malignancies, the contention that a minimum number of treatment courses are necessary to cure is defensible.

For Hodgkin's disease, MOPP chemotherapy is curative in approximately 50% of patients with advanced disease. The median time to the attainment of a complete remission is 3 months, which is equivalent to three cycles of therapy. Thus, few if any patients would have been cured if their treatment consisted of only one course of this combination. Four courses of cisplatin and etoposide will be curative in the majority of patients with testicular carcinoma (Bajorin et al., 1993). However, three courses of this two-drug regimen produced results (in the context of a prospective randomized comparison against a three-drug regimen), that appeared to be inferior to those achieved historically with four courses of the doublet (Loehrer et al., 1991). There is also anecdotal evidence that patients who default following one course of cisplatin-based therapy have poor outcomes (Bosl, Geller and Bajorin, 1988; Canellos et al., 1992; DeVita and Hubbard, 1993). Even patients with gestational trophoblastic disease – known to be highly responsive to chemotherapy – properly receive repeated courses of therapy until their serum chorionic gonadotrophin level has become normal (Berkowitz, Goldstein and Bernstein, 1986).

Hence, the inability of single courses of high-dose chemotherapy to cure most patients with advanced 'solid' tumors should not be regarded as evidence against the potential value of dose escalation. This point is of major importance as we await the results of trials using a single course of late-intensification in the treatment of high-risk stage II breast cancer (Peters et al., 1993). Given the value of multiple cycle regimens, we are left with the important question of how to design such treatments. Is dose escalation the key feature of multicycle therapies, even if we must compromise the rapidity with which such chemotherapy can be recycled? That is, if it takes many weeks for a patient to recover from a high-dose exposure, is this still preferable to lower doses given more frequently? If we have more agents than can be delivered concurrently, how should we combine their combinations to achieve optimal cancer cell kill?

The Goldie–Coldman Hypothesis predicts that if one were to use two treatments, which we may label A and B, in the design of a multicycle regimen, then ABABAB will be superior to AAABBB. Either A or B may be single agents or combinations of agents given simultaneously. The reason they propose this alternation is that ABABAB will deliver treatment B sooner than AAABBB. According to the hypothesis, were AAABBB used, then cells resistant to A would stand a great chance of mutating to resistance to B during the AAA portion of the regimen.

This concept has been highly influential. Yet clinical experience actually contradicts these predictions. In patients with advanced breast cancer there is no advantage to CMFVP alternating with VATH over CAF with VATH alone (Aisner et al., 1995). Similarly, in patients with node-positive primary breast cancer, a sequential chemotherapy regimen was found to be superior to an alternating one (Buzzoni et al., 1991). The sequential regimen used was four 3-week courses of adjuvant doxorubicin (A) followed by eight 3-week courses of intravenous CMF (C). This may be symbolized as

AAAACCCCCCCC

The alternating regimen that was compared with the above was two courses of CMF alternating with one course of doxorubicin, this grouping repeated four times for a total of 12 courses. This regimen may be symbolized as

CCACCACCACCA

The superiority of the sequential regimen over the alternation one casts serious doubt about the therapeutic applicability of the Goldie–Coldman Hypothesis to the treatment of breast cancer. We will return to this issue below in our consideration of the concept of dose density. However, before we enter that discussion, it may be profitable to return to the issue of the clinical impact of the magnitude of dose escalation of chemotherapy drugs.

Dose escalation (with hematopoietic support)

One of the major impediments to dose escalation to a truly meaningful level has always been hematological toxicity. Prolonged severe myelosuppression produces morbidity and mortality from infection and hemorrhage, and also contributes to organ toxicity by two mechanisms: first, bleeding may damage organs (i.e. pulmonary hemorrhage); second, organ damage may ensue from multiple transfusions of erythrocytes and platelets or the protracted administration of toxic antibiotics. One of the most important developments in modern medical oncology has been in the technology of hematopoietic support. Granulocyte colony stimulating factor, G-CSF, and granulocyte–macrophage colony stimulating factor, GM-CSF, accelerate leukocyte recovery following chemotherapy, resulting in the amelioration of associated morbidity (Taylor et al., 1989; Gulati and Bennett, 1992). These observations have prompted extensive investigations of these agents as facilitators of dose escalation (Jones et al., 1987). A general result has been a substantial reduction in the need for attenuations of dose in conventional combination regimens.

However major dose escalations of single courses have proven more difficult to achieve.

As an example, for metastatic breast cancer the Dana-Farber group tried use of G-CSF to increase the doses of the CAF regimen (Younger et al., 1992). Mucositis emerged as a major dose-limiting toxicity of CAF. In a similar study in the Netherlands, the use of GM-CSF permitted the use of moderately escalated doses of cyclophosphamide and doxorubicin. However, acute hematologic toxicity was considerable, and cumulative myelosuppression was observed (Hoekman et al., 1991). In a prospective Italian study, patients with metastatic breast cancer were treated with epirubicin, cyclophosphamide and 5-fluorouracil, randomized to receive GM-CSF or not. All patients were re-treated promptly on recovery from the previous cycle (Venturini et al., 1992). The GM-CSF facilitated dose escalation, but only by approximately 130% of the doses achieved in the control group.

For many other chemotherapy agents, hematopoietic cytokines have provided even less protection from myelosuppression. A reason is that both G-CSF and GM-CSF are active primarily in leukocyte pathways. While some accelerated platelet recovery has been reported, this has not been a consistent finding (Advani et al., 1992). For example, an attempt to escalate the dose of thiotepa by the administration of GM-CSF was not successful because of thrombocytopenia (O'Dwyer et al., 1992). Thrombocytopenia and cumulative myelosuppression have also limited dose-escalation strategies for carboplatin.

However, the use of CSFs as the only means of hematopoietic support has been reported to be successful in two studies. Neidhart and colleagues have been able to administer multiple cycles of high-dose cisplatin plus cyclophosphamide plus etoposide by the use of G-CSF alone, without autologous marrow reinfusion (Neidhart et al., 1990). It is important to note – relevant to the concept of dose-density discussed below – that in this study cycles could be repeated only with long inter-treatment intervals of more than 4 weeks. In another study using GM-CSF, the CALGB demonstrated that multiple cycles of high-dose cyclophosphamide could be administered to patients with various cancers, but here the inter-treatment interval was short at approximately 2 weeks (Lichtman et al., 1990).

The general failure of the CSFs to permit major dose escalations may be because some chemotherapy drugs influence very early hematopoietic progenitors. We therefore look forward to the thrombopoietic effects of growth factors that act earlier in bone marrow maturation (Crown et al.,

1991). Interleukin-1, for example, may shorten the duration of carbopla-tin-induced thrombocytopenia (Smith et al., 1992; Vadban-Raj et al., 1992). While this field develops investigators have turned to the use of CSFs plus the reinfusion of hematopoietic progenitor cells as a means of promoting both dose-escalation and the achievement of dose-density.

High-dose chemotherapy to a degree requiring autologous bone mar-row reinfusion has been able to produce a very high rate of overall and complete response in patients with a variety of tumors. The use of marrow-supported high-dose chemotherapy has produced long-term dis-ease-free survivals, which for practical purposes may be tantamount to cure, for patients with lymphomas (Gulati et al., 1992) and germ-cell cancers (Motzer et al., 1992) who have had diseases refractory to stan-dard-dose therapy. In the treatment of metastatic breast cancer, such therapy has produced high objective response rates. Some regimens have used high doses of the single agents melphalan, cyclophosphamide, and thiotepa (Jones et al., 1990; Kennedy et al., 1991; Antman et al., 1992; Bezwoda, Seymour and Vorobiof, 1992). Because of its limited non-hematological toxicity, thiotepa has particular potential for dose escal-ation. A phase I study published in 1992 recommended that 75 mg/m^2 be considered the phase II dose, but the dose of 30 mg/m^2 had been in use for decades (Neidhart et al., 1990). GM-CSF alone does not provide adequate protection from cumulative myelosuppression (Neidhart et al., 1990), but the reinfusion of autologous marrow allows for the use of a substantially higher dose. High-dose thiotepa with autologous marrow rescue has produced response and survival data similar to those reported for combination regimens (Crown et al., 1994). Above a dose of approxi-mately 700 mg/m^2 mucosal toxicity becomes prominent (Wolff et al., 1990), and doses above 1200 mg/m^2 produce neurological toxicity in approximately 10% of patients.

The combination of the alkylating agents cyclophosphamide, cisplatin, and carmustine (CPB) has produced a complete response rate of approximately 25% in breast cancer patients with otherwise refractory disease (Eder et al., 1986). These responses were not durable, for theor-etical reasons discussed above, but the results prompted a phase II evaluation of this same combination in patients with more favorable disease status. Accordingly, 22 patients without prior chemotherapy for metastatic disease, who were nevertheless regarded as having a poor prognosis because their tumors were hormone receptor negative, or who had failed prior endocrine therapies, were treated with a single applica-tion of CPB. Toxicity was substantial but complete responses were achieved in more than half of the patients. Three of the original 22 remained in unmaintained complete remissions for more than 5 years (Peters et al., 1988). Many other single-course combinations of chemotherapy drugs with marrow support have been studied: they differ somewhat in their spectrum of toxicities, but no one regimen has emerged as clearly superior.

Exploiting the idea of multicycle regimens, some investigators have used induction chemotherapy at conventional dose levels followed by a single course of high-dose combination chemotherapy with autologous bone marrow rescue (Antman et al., 1992). Others have tried to use repeated cycles of high-dose chemotherapy. At the M. D. Anderson Hospital interesting results were achieved with double applications of such high-dose chemotherapy (Dunphy and Spitzer, 1992). However, toxicity necessitated substantial inter-treatment delays averaging 6–8 weeks. Bezwoda and colleagues have reported preliminary findings from a prospective randomized trial in which two courses of very high doses of mitoxantrone, etoposide, and cyclophosphamide were administered with autologous marrow or peripheral blood-derived hematopoietic progenitor cell support (*vide infra*). The control arm was conventional chemotherapy, which yielded a 70% response rate, 6% complete (Bezwoda et al., 1992). The experimental arm, in contrast, produced a 100% response rate including a 50% complete response rate in patients who received the treatment as first chemotherapy for stage IV disease.

The CSFs are an important component of therapies using autologous marrow reinfusions since they contribute to more rapid leukocyte recovery (Taylor et al., 1989). Another role for the CSFs is in the generation of hematopoietic progenitor cells to be obtained from the peripheral blood. Investigators at the Dana-Farber Cancer Institute reported that the administration of GM-CSF to cancer patients enriched the pool of peripheral blood-derived hematopoietic progenitor cells (PBPC) (Socinski et al., 1988). An increase in peripheral progenitors was also noted during the recovery phase from myelosuppressive chemotherapy. Administration of hematopoietic growth factor during recovery phase markedly augmented the effect. Gianni et al. (1989), Peters, Kurtzberg and Kirkpatrick (1989), and others subsequently found that these PBPC, when reinfused simultaneously with autologous marrow, accelerated hematological – especially platelet – recovery from high-dose chemotherapy. This resulted in decreased morbidity and mortality. The combination of cyclophosphamide and CSF increases the peripheral blood CFU count by up to a thousand-fold (Ozols et al., 1987). Similarly the addition of escalated doses of paclitaxel to cyclophosphamide has been shown not to compromise, and perhaps augment, the progenitor cell yield (Fennelly et al., 1994). Gianni has also reported that a sequence of high-dose single agents could be delivered, with PBPC plus CSF after the last high-dose course, and that this therapy seems promising in the treatment of lymphoma and in breast cancer (Frei et al., 1985). We will discuss below our use of PBPC technology to improve dose density as well as dose escalation.

In the treatment of ovarian carcinoma, the use of high-dose chemo-therapy with autologous bone marrow support has been demonstrated to be capable of achieving high rates of response in patients failing conventional treatment regimens. This is an area of considerable interest for a number of reasons. First, ovarian cancer is a tumor with demon-strated chemosensitivity, although clearly less sensitivity than the hema-tological malignancies. Second, patients failing conventional therapy have a universally poor prognosis. Additionally, as described above, there is a rising dose–response relationship for both the platinum com-pounds and the alkylating agents in general (Frei et al., 1985; Ozols et al., 1987). Agents such as melphalan, cyclophosphamide and thiotepa are active in ovarian cancer, and can be substantially dose-escalated with the use of autologous bone marrow support (Mulder et al., 1989; Shea et al., 1989). Using high-dose melphalan in patients who had failed prior cisplatin therapy, Stoppa et al. reported a 75% overall response rate. At a median follow-up of 23 months, 15 of 35 patients were alive, and disease-free. Dauplat et al. (1989), utilizing a similar regimen, obtained a 36% 2-year disease-free survival rate, also in patients failing induction cisplatin regimens. Pre-clinical studies by Lidor et al. have demonstrated synergy between cisplatin and cyclophosphamide and cis-platin plus thiotepa. Shpall et al. evaluated in a phase I setting the combination of high-dose cyclophosphamide, thiotepa and cisplatin fol-lowed by autologous bone marrow supporting patients with advanced ovarian cancer. Cisplatin was delivered by the intraperitoneal route in an escalating dose schedule commencing at 90 mg/m^2 divided over 3 days. They reported an overall response rate of 75% in a group of patients, all of whom had progressive disease on platinum based therapy (Shpall et al., 1990).

Based on the demonstrated activity of doxorubicin in advanced ovarian cancer, and the limited potential of this agent for dose escalation (because of dose-limiting mucositis and cardiotoxicity), investigators have turned to mitoxantrone for incorporation into dose-escalated approaches (Wallerstein et al., 1990). Mitoxantrone is an anthracene derivative, with an intercalative and non-intercalative effect on DNA (Lown et al., 1984; Bowden et al., 1985), which is cytotoxic to proliferating and non-proliferating cells in vitro (Wallace, Citarella and Durr, 1979; Drewinko et al., 1981). Clinical congestive heart failure occurs in less than 3% of patients with conventional dosing of mitoxantrone, up to cumulative doses of 100 mg/m^2 in patients previously treated with anthracyclines, and up to 160 mg/m^2 in previously untreated patients (Shenkenberg and Von Hoff, 1986). In experimental systems, mitoxantrone showed some lack of cross-resistance to anthracyclines (Hill et al., 1989). In the human tumor colony forming assay, mitoxantrone has been demonstrated to be highly cytotoxic to ovarian cancer cells (Alberts et al., 1985). It has also demonstrated activity against ovarian cancer, when delivered by either the intravenous (Lawton et al., 1987) or intraperitoneal routes (Markman et al., 1991a). Mitoxantrone is an unusual drug to dose-escalate because it is not an alkylating agent (Lawton et al., 1987). Yet a number of investigators have evaluated mitoxantrone in the setting of autologous marrow reinfusion. Shea et al. (1992, 1993) have evaluated escalated-dose mitoxantrone in addition to high-dose intraperitoneal carboplatin and intravenous thiotepa and etoposide. The dose of mitoxantrone used was 42 mg/m^2. The Southwest Oncology Group is currently evaluating mitoxantrone at a dose of 75 mg/m^2 in a phase II study of high-dose chemotherapy with marrow support for patients with advanced ovarian cancer. Mulder et al. (1989b) combined either cyclophosphamide or melphalan with high-dose mitoxantrone and obtained a 66% complete response rate.

Many other single-course dose-escalated combinations have been tested against advanced ovarian carcinoma. Legros et al. (1992) evaluated the long-term results achieved with high-dose chemotherapy and autologous bone marrow transplant in 31 patients. All patients had received induction therapy with a cisplatin-containing regimen followed by debulking surgery and consolidation with high-dose chemotherapy with autologous bone marrow support. Patients received either high-dose melphalan (140 mg/m^2) or a combination of carboplatin (1000–1500 mg/m^2) with cyclophosphamide 6 g/m^2. With a median follow-up of 52 months 18 of 31 patients were alive, 11 free of disease. Overall disease-free survival at 3 years was 35%. Stiff et al. (1992) published a survey of 11 autologous bone marrow transplant centers in the United States. The survey included 153 ovarian carcinoma patients of whom 95% were transplanted with relapsed or refractory disease. Only 5%

of patients were transplanted in their first remission. Twenty different transplant preparative regimens were identified. The overall response rate was 71%, with a 43% complete response rate. In patients with platinum-sensitive disease by conventional criteria, overall response rate was 87% with a 73% clinical complete response rate. In patients with documented platinum-resistant disease, the overall response rate was 85%, with a 34% clinical complete response rate. The median time to progression was 6 months, with 14% of patients disease-free at one year. An ongoing randomized study by the South-West Oncology Group (SWOG) is evaluating two different high-dose chemotherapy regimens with autologous bone marrow support in patients with either progressive disease, responding-but-persistent disease (residual disease at second-look of more than five millimeters in diameter), or disease recurrent after platinum-based therapy. Patients are treated with either high-dose cyclophosphamide, mitoxantrone, and carboplatin or high-dose thiotepa, cyclophosphamide, and cisplatin. In both cases hematological support is being provided by autologous bone marrow reinfusion.

Dose density

We have described clinical data suggesting that dose-escalation of many chemotherapeutic agents can kill more cancer cells than conventional doses, and that multiple cycles of chemotherapy seem to be associated with better clinical results. We have also examined some implications of the Goldie–Coldman Hypothesis, and have found them lacking in empirical support. To use these observations in the design of improved chemotherapy regimens, it is necessary to re-examine the pattern of growth of human cancer. There is an increasing body of evidence that many cancers grow not exponentially but by Gompertzian kinetics (Gilewski and Norton, 1995). In this pattern of growth smaller tumors are more sensitive – in terms of the fraction of cells killed – than larger tumors, but the regrowth rate is faster as well. Therefore, the overall impact of treatment will be modest even in the face of very large cell-kills, unless the tumor is precluded from regrowing. One path to the permanent prevention of regrowth is the elimination of all cancer cells. This conclusion is relevant to the practical design of treatment regimens because of the concepts of drug resistance. If a whole cancer is a collection of different sublines with different proliferation rates and different sensitivities to treatment, eradicating some sublines by chemotherapy would leave others to grow. By Gompertzian kinetics the residual sublines would have a tendency to regrow rapidly. Hence, partially effective therapies, even those killing most of the cells present, might produce only small increases in disease-free survival.

One subline that may be particularly difficult to eradicate with chemotherapy are the stem cells. These cells are an important class of undifferentiated cells that constitute less than 1% of the cells present in a cancer. They can form colonies in soft agar (Hamburger and Salmon, 1977), and are thought to be able to react to the death of adjacent cells to reproduce the entire spectrum of subtypes that make up a mature tumor (Bruce and Valeriote, 1968; Till et al., 1968). Hence, they could be a major source of therapeutic failure (Look, Douglass and Meyer, 1988). An optimistic side of this consideration is that some of our current chemotherapy treatments might actually be bringing us closer to total cellular eradication than we might otherwise be led to suspect by their modest impact on disease-free and overall survival.

How do we eradicate residual sublines, particularly those that are slowly growing, slowly regressing, and therefore harder to kill (Norton and Simon, 1986)? Slower-growing cells should constitute a minority of the cells in a cancer because by the time of diagnosis they should have been overgrown by faster-growing cells. We have hypothesized that the best way to cure a population of cells heterogeneous in growth rate and drug sensitivity is to eradicate the more numerous, faster-growing cells first, then the more resistant, slower-growing cells (Norton, 1985). To eradicate any population of cells, it should be treated with drugs to which they are sensitive, with minimal time between treatments so as to minimize their opportunities to recover. Conventional combination chemotherapy does not accomplish this goal since doses are reduced to permit the construction of tolerable combinations. Also, little attention is usually directed to the speed of recycling, i.e. minimizing the inter-treatment intervals.

These concepts might explain the superiority of A A A A C C C C C C C C over C C A C C A C C A C C A in the adjuvant treatment of breast cancer as described above (Buzzoni et al., 1991). The sequential regimen gave eight cycles of CMF over 33 weeks counting from the beginning of treatment, and four cycles of doxorubicin over 9 weeks. This means that the dose-density of the doxorubicin was very high compared with the alternating regimen, which gave eight cycles of CMP over a similar 30 weeks, but four cycles of adriamycin over a much longer 33 weeks. In the sequential regimen, dose-density is achieved by *cross-over scheduling*, A A A A crossing over to C C C C C C C. It is important to note that the concept of cross-over scheduling is supported by several theoretical models. Goldie and Coldman's prediction of the superiority of alternating chemotherapy, CCACCACCACCA, was dependent on the assumption of 'symmetry', which means the presence of sublines with equal numbers of cells, equal proliferation rates, and equal mutation rates. Roger Day reconsidered the Goldie–Coldman model, but performed computer simulations of mutation to drug resistance under asymmetrical conditions (Day, 1986). From this he predicted that the alternating plan would be inferior (Norton and Day, 1991). In the laboratory, the cure of advanced murine leukemia is best accomplished by using cytosine arabinoside plus 6-thioguanine for two or three courses, followed by one high-dose treatment with cyclophosphamide plus BCNU (Skipper, 1986). Hence, the high-dose regimens described above that use conventional-dose induction followed by a short late-intensification are supported by experimental as well as clinical evidence. As another laboratory example, the complete remission rate and the median survival time of BDF1 mice bearing the M5076 tumor may be doubled by using four doses of methyl-CCNU first, then crossing over to a single dose of L-phenylalanine mustard, as compared to the use of methyl-CCNU alone (Griswold et al., 1982). In this experimental setting, L-phenylalanine mustard by itself has very weak activity because only a small subpopulation of cells is sensitive just to this drug. Yet this is the subpopulation that leads to relapse if methyl-CCNU is used alone.

Cross-over scheduling is just one way of applying these concepts. We recall that dose intensity is total amount of drug divided by time. In the past, we have been able to increase dose intensity only by increasing dose level. However, the major improvements in hematopoietic technology described above and elsewhere in this volume now allow us to shorten the inter-treatment time as well. We have combined the notions of cross-over scheduling and dose-density in the design of pilot studies in patients with high-risk stage II–III breast cancer (Hudis et al., 1994). We used four cycles of a conventional dose of doxorubicin followed by dose-dense, dose-intense cyclophosphamide, a strategy permitted by the use of G-CSF (Lichtman et al., 1993). We have studied 74 patients with primary resected breast cancer who had four or more axillary lymph nodes involved with metastatic cancer (Hudis et al., 1996). The median number of involved nodes was ten. Radiation therapy was delivered to all conserved breasts or to the chest wall of patients with mastectomies but ten or more involved nodes. Amenorrheic patients with estrogen or progesterone receptor positive cancers were advised to take tamoxifen 20 mg p.o. daily for 5 years after the completion of chemotherapy. This regimen, which we have termed A-to-C, was shown to be tolerable. At the median follow-up of more than 2 years 70% of patients are disease-free. This was felt to be sufficiently interesting to merit the randomized comparison of A-to-C with a more traditional doxorubicin plus cyclophosphamide combination in an intergroup trial coordinated by the SWOG.

To improve the A-to-C regimen we have explored the activity of paclitaxel (Taxol, T) against stage IV disease (Reichman, Seidman and Crown, 1993). We have treated 25 patients with paclitaxel (250 mg/m^2 over 24 hours) as second chemotherapy for stage IV disease and 52 patients with paclitaxel (200 mg/m^2 over 24 hours) as third or higher stage IV treatment. All patients had had breast cancers that grew on prior anthracycline. The response rate to paclitaxel was 32% in this setting, with a median response duration of 7 months. Patients with de novo anthracycline-resistant disease experienced a response rate of 30%; those with acquired resistance (initial response to anthracycline, followed by progressive disease) had an almost identical 32% response rate (Seidman, Reichman and Crown, 1997). Hence, paclitaxel seems an excellent agent to use against cells resistant to doxorubicin. For this reason we have evaluated sequential doxorubicin–paclitaxel–cyclophosphamide (A–T–C) in the high-risk adjuvant setting, and are currently involved in a randomized comparison with a regimen composed of doxorubicin followed by cyclophosphamide plus paclitaxel (Hudis et al., 1996). In all cases, G-CSF is used to assure high dose-density.

These concepts are also applicable to patients with stage IV breast cancer responsive to conventional chemotherapy. In this setting we have exploited the ability of PBPC to promote thrombocyte as well as granulocyte recovery (Kritz et al., 1993). In a series of trials we have confirmed the activity of this approach and the relative tolerability of high-dose alkylating agents given each 2 weeks with hematopoietic support (Crown et al., 1993). In a preliminary trial at MSKCC, patients receiving high dose carboplatin (1500 mg/m^2), etoposide (1200 mg/m^2), cyclophosphamide (5000 mg/m^2) with GM-CSF were randomized to receive, or not to receive, PBPC. The initial cohort of five patients receiving PBPC had approximately seven fewer days of neutropenia (ANC $< 0.5 \times 10^9$/L) and nine fewer days of thrombocytopenia (PLT < 50), compared to the cohort of five patients receiving only GM-CSF (Kritz et al., 1991). As there was such a marked difference early in this randomization, further patients were accrued only to receive PBPC and HGF. At a median follow-up of 40 months 7/18 patients (39%) remained progression free. This study established the superiority of PBPC HGF over HGF alone in providing rapid hematologic recovery. In an attempt to sequence HDC rapidly and to investigate the efficacy of HGF chemotherapy mobilization of PBPC, a subsequent trial was conducted in which patients received tandem cycles of cyclophosphamide (3000 mg/m^2) G-CSF for mobilization of PBPC followed by a course of high dose carboplatin (1200 mg/m^2), etoposide (1200 mg/m^2) and cyclophosphamide (5000 mg/m^2) with PBPC G-CSF for hematologic rescue. The median inter-treatment interval for cyclophosphamide courses was 14 days and following the third course of HDC an ANC > 500 was achieved at a median of 12 days following PBPC infusion (Shea et al., 1993). The PR-CR conversion rate was 3/8 (38%) with 4/17 patients (24%) remaining progression free at a median follow-up of 31 months. This trial established the feasibility of rapidly sequenced HDC and the efficacy of chemotherapy HGF mobilization of PBPC and enabled us to develop a reliable threshold number of CD34 PBPC to support cycles of HDC. Consequently we conducted a trial to evaluate the feasibility and efficacy of rapidly administered, sequential high-dose alkylator therapy in patients with responding metastatic breast cancer. PBPC were collected following tandem cycles of cyclophosphamide (3000 mg/m^2) G-CSF to support tandem cycles of escalating dose thiotepa ($500-700 \text{ mg/m}^2$) with a median inter-treatment interval of 16 days (Fennelly et al., 1993). Of 42 patients entered, 38 received all four planned cycles of chemotherapy (four had insufficient PBPC). The median inter-treatment interval was 15 days with a PR–CR conversion in 9/21 (43%) patients. At a median follow-up of 22 months, 11/42 (26%) patients remained progression free. In a recently completed study in metastatic breast cancer patients, PBPC were collected prior to and following cyclophosphamide (5000 mg/m^2) G-CSF to support sequential cycles of high-dose melphalan (180 mg/m^2) and thiotepa (700 mg/m^2) given once or twice. The median inter-treatment interval was 18 days with a PR–CR conversion in 12/15 (80%) (Raptis et al., 1994). With a median follow-up of 13 months, 20/31 (65%) of evaluable patients remained progression free.

Our current regimen is cyclophosphamide plus paclitaxel twice, then thiotepa plus paclitaxel twice, for an intense, multi-agent, multi-cycle program given over 8 weeks, largely in the outpatient setting. It is important to note that these plans differ from the conventional single-bolus intensification plans that have traditionally been associated with the use of autologous bone marrow reinfusions. Single-bolus plans increase dose level, but dose density is dependent on multiple cycles.

We have also applied these concepts to the treatment of advanced ovarian carcinoma. Previously, Shea and colleagues (1992) have demonstrated the feasibility of a strategy of sequential leukapheresis and reinfusion of peripheral blood progenitors to support patients through three courses of carboplatin at a dose of 1200 mg/m^2. Investigators at the Dana-Farber Cancer Institute treated patients with a single course of high-dose cyclophosphamide 4.0 g/m^2 plus G-CSF and multiple leukapheresis, followed by four courses of cyclophosphamide 600 mg/m^2 (a standard dose) plus carboplatin 600 mg/m^2 (approximately 50% higher than standard dose), supported by the previously collected PBPC (Tepler et al., 1992). These investigators have shown that PBPC plus GM-CSF leads to faster hematological recovery than GM-CSF alone.

Our initial studies addressed patients with advanced ovarian and other cancers. Patients were treated with two to three courses of high-dose cyclophosphamide (3.0 g/m^2) plus G-CSF and underwent multiple peripheral blood leukaphereses. They subsequently were treated with a sequence of four courses of high-dose carboplatin (500–1200 mg/m^2, with no intrapatient dose escalation) rescued with PBPC. The planned inter-treatment interval was 14 days (Fennelly et al., 1993). We reached a maximum tolerated dose of 1000 mg/m^2 with ototoxicity being dose-limiting at a carboplatin dose of 1200 mg/m^2. The median interval between carboplatin treatments was 15 days. We have now rescued over 100 courses of high-dose chemotherapy with PBPC without marrow reinfusion. In only two instances has reinfusion of back-up marrow been necessary, and in both the count of hematopoietic stem cells (CD34) was less than 0.4 × 10^6 cells/kg. We have recently completed a phase I dose-escalation study of taxol administered with high-dose cyclophosphamide. Patients received two cycles of high-dose cyclophosphamide (3 g/m^2) followed by escalating doses of paclitaxel from 150 to 200, 250, and eventually 300 mg/m^2 as a 24 hour continuous infusion, followed by four cycles of carboplatin 1000 mg/m^2 plus cyclophosphamide 1.5 g/m^2. We demonstrated the feasibility of administering taxol 300 mg/m^2 with high-dose cyclophosphamide as induction therapy. Additionally, we identified taxol as an agent that did not compromise the progenitor cell yield following high-dose cyclophosphamide (Fennelly et al., 1995). We are currently addressing in a phase I study high-dose cyclophosphamide (3 g/m^2) paclitaxel 300 mg/m^2, followed by four cycles of carboplatin

1000 mg/m^2 plus escalating doses of paclitaxel from 150 to 200, 250, and 300 mg/m^2.

Conclusion

Regarding the clinical potential of dose-intensity (via dose-escalation, dose-density, or both) to overcome drug resistance, we can at this early stage of clinical development draw a few conclusions from the available published data. The inability of chemotherapy to eradicate tumors is in general related to the emergence of drug resistance. This drug resistance appears to be relative, in that by increasing the dose of drug delivered, more cancer cells are often killed. Single courses of high-dose chemotherapy, such as those rescued with autologous bone marrow reinfusions, have achieved high rates of response in patients whose cancers grew in spite of conventional chemotherapy. These responses however are frequently of short duration. However, the use of hematopoietic progenitor cells plus G-CSF has enabled us to deliver repeated cycles of high-dose chemotherapy at short inter-treatment intervals. Based on our experience with curative standard chemotherapy for Hodgkin's and other diseases, we might expect that repeated application of regimens capable of producing such high response rates will improve long-term survival.

A remaining and critical issue is to identify the patients who will derive maximum benefit from dose-intense chemotherapy. The true efficacy of this approach will require its testing as first chemotherapy, without extensive prior treatment for advanced disease. For conventionally dosed as well as dose-intense regimens, bulky disease is a negative prognostic factor, so the best test may be in patients with small-volume disease. Another important field of research concerns improved methods of hematopoietic support. Efforts to expand the population of true stem cells in PBPC collections could lead to greater efficacy in marrow reconstitution and reduced costs (Shapiro et al., 1994). As important will be methods of reducing toxicity to organs other than the marrow. These include pulmonary toxicity (e.g. from melphalan and BCNU), hemorrhagic myocarditis (e.g. from cyclophosphamide), neurological damage (e.g. from cisplatin and thiotepa), and renal impairment (e.g. from cisplatin). In addition, efforts to improve chemotherapeutic cell-kill by the joint use of biological therapies are under investigation (Baselga et al., 1993, 1994). Laboratory and clinical research will continue to expand the potential of high-dose chemotherapy in the management of malignant disease.

References

Advani, R., Chao, N. J., Horning, S. J. et al. (1992). Granulocyte-macrophage colony-stimulating factor (GM-CSF) as an adjunct to autologous hemopoietic stem cell transplantation for lymphoma. *Ann. Int. Med.*, **116**, 183–9.

Aisner, J., Weinberg, V., Perloff, M. *et al.* (1987). Chemotherapy versus chemoimmuno-therapy (CAF, CAFVP, CMF each ± MER) for metastatic carcinoma of the breast: a CALGB study. Cancer and Leukemia Group B. *J. Clin Oncol.*, **5**, 1523–33.

Aisner, J., Cirrincione, C., Perloff, M. et al. (1995). Combination chemotherapy for metastatic or recurrent carcinoma of the breast – a randomized phase III trial comparing CAF versus VATIII alternating with CMFVP: Cancer and Leukemia Group B study 8281. *J. Clin. Oncol.*, **13**, 1443 –52.

Alberts, D. S., Young, L., Mason, N. L. et al. (1985). In vitro evaluation of anti-cancer against ovarian cancer at concentrations achievable by intraperitoneal administration. *Semin. Oncol.*, **12**, 38–42.

Antman, K., Ayash, L. J., Elias, A. et al. (1992). A phase II study of high dose cyclophosphamide, thiotepa and carboplatin with autologous bone marrow support in patients with measurable advanced breast cancer responding to standard-dose therapy. *J. Clin. Oncol.*, **10**, 102–10.

Bajorin, D. F., Sarosdy, M. F., Pfister, G. et al. (1993). Randomized trial of etoposide and cisplatin versus etoposide and carboplatin in patients with good-risk germ-cell tumors: A multiinstitutional study. *J. Clin. Oncol.*, **11**, 598–606.

Barker, G. H. et al. (1981). Use of high dose cisplatin following failure on previous chemotherapy for advanced carcinoma of the ovary. *Brit. J. Obstet. Gynecol.*, **88**, 1192–9.

Baselga, J., Norton, L., Masui, H. et al. (1993). Anti-tumor effects of doxorubicin in combination with anti-epidermal growth factor receptor monoclonal antibody. *J. Natl. Cancer Inst.*, **85**, 1327–33.

Baselga, J., Norton, L., Shalaby, R. and Mendelsohn, J. (1994). Anti HER2 humanized monoclonal antibody alone and in combination with chemotherapy against human breast carcinoma xenografts. *Proc. Am. Soc. Clin. Oncol.*, **13**, 53.

Behrens, B. C., Hamilton, T. C., Masuda, H. et al. (1987). Characteristics of cisdiamminedochloroplatinum(II)-resistant human ovarian cancer cell line and its evaluation of platinum analogues. *Cancer Res.*, **47**, 414–18.

Bella, M., Cocconi, G., Lotticci, R. et al. (1992). Conventional versus high dose intensity regimen of cisplatin in advanced ovarian carcinoma. A prospective randomized study. *Proc. Am. Soc. Clin. Oncol.*, **11**, 223.

Berkowitz, R. S., Goldstein, G. P. and Bernstein, M. R. (1986). Ten years experience with methotrexate and folinic acid as primary therapy for gestational trophoblastic disease. *Gynecol. Oncol.*, **23**, 111–18.

Bezwoda, W. R., Seymour, L. and Vorobiof, D. A. (1992). High dose cyclophosphamide, mitoxantrone and VP-16 as first line treatment for metastatic breast cancer. *Proc. Am. Soc. Clin. Oncol.*, **11**, 64 (abst.).

Bosl, G. J., Geller, N. L. and Bajorin, D. (1988). A randomized trial of etoposide cisplatin versus vinblastine bleomycin cisplatin cyclophosphamide dactinomycin in patients with good prognosis germ-cell tumors. *J. Clin. Oncol.*, **6**, 1231–8.

Bowden, G. T., Roberts, R., Alberts, D. S. et al. (1985). Comparative molecular pharmacology in leukemic L1210 cells of the anthracene anticancer drugs mitoxantrone and bisanthracene. *Cancer Res.*, **45**, 4915–20.

Bruce, W. R. and Valeriote, F. A. (1968). Normal and malignant stem cells and chemotherapy. In *The Proliferation and Spread of Neoplastic Cells, 21st Annual Symposium on Fundamental Cancer Research 1967*, pp. 409–22. Williams and Wilins, Baltimore.

Bruckner, H. et al. (1984). High dose platinum for the treatment of ovarian cancer. *Gynecol. Oncol.*, 12, 64–7.

Budman, D. R., Korzun, A. H., Cooper, M. R. et al. (1997). Dose and dose intensity trial of adjuvant chemotherapy for stage II, node-positive breast carcinoma. *New Engl. J. Med.*, in press.

Burchenal, J. H., Cramer, M. A., Williams, B. S. and Armstrong, R. A. (1951). Sterilization of leukemic cells in vivo and in vitro. *Cancer Res.*, 11, 700–5.

Buzzoni, R., Bonadonna, G., Valagussa, P. and Zambetti, M. (1991). Adjuvant chemotherapy with doxorubicin plus cyclophosphamide, methotrexate, and fluorouracil in the treatment of resectable breast cancer with more than three positive axillary nodes. *J. Clin. Oncol.*, 9, 2134.

Canellos, G. P., Anderson, J. R., Propert, K. et al. (1992). Chemotherapy of advanced Hodgkin's disease with MOPP, ABVD or MOPP alternating with ABVD. *N. Engl. J. Med.*, 327, 1478–84.

Coates, A., Gebski, V. and Bishop, J. F. (1987). Improving the quality of life during chemotherapy for advanced breast cancer. A comparison of intermittent and continuous treatment strategies. *New Engl. J. Med.*, 317, 1490–5.

Coldman, A. J. and Goldie, J. H. (1982). A mathematical model of drug resistance in neoplasms. In *Drug and Hormone Resistance in Neoplasia* (ed. N. Bruchovsky and J. H. Goldie), pp. 55–78. CRC Press, Boca Raton.

Colombo, N., Pittelli, M. R., Parma, G. et al. (1993). Cisplatin dose-intensity in advanced ovarian cancer: a randomized study of dose-intense versus standard dose cisplatin monochemotherapy. *Proc. Amer. Soc. Clin. Oncol.*, 12, 255.

Conte, P. F., Bruzzone, M., Gadducci, A. et al. (1993). High doses versus standard doses of cisplatin in combination with epidoxorubicin and cyclophosphamide in advanced ovarian cancer patients with bulky residual disease: a randomized trial. *Proc. Am. Soc. Clin. Oncol.*, 12, 273.

Crown, J., Jakubowski, A., Kemeny, N. et al. (1991). A phase I trial of recombinant human interleukin-1B alone and in combination with myelosuppressive doses of 5-fluorouracil in patients with gastrointestinal cancer. *Blood*, 78, 1420–7.

Crown, J., Kritz, A., Vahdat, L. et al. (1993). Rapid administration of multiple cycles of high-dose myelosuppressive chemotherapy in patients with metastatic breast cancer. *J. Clin. Oncol.*, 11, 1144–9.

Crown, J., Raptis, G., Vahdat, L. et al. (1994). Sequential high-dose cyclophosphamide, L-PAM and thiotepa in patients with metastatic breast cancer. *Ann. Oncol.*, 5 (suppl. 8).

Dauplat, J., Legros, M., Condat, P. et al. (1989). High-dose melphalan and autologous bone marrow support for treatment of ovarian carcinoma with positive second-look operation. *Gynecol. Oncol.*, 34(3), 294–8.

Day, R. S. (1986). Treatment sequencing, asymmetry, and uncertainty: protocol strategies for combination chemotherapy. *Cancer Res.*, 46, 3876.

Dedrick, R. L. (1978). Pharmacokinetic rationale for peritoneal drug administration in the treatment of ovarian cancer. *Cancer Treat. Rep.*, 62, 1–9.

DeVita, V. T. Jr. (1986). Dose-response is alive and well. *J. Clin. Oncol.*, 4, 1157.

DeVita, V. T. (1988). Principles of chemotherapy. In *Cancer: Principles and Practice*, 3rd Edition (ed. V. T. Devita, Jr, S. Hellman and S. A. Rosenberg), p. 279. J. B. Lippincott, Philadelphia.

DeVita, V. T. and Hubbard, S. M. (1993). Hodgkin's disease. *N. Engl. J. Med.*, **328**, 560–5.

DeVita, V. T., Young, R. C. and Cannellos, G. P. (1975). Combination vs. single agent chemotherapy: A review of the basis for selection of drug treatment of cancer. *Cancer*, **35**, 98.

Dimitrov, N., Anderson, S., Fisher, B. et al. (1994). Dose intensification and increased total dose of adjuvant chemotherapy for breast cancer (BC): findings from NSABP B-22. *Proc. Am. Soc. Clin. Oncol.*, **13**, 64.

Dittrich, C., Sevelda, P., Baur, M. et al. (1993). In vitro and in vivo evaluation of the combination of cisplatin and its analogue carboplatin for platinum dose intensification in ovarian carcinoma. *Cancer*, **71**, 3082–90.

Drewinko, B., Patchen, M., Yang, L.-Y. et al. (1981). Differential killing efficacy of twenty anti-tumor drugs on proliferating and non-proliferating human tumor cells. *Cancer Res.*, **41**, 2329–33.

Dunphy, F. and Spitzer, G. (1992). Use of very high-dose chemotherapy with autologous bone marrow transplantation treatment of breast cancer. *J. Natl. Cancer Inst.*, **84**, 129–9.

Early Breast Cancer Trialists' Collaborative Group (1992). Systemic treatment of early breast cancer by hormonal, cytotoxic, or immune therapy. *Lancet*, **339**, 71–85.

Eddy, D. M. (1992). High-dose chemotherapy with autologous bone marrow transplantation for the treatment for metastatic breast cancer. *J. Clin. Oncol.*, **10**, 657–70.

Eder, J. P., Antman, K., Peters, W. P. et al. (1986). High-dose combination alkylating agent chemotherapy with autologous marrow support for metastatic breast cancer. *J. Clin. Oncol.*, **4**, 1592–7.

Ehrlich, C. E., Einhorn, L., Stehman, F. B. and Blessing, J. (1983). Treatment of advanced epithelial ovarian cancer using cisplatin, adriamycin and cytoxan, the Indiana University experience. *Clin. Obstet. Gynecol.*, **10**(2), 325–35.

Fennelly, D., Crown, J., Hakes, T. et al. (1993). Accelerated delivery of multiple cycles of high-dose chemotherapy: a new role for peripheral blood progenitor cells. *Proc. Am. Soc. Clin. Oncol.*, **12**, 260.

Fennelly, D., Bengala, C., Schneider, J. et al. (1994). Taxol in combination with cyclophosphamide and GCSF, a novel peripheral blood progenitor cell mobilizing regimen. *Proc. Am. Assoc. Cancer Res.* **35**, 247.

Fennelly, D., Schneider, J., Spriggs, D. et al. (1995). Dose escalation of paclitaxel with high-dose cyclophosphamide, with analysis of progenitor-cell mobilization and hematologic support of advanced ovarian cancer patients receiving rapidly sequenced high-dose carboplatin/cyclophosphamide courses. *J. Clin. Oncol.*, **13**, 1160–6.

Forastiere, A. A., Hakes, T. B., Wittes, J. T. et al. (1982). Cisplatin in the treatment of metastatic breast carcinoma. A prospective randomized trial of two dosage schedules. *Am. J. Clin. Oncol.*, **5**, 243–7.

Frei, E. III and Canellos, G. P. (1980). Dose: A critical factor in cancer chemotherapy. *Am. J. Med.*, **69**, 585.

Frei, E. III, Freireich, E. J., Gehan, E. et al. (1961). Studies of sequential and combination antimetabolite therapy in acute leukemia: 6-mercaptopurine and methotrexate. *Blood*, **18**, 431.

Frei, E. III, Cucchi, C., Rosowsky, A. et al. (1985). Alkylating agent resistance: *in vitro* studies with human cell lines. *Proc. Natl. Acad. Sci. USA*, **82**, 2158–62.

Frei, E. III, Antman, K., Teicher, B. et al. (1989). Bone marrow autotransplantation for solid tumors – Prospects. *J. Clin. Oncol.*, **7**, 515–26.

Gianni, A., Bregni, M., Stern, A. et al. (1989). Granulocyte-macrophage colony-stimulating factor to harvest circulating haemopoietic stem cells for autotransplantation. *Lancet*, 11, 580–5.

Gilewski, T. and Norton, L. (1995). Cytokinetics of Neoplasia. In *The Molecular Basis of Cancer* (ed. J. Mendelsohn, P. Howley, M. A. Israel and A. Liotta), pp. 143–59. W. B. Saunders, Philadelphia.

Gill, J., Muggia, F. M., Terheggan, P. M. et al. (1991). Dose escalation study of carboplatin (day 1) and cisplatin (day 3): tolerance and relation to leukocyte and buccal cell platinum DNA adducts. *Ann. Oncol.*, 2, 115–21.

Goldie, J. H. (1987). Scientific basis for adjuvant and primary (neoadjuvant) chemotherapy. *Semin. Oncol.*, 14, 1.

Goldie, J. H. and Coldman, A. J. (1979). A mathematic model for relating the drug sensitivity of tumors to their spontaneous mutation rate. *Cancer Treat. Rep.*, 63, 1727.

Goldie, J. H. and Coldman, A. J. (1986). Application of theoretical models to chemotherapy protocol design. *Cancer Treat. Rep.*, 70, 127.

Griswold, D. P., Schabel, F. M. Jr, Corbett, T. H. and Dykes, D. J. (1982). Concepts for controlling drug-resistant tumor cells. In *Design of Models for Testing Cancer Therapeutic Agents* (ed. I. J. Fidler and R. J. White), pp. 215–24. Reinhold, New York.

Gulati, S. C. and Bennett, C. L. (1992). Granulocyte-macrophage colony-stimulating factor as adjunct therapy in relapsed Hodgkin's Disease. *Ann. Int. Med.*, 116, 177–82.

Gulati, S., Yahalom, Y., Acaba, L. et al. (1992). Treatment of patients with relapsed and resistant non-Hodgkin's lymphoma using total body irradiation, etoposide, cyclophosphamide and autologous bone marrow transplantation. *J. Clin. Oncol.*, 10, 936–41.

Hamburger, A. and Salmon, S. E. (1977). Primary bioassay of human myeloma stem cells. *J. Clin. Invest.*, 60, 846.

Hardy, J. R., Wiltshaw, E., Blake, P. R. et al. (1991). Cisplatin and carboplatin in combination for the treatment of stage IV ovarian carcinoma. *Ann. Oncol.*, 2, 131–6.

Hill, B. T., Hoskins, L. K., Shellard, S. A. et al. (1989). Comparative effectiveness of mitoxantrone and doxorubicin in overcoming experimentally induced drug resistance in murine and human tumor cell lines *in vitro*. *Cancer Chemother. Pharmacol.*, 23, 140–4.

Hoekman, K., Wagstaff, F., van Groeningen, J. et al. (1991). Effects of recombinant human granulocyte-macrophage colony-stimulating factor on myelosuppression induced by multiple cycles of high-dose chemotherapy in patients with advanced breast cancer. *J. Natl. Cancer Inst.*, 83, 1546–53.

Hreschyshyn, M. M. (1973). Single agent therapy in ovarian cancer. Factors influencing response. *Gynecol. Oncol.*, 1, 220.

Hudis, C., Lebwohl, D., Yao, T. J. et al. (1994). Results of sequential dose intensive adjuvant therapy with doxorubicin and cyclophosphamide. *Breast Cancer Res. Treat.*, 32, 37.

Hudis, C. (1996). New approaches to adjuvant chemotherapy for breast cancer. *Pharmacotherapy*, 16, 88S–93S.

Jaffe, N., Frei, E., Watts, H. and Traggis, D. (1978). High dose methotrexate in osteogenic sarcoma: a five year experience. *Cancer Treat. Rep.*, 62, 259–64.

Jones, A., Wiltshaw, E. and Harper, P. (1992). A randomized study of high- versus conventional-dose carboplatin for previously untreated ovarian cancer. *Proc. BACR/ACP*, 15(C8).

Jones, R. B., Holland, J. F., Bhardwal, S. et al. (1987). A phase I–II study of intensive-dose adriamycin for advanced breast cancer. *J. Clin. Oncol.*, **5**, 172–7.

Jones, R. B., Shpall, E. J., Ross, M. et al. (1990). AFM induction chemotherapy followed by intensive alkylating agent consolidation with autologous bone marrow support for advanced breast cancer. Current results. *Proc. Am. Soc. Clin. Oncol.*, **9**, 9.

Kaiser, H., Ghalle, R., Adler, S. S. et al. (1990). High-dose chemotherapy and autologous bone marrow transplantation in the treatment of metastatic breast cancer. *J. Cell. Biochem.*, **14a**, 321.

Kardinal, C. G., Perry, M. C., Korzun, A. H. et al. (1988). Responses to chemotherapy or chemohormonal therapy in advanced breast cancer patients treated previously with adjuvant chemotherapy: A subset analysis of CALGB study 8081. *Cancer*, **61**, 415.

Kaye, S. B., Lewis, C. R., Paul, J. et al. (1992). Randomized study of two doses of cisplatin and cyclophosphamide in epithelial ovarian cancer. *Lancet*, **340**, 329–33.

Kendal, W. S. and Frost, P. (1986). Metastatic potential and spontaneous mutation rates: studies with two murine cell lines and their recently induced metastatic variants. *Cancer Res.*, **46**, 6131.

Kennedy, M. J., Beveridge, R. A., Rowley, S. D. et al. (1991). High-dose chemotherapy with reinfusion of purged autologous bone marrow following dose-intense induction as initial therapy for metastatic breast cancer. *J. Natl. Cancer Inst.*, **83**, 920–6.

Kritz, A., Crown, J., Motzer, R. et al. (1991). Prospective randomized trial of recombinant human GM-CSF with or without autologous peripheral blood stem cells in patients receiving high dose chemotherapy for metastatic breast cancer. *Blood*, **78**, 19 (abst.).

Kritz, A., Crown, J. P., Motzer, R. J. et al. (1993). Beneficial impact of peripheral blood progenitor cells in patients with metastatic breast cancer treated with high-dose chemotherapy plus granulocyte-macrophage colony-stimulating factor. *Cancer*, **71**, 2515–21.

Law, L. W. (1952). Origin of resistance of leukaemic cells to folic acid antagonists. *Nature*, **169**, 628.

Lawton, L., Blackledge, G., Mould, J. et al. (1987). A phase II study of mitoxantrone in epithelial ovarian cancer. *Cancer Treat. Rep.*, **71**, 627–9.

Legros, M., Fleury, J., Cure, P. et al. (1992). High-dose chemotherapy and autologous bone marrow transplant in 31 advanced ovarian cancers. Long-term results. *Proc. Amer. Soc. Clin. Oncol.*, **11**, 222.

Levin, L. and Hryniuk, W. M. (1987). Dose intensity analysis of chemotherapy regimens in ovarian carcinoma. *J. Clin. Oncol.*, **5**, 756.

Lichtman, S., Ratain, M., Budner, D. et al. (1990). Phase I trial of recombinant granulocyte-macrophage colony-stimulating factor plus high-dose cyclophosphamide. *Proc. Am. Soc. Clin. Oncol.*, **9**, 66 (abst.).

Lichtman, S. M., Ratain, M. J., Van Echo, D. A. et al. (1993). Phase I trial of granulocyte-macrophage colony stimulating factor (GM-CSF) plus high dose biweekly cyclophosphamide: a CALGB study. *J. Natl. Cancer Inst.*, **85**, 1319–26.

Loehrer, P. J., Elson, P., Johnson, D. H. et al. (1991). A randomized trial of cisplatin plus etoposide with or without bleomycin in favorable prognosis disseminated germ-cell tumors. *Proc. Am. Soc. Clin. Oncol.*, **5**, 97.

Look, A. T., Douglass, E. C. and Meyer, W. II. (1988). Clinical importance of near-diploid tumor stem lines in patients with osteosarcoma of an extremity. *N. Engl. J. Med.*, **318**, 1567.

Lown, J. W., Hanstock, C. C., Bradley, R. D. et al. (1984). Interactions of the antitumor mitoxantrone and bisantrene with deoxyribonucleic acids studies by electron microscopy. *Mol. Pharmacol.*, **25**, 178–84.

Ludwig Breast Cancer Study Group. (1988). Combination adjuvant chemotherapy for node positive breast cancer. *N. Engl. J. Med.*, **319**, 677.

Lund, B., Hansen, M., Hansen, O. P. et al. (1989). High-dose platinum consisting of combined carboplatin and cisplatin in previously untreated ovarian cancer patients with residual disease. *J. Clin. Oncol.*, **7**, 1469–73.

Lund, B., Hansen, M., Hansen, O. P. et al. (1990). Combined high-dose carboplatin and cisplatin, and ifosfamide in previously untreated ovarian cancer patients with residual disease. *J. Clin. Oncol.*, **8**, 1226–30.

Luria, S. E. and Delbruck, M. (1943). Mutations of bacteria from virus sensitivity to virus resistance. *Genetics*, **28**, 491.

Markman, M. (1991). Intraperitoneal chemotherapy. *Semin. Oncol.*, **18**(3), 248–54.

Markman, M. et al. (1985). Intraperitoneal chemotherapy for ovarian carcinoma. In *Gyn Oncology* (ed. D. Alberts and E. Surwitt), pp. 179–212. Martinus Nijhoff, Boston.

Markman, M., Hakes. T., Reichman, B. et al. (1991a). Phase II trial of weekly or bi-weekly intraperitoneal mitoxantrone in epithelial ovarian cancer. *J. Clin. Oncol.*, **9**(6), 978–82.

Markman, M. et al. (1991b). Responses to second-line cisplatin-based intraperitoneal therapy in ovarian cancer: influence of a prior response to intravenous cisplatin. *J. Clin. Oncol.*, **9**, 1801–5.

McGuire, W. P., Hoskins, W. J., Brady, M. F. et al. (1996). Cyclophosphamide and cisplatin compared with paclitaxel and cisplatin in patients with stage III and stage IV ovarian cancer. *N. Engl. J. Med.*, **334**, 1–6.

McGuire, W. P. (1993). Dose intensity in ovarian cancer, pp. 31–6. Am. Soc. Clin. Oncol. Educational Book.

Motzer, R., Gulati, S., Crown, J. et al. (1992). High dose chemotherapy and autologous bone marrow rescue for patients with refractory germ cell tumors. *Cancer*, **69**, 550–6.

Mulder, P. O. M., Willemse, P. H. B., Azalders, J. G. et al. (1989a). High-dose chemotherapy with autologous bone marrow transplantation in patients with refractory ovarian cancer. *Eur. J. Clin. Oncol.*, **25**, 645–9.

Mulder, P. O. M., Sleijfer, D. T., Willemse, P. H. B. et al. (1989b). High-dose cyclophosphamide or melphalan with escalating doses of mitoxantrone and autologous bone marrow transplantation for refractory solid tumors. *Cancer Res.*, **49**, 4654–8.

Neidhart, J. A., Kohler, W., Stidley, C. et al. (1990). Phase I study of repeated cycles of high dose cyclophosphamide, etoposide and cisplatin administered without bone marrow transplantation. *J. Clin. Oncol.*, **8**, 1728–38.

Ngan, H. Y. S., Choo, Y. C., Cheung, M. et al. (1989). A randomized study of high-dose versus low-dose cisplatinum combined with cyclophosphamide in the treatment of advanced ovarian cancer. *Chemotherapy*, **35**, 221–7.

Norton, L. (1985). Implications of kinetic heterogeneity in clinical oncology. *Semin. Oncol.*, **12**, 231.

Norton, L. and Simon, R. (1977). Tumor size, sensitivity to therapy and the design of treatment protocols. *Cancer Treat. Rep.*, **61**, 1307–17.

Norton, L. and Simon, R. L. (1986). The Norton–Simon hypothesis revisited. *Cancer Treat. Rep.*, **70**, 163.

Norton, L. and Day, R. (1991). Potential innovations in scheduling in cancer chemotherapy. In *Important Advances in Oncology* (ed. V. T. DeVita Jr, S. Hellman and S. A. Rosenberg), pp. 57–72. J. B. Lippincott, New York.

O'Dwyer, P. J., LaCreta, F., Schilder, R. et al. (1992). Phase I trial of thiotepa in combination with recombinant human granulocyte-macrophage colony-stimulating factor. *J. Clin. Oncol.*, **10**, 1352–8.

Ozols, R. F., Ostchega, Y., Myers, C. E. et al. (1987). Cisplatin in hypertonic saline in refractory ovarian cancer. *J. Clin. Oncol.*, **5**, 1246–50.

Peters, W. P., Shpall, E. J., Jones, R. B. et al. (1988). High-dose combination alkylating agents with bone marrow support as initial treatment for metastatic breast cancer. *J. Clin. Oncol.*, **6**, 1368–76.

Peters, W. P., Kurtzberg, J. and Kirkpatrick, G. (1989). GM-CSF primed peripheral blood progenitor cells coupled with autologous bone marrow transplantation will eliminate absolute leukopenia following high dose chemotherapy. *Blood*, **74**, 178 (abst.).

Peters, W. P., Ross, M. and Vredenburgh, J. J. (1993). High-dose chemotherapy and autologous bone marrow support as consolidation after standard-dose adjuvant therapy for high-risk primary breast cancer. *J. Clin. Oncol.*, **11**, 1132–43.

Piccart, M. J., Nogaret, J. M., Marcelis, L. et al. (1990). Cisplatin combined with carboplatin: a new way of intensification of platinum dose in the treatment of advanced ovarian cancer. *J. Natl. Cancer Inst.*, **82**, 703–7.

Raptis, G., Crown, J., Vahdat, L. et al. (1994). Rapidly administered sequential high-dose cyclophosphamide, melphalan, thiotepa, supported by filgrastim plus peripheral blood progenitors in metastatic breast cancer patients. *17th International Breast Cancer Symposium*, pp. 15–145.

Reichman, B. S., Seidman, A. S. and Crown, J. P. A. (1993). Paclitaxel and recombinant human granulocyte colony stimulating factor as initial chemotherapy for metastatic breast cancer. *J. Clin. Oncol.*, **11**, 1943–51.

Rudnick, S. A., Cadman, E. C., Capizzi, R. L. et al. (1979). High dose cytosine arabinoside (HDARAC) in refractory acute leukemia. *Cancer*, **44**, 1189–93.

Seidman, A. D., Reichman, B. S., Crown, J. P. A. et al. (1997). Paclitaxel as second and subsequent therapy for metastatic breast cancer: activity independent of prior anthracycline response. *J. Clin. Oncol.*, in press.

Shapiro, F., Yao, T.-J., Raptis, G. et al. (1994). Optimization of conditions for *ex-vivo* expansion of peripheral blood progenitors from patients with breast cancer. *Blood*, **84**, 3567–74.

Shea, T. C., Flaherty, M., Elias, A. M. et al. (1989). A phase I clinical and pharmacokinetic study of carboplatin and autologous bone marrow support. *J. Clin. Oncol.*, **7**, 651–61.

Shea, T. C., Mason, J. R., Storniolo, A. M. et al. (1992). Sequential cycles of high-dose carboplatin administered with recombinant human granulocyte-macrophage colony-stimulating factor and repeated infusions of autologous peripheral-blood progenitor cells: a novel and effective method for delivering multiple courses of dose-intensive therapy. *J. Clin. Oncol.*, **10**, 464–73.

Shea, T. C., Mason, J. R., Stornido, A. M., et al. (1993). High-dose carboplatin chemotherapy with GM-CSF and peripheral blood progenitor cell support: a model for delivering repeated cycles of dose-intensive therapy. *Cancer Treat. Rev.*, **19**, 11–20.

278   D. Fennelly, G. Raptis, J. P. A. Crown & L. Norton

Shenkenberg, T. D. and Von Hoff, D. D. (1986). Mitoxantrone: a new anti-cancer drug with significant clinical activity. *Ann. Int. Med.*, **105**, 67–81.

Shpall, E., Clarke-Peterson, D., Soper, J. et al. (1990). High-dose alkylating agent chemotherapy with autologous bone marrow support in patients with stage III/ IV epithelial ovarian cancer. *Gynecol. Oncol.*, **38**, 386–91.

Silverberg, E., Boring, C. and Squires, T. S. (1990). *Cancer Statistics 1990, Ca – A Cancer Journal for Clinicians*, **40**, 9–26.

Skipper, H. E. (1967). Criteria associated with destruction of leukemia and solid tumor cells in animals. *Cancer Res.*, **27**, 2636–45.

Skipper, H. E. (1986a). Laboratory models: the historical perspective. *Cancer Treat Rep.*, **70**, 3.

Skipper, H. E. (1986b). Analyses of multiarmed trials in which animals bearing different burdens of L1210 leukemia cells were treated with two, three, and four drug combinations delivered in different ways with varying dose intensities of each drug and varying average dose intensities. *Southern Research Institute Booklet*, **7**, 42–87.

Smith, I. E., Evans, B. D., Harland, S. J. and Millar, J. L. (1983). Autologous bone marrow rescue is unnecessary after very-high-dose cyclophosphamide. *Lancet*, **1**, 76.

Smith II, J., Longo, D., Alvord, W. et al. (1992). Thrombopoietic effects of IL-1α in combination with high-dose carboplatin. *Proc. Am. Soc. Clin. Oncol.*, **11**, 252 (abst.).

Socinski, M. A., Cannesta, S. A., Elias, A. et al. (1988). Granulocyte-macrophage colony-stimulating factor expands the circulating haemopoietic progenitor cell compartment in man. *Lancet*, 1194–8.

Stiff, P., Antman, K., Randolph Broun, E. et al. (1992). Bone marrow transplantation for ovarian carcinoma in the United States: a survey of active programs. *Proc. 6th International Autologous Bone Marrow Transplant Symposium*, 1–9.

Tannock, I. F., Boyd, N. F., DeBoer, G. et al. (1988). A randomized trial of two dose levels of cyclophosphamide, methotrexate and fluorouracil chemotherapy for patients with metastatic breast cancer. *J. Clin. Oncol.*, **6**, 1377–87.

Taylor, K., Jagannath, S., Spitzer, G. et al. (1989). Recombinant human granulocytes colony-stimulating factor hastens granulocyte recovery after high-dose chemotherapy and autologous bone marrow transplantation in Hodgkin's disease. *J. Clin. Oncol.*, **7**, 1791–9.

Teicher, B. A., Holden, S. A., Cucchi, C. A. et al. (1988). Combination thiotepa and cyclophosphamide in vivo and in vitro. *Cancer Res.*, **48**, 94–100.

Tepler, I., Cannistra, S., Anderson, K. et al. (1992). Use of peripheral blood progenitor cells (PBPC) for support of repetitive high-dose carboplatin chemotherapy (X4) in previously untreated outpatients with cancer. *Blood*, **80** (suppl. 1), 71a (abst. 275).

Till, J. E., McCullock, G. A., Phillips, R. A. and Siminovitch, L. (1968). Aspects of the regulation of stem cell function. In *The Proliferation and Spread of Neoplastic Cells, 21st Annual Symposium on Fundamental Cancer Research 1967*, pp. 235–44. Williams and Wilkins, Baltimore.

Trump, D. L., Grem, J. L., Tutsch, K. D., et al. (1987). Platinum analog combination chemotherapy: cisplatin and carboplatin: a phase I trial with pharmacokinetic assessment of the effect of cisplatin administration on carboplatin excretion. *J. Clin. Oncol.*, **5**, 1281–9.

Vadban-Raj, S., Kudelka, A., Garrison, L. et al. (1992). Interleukin-1α (IL-1α) increases circulating platelet (PLT) counts and reduces carboplatin

(CBDCA)-induced thrombocytopenia. *Proc. Am. Soc. Clin. Oncol.*, **11**, 224.

Valagussa, P., Tancini, G. and Bonadonna, G. (1986). Salvage treatment of patients suffering relapse after adjuvant CMF chemotherapy. *Cancer*, **58**, 1411.

Valagussa, P., Brambilla, C., Zambetti, M. and Bonadonna, G. (1988). Salvage treatment after first relapse of breast cancer: a review. In *Proceedings of the Third International Conference on Adjuvant Therapy of Primary Breast Cancer*, St Gallen, Switzerland, p. 9.

Venturini, M., Sertoli, M. R., Ardizzoni, A. et al. (1992). Prospective randomized trial of accelerated FEC chemotherapy (CT) with or without GM-CSF in advanced breast cancer (ABC). *Proc. Am. Soc. Clin. Oncol.*, **11**, 52.

Wallace, R. E., Citarella, R. V. and Durr, F. E. (1979). The inhibitory effects of 1,4-dihydroxy-5,8-bis (2-(2-hydroxyethyl)amino)-9,10 anthracene-dione (CL232315; NSC 301739D) on dividing and non-dividing cells in vitro. *Proc. Am. Assoc. Cancer Res.*, **20**, 12.

Wallerstein, R., Spitzer, G., Dunphy, F. et al. (1990). A phase II study of mitoxantrone, etoposide, and thiotepa with autologous marrow support for patients with relapsed breast cancer. *J. Clin. Oncol.*, **8**(11), 1782–8.

Waterhouse, D. M., Reynolds, R. K. and Natale, R. B. (1993). Combined carboplatin and cisplatin. Limited prospects for dose intensification. *Cancer*, **71**, 4060–6.

Williams, S. F., Gilewski, T., Mick, R. and Bitran, J. D. (1992). High-dose consolidation therapy with autologous stem-cell rescue in stage IV breast cancer: follow-up report. *J. Clin. Oncol.*, **10**, 1743–7.

Wolff, S. N., Herzig, R. H., Fay, J. W. et al. (1990). High-dose *N,N,N*''-triethylenethiophosphoramide (thiotepa) with autologous bone marrow transplantation: phase I studies. *Semin. Oncol.*, **17** (suppl. 3), 2–6.

Younger, J., Shapiro, C., Douville, L. et al. (1992). A phase I study of dose-intensified CAF chemotherapy with adjunctive r-metHug-CSF (GCSF) in patients with advanced breast cancer. *Proc. Am. Soc. Clin. Oncol.*, **11**, 108.

Zittoun, R. A., Mandelli, F., Willemze, R. et al. (1995). Autologous or allogeneic bone marrow transplantation compared with intensive chemotherapy in acute myelogenous leukemia. *N. Engl. J. Med.*, **332**, 217–33.

9

Circumvention of drug resistance by high-dose chemotherapy in solid tumors

ELISABETH G. E. DE VRIES, WIL V. DOLSMA, GEKE
A. P. HOSPERS and NANNO H. MULDER

Introduction

Drug resistance is a major problem in the treatment of patients with chemotherapeutic drugs. The roots of this problem lie in part in the presence of tumor cells that are intrinsically resistant to chemotherapeutic drugs, or that have become so in the course of treatment. One of the ways to circumvent drug resistance is to administer the chemotherapeutic drugs in a higher dose. Initially, studies on the treatment of breast cancer and ovarian cancer with high-dose chemotherapy and bone marrow support dealt with patients having a large tumor load at the time of treatment. In similar situations of high tumor load, other malignancies including acute leukemia, germ cell tumors, small cell lung cancer and ovarian cancer have been shown to be incurable with standard dose chemotherapy. Several malignancies in complete remission, however, can be cured by high-dose therapy. These include acute leukemia, aggressive non-Hodgkin's lymphoma and occasional germ cell tumors. The fact that supportive care improved has made this procedure less dangerous. Therefore, it is more acceptable to enter this type of treatment earlier in the stage of disease of solid tumors.

Myelo-, cardio-, pulmonal- and neurotoxicity are the main toxicities that make dose intensification difficult. Cardio-, pulmonal- and neurotoxicity are difficult to circumvent. It is however possible to circumvent bone marrow toxicity without long-term untoward effects for the patient. With the help of bone marrow or peripheral stem cell reinfusion and hematopoietic growth factors it is possible to increase chemotherapy dose by a 10-fold factor for certain chemotherapeutic drugs.

280

Circumvention of chemotherapeutic related toxicity

Bone marrow and peripheral stem cell reinfusion

In the earlier nineties it was shown that the hematopoietic growth factors granulocyte–macrophage-colony stimulating factor (GM-CSF) and granulocyte-colony stimulating factor (G-CSF) had a positive effect on leucocyte recovery in autologous bone marrow transplant patients (Brandt et al., 1988; Sheridan et al., 1989; Taylor et al., 1989; Nemunaitis et al., 1991; Gorin et al., 1992; Gulati and Bennett, 1992; Link et al., 1992; Rabinowe et al., 1993; Gisselbrecht et al., 1994; De Vries et al., 1995). However, over the last years, apart from bone marrow reinfusion plus growth factor, the use of peripheral stem cells has gained a special place in the high-dose chemotherapy schedules in solid tumors. After a hematopoietic growth factor, chemotherapy or a combination of both, stem cells can be harvested from the peripheral blood with pheresis (De Vries et al., 1995). The advantage of peripheral blood stem cells compared to bone marrow reinfusion is the fact that if administered in a sufficient amount, does result in a faster leucocyte as well as platelet recovery. We wanted to evaluate the additive effect of peripheral blood stem cells to autologous bone marrow transplantation of hematopoietic reconstitution after ablative chemotherapy in patients with locally advanced breast cancer. Twenty-five patients were treated with induction chemotherapy, followed by ablative chemotherapy consisting of mito-xantrone 50 mg/m^2 and thiotepa 800 mg/m^2. The first 14 patients received autologous bone marrow reinfusion and GM-CSF (group I). The following 11 patients received autologous bone marrow reinfusion, peripheral blood stem cells and G-CSF (group II). Peripheral blood stem cells were harvested after a low-dose cyclophosphamide (750 mg/m^2), followed by G-CSF. Stem cell harvest was routinely started 12 days after cyclophosphamide. Compared to group I, group II showed a significant reduction of median days of leucocytes: $< 0.5 \times 10^9/\text{L}$ from 14.5 to 10 days, leucocytes $< 1.0 \times 10^9/\text{L}$ from 16.5 to 11 days, platelets $< 20 \times 10^9/\text{L}$ from 25 to 16 days and platelets $< 40 \times 10^9/\text{L}$ from 32.5 to 20 days. The median number of platelet transfusions fell from 11.5 to 7 and of red blood cell transfusions from 8.5 to 6. The median hospitalization duration declined from 40.5 to 30 days, fever above 38°C from 11.5 to 3 days, fever above 38.5°C from 4 to 0 days and antibiotic treatment from 19.5 to 11 days in group I versus group II. We thus observed an improvement of hematologic recovery, duration of fever and hospitalization by the addition of peripheral blood stem cells, obtained after a relatively low-dose cyclophosphamide and G-CSF and stem cell pheresis on fixed days, compared to autologous bone marrow and growth factor in the period after ablative chemotherapy (De Graaf et al., 1995).

A number of studies also suggest that, apart from a more rapid recovery of blood count, less transfusions of red blood cells and platelets, and less use of antibiotics with a shorter hospitalization ensue (Gianni et al., 1989; Peters et al., 1993a; Bensinger et al., 1995; De Vries et al., 1995; Schmitz et al., 1996).

Bone marrow as well as peripheral blood, although probably to a lesser extent, can contain tumor cells. The clinical significance of the presence of these tumor cells in the stem cell harvest is not yet clear for solid tumors. Immunocytochemistry as well as reverse-transcriptase PCRs are now available to detect low amounts of tumor cells (Ross et al., 1993; Brugger et al., 1994; Datta et al., 1994). This should help as part of a larger phase III study to define the prognostic role of tumor cell contamination.

The above-mentioned results from phase II studies seem to be strongly in favor of the use of peripheral stem cells. Bensinger et al. (1995) showed that a number of factors affected the collection of peripheral blood stem cells. The best yield of CD34 cells was obtained with mobilization with chemotherapy plus growth factor, in patients with breast cancer, in the absence of marrow disease, without prior radiation therapy and after fewer cycles of chemotherapy. They observed also that the CD34 dose was the predictor of engraftment kinetics after peripheral stem cell reinfusion and that the addition of G- or GM-CSF gave a faster neutrophil recovery but a slower platelet recovery in the case of $< 5 \times 10^6$ CD34 cells/kg body weight reinfused (Bensinger et al., 1995). The long-term effects on bone marrow capacity are as yet not available for peripheral stem cells. Results from a phase III study comparing bone marrow versus peripheral stem cells are now available. Lymphoma patients treated with high-dose chemotherapy, who received filgrastim-mobilized peripheral stem cells, had a reduced number of platelet transfusions, time to platelet recovery and neutrophil recovery, and an earlier hospital discharge than patients who received autologous bone marrow (Schmitz et al., 1996). Preliminary data suggest that bone marrow of patients who received high-dose chemotherapy is more vulnerable to further attacks.

Concerning the purging of peripheral stem cells and in vitro culturing of hematopoietic stem cells to upscale them and then reinfuse, a lot of research is ongoing (De Vries et al., 1995).

Tissue protection with drug resistant genes

A new approach to protect tissue against chemotherapeutic drugs is the transfer of drug resistant genes. In Table 9.1 a list of drug resistant genes that could be used is given. Another approach is the insertion of drug resistant genes in the bone marrow, which will theoretically result in prevention of toxicity. This approach has been investigated with the *MDR1* gene. The product of this gene, the so-called P-glycoprotein, is a multidrug transporter. Pastan et al. showed in 1988 that transduction of this gene in non-resistant MDCK cells transfers resistance to *MDR1* related chemotherapeutic drugs and not to the MDR unrelated drugs. In 1992, Sorrentino et al. succeeded in the transfer of the *MDR1* gene in bone marrow stem cells of mice. This results in a prevention of the *MDR1* drug-related bone marrow toxicity. These experiments introduced the *MDR1* gene in bone marrow by the use of a retroviral transduction system. This system has shown to be safe when there is no contamination with competent retroviruses (also called helper viruses). It has been shown that competent retroviruses are able to induce lymphoma in monkeys (Vanin et al., 1994). Based on these results and the knowledge that careful testing for the presence of competent retroviruses is necessary, a clinical trial has been started in the USA (O'Slaughnessy et al., 1994) and efforts are being made to start also in the Netherlands. Based on the same principle, other drug resistant genes with another drug resistance profile can be used to prevent bone marrow toxicity (Table 9.1). To widen the area of drug resistant genes, fungal and bacterial drug resistant genes can also be used. These genes, some related to the MDR gene family, may have a different spectrum of resistance to certain chemotherapeutic drugs. An example of such a resistant gene is the *PDR5* (Pleomorphic Drug Resistant) gene found in *Saccharomyces cerevisiae* (Decottignies et al., 1994a,b). Apart from the nucleotide structure of this gene transcriptional control factors have also been identified (Katzmann et al., 1994). The information on the regulation of drug resistant genes is useful from the point of view of counteracting drug resistance as well as to get information on how these genes can be stimulated to achieve a higher level of resistance in the tissue that has to be protected.

As yet there are no experiments described where drug resistant genes

Table 9.1. *Drug-resistant genes*

MDR genes
MRP gene(s)
O^6-methylguanine DNA methyl transferase gene(s)
Aldehyde dehydrogenase gene(s)
Thymidylate synthase gene(s)
Glutathione-S-transferase gene(s)
Metallothionein gene(s)
Dihydrofolate reductase gene(s)

Table 9.2. *Possible ways of achieving tissue-specific transduction*

1. Viruses with a tissue specific tropism
2. Liposomes with tissue specific antibodies
3. The gene under the transcriptional control of a tissue specific promotor
4. In vitro cell purification (e.g. stem cell purification)

are used for the prevention of cardio-, pulmonary- and neurotoxicity. On counteracting these toxicities with the use of resistant genes one encounters the problem of gene delivery to these selected tissues. To transduce these tissues with genes, an in vivo transduction system is needed. An in vivo transduction system has to be tissue specific, therefore in the future gene targeting is a very important issue to study. In Table 9.2 some possibilities are listed that might allow achievement of tissue specificity.

The use of drug resistant genes will coincide with a lot of technical problems. It also poses the risk of introducing drug resistant genes in tumor cells. In the clinical trial where bone marrow is transduced with the *MDR1* gene patients without macroscopic bone marrow infiltration will be especially eligible for future study. Stem cell purification will also contribute in a selection for bone marrow cells. But the existence of micro metastasis in the bone marrow cannot be excluded. This underscores the relevance of detecting microscopic disease with the help of immunocytochemistry or sensitive polymerase chain reactions. This problem is even greater in the case of the use of resistant genes for pulmonary-, cardio- and neurotoxicity, where gene delivery has to be performed in vivo. Thus, the use of drug resistant genes for the circumvention of chemotherapy-induced toxicity may be useful in the future. Preliminary data from clinical studies showing successful engraftment of *MDR1* modified cells are just becoming available (Hanania et al., 1996).

Indications for high-dose chemotherapy in solid tumors

High-dose chemotherapy is potentially interesting in the treatment of germ cell carcinomas, breast carcinoma, ovarian carcinoma and tumors of young adults, such as Ewing sarcoma (Coiffier et al., 1994).

Germ cell carcinomas

Germ cell carcinomas are, compared to most other solid tumors, extremely sensitive to chemotherapy. Most of the patients with metastatic germ cell carcinomas are cured with first line chemotherapy. Patients who relapse after chemotherapy or who do not achieve a complete remission on first line chemotherapy have a bad prognosis. Based on a retrospective study it appears that less than 25% of these patients can be cured with additional chemotherapy (Motzer et al., 1991). Patients who do not achieve a complete remission on first line cisplatin- or carboplatin-based chemotherapy are an especially bad prognostic group with a very low survival chance on standard chemotherapy (Levi et al., 1988; Stoter et al., 1989). Potentially interesting drugs for chemotherapy dose escalation for this tumor type are etoposide, cyclophosphamide, ifosfamide and carboplatin. These drugs have antitumor activity in germ cell carcinomas and are especially toxic to bone marrow. High-dose chemotherapy (carboplatin and etoposide) can result in about 10–15% long lasting disease free survival (Mulder et al., 1988; Nichols et al., 1989; Broun et al., 1992; Motzer and Bosl, 1992; Motzer et al., 1992). Patients with a relapse after an earlier complete remission have a somewhat better prognosis with 'non-crossresistant' second-line chemotherapy (cisplatin, ifosfamide, vinblastine), and a survival of 25–30% (Borge et al., 1988; Motzer et al., 1992; Horwich et al., 1993). A study of the Dutch Cancer Institute (Rodenhuis et al., 1995) suggests a 'salvage rate' of 63% in this patient group ($n = 11$) with one or two courses of carboplatin and etoposide on days 1, 3 and 5, followed by one or two courses of high-dose carboplatin, cyclophosphamide and thiotepa with stem cell support. Currently, there is in The Netherlands an ongoing phase II study with high-dose chemotherapy followed after each cycle by peripheral stem cells. A phase III trial including high-dose chemotherapy for high-risk patients in the first line is being performed in the USA.

Breast carcinoma

Metastatic breast carcinomas often respond to chemotherapy. From studies in patients with metastatic disease, data suggest a trend that more chemotherapy results in a better chance to obtain remission and a longer survival. The prognosis of patients with metastatic breast cancer has, however, hardly improved over the last decade. The median survival of these patients is, with conventional combination chemotherapy, 18–24 months. The survival of these patients at 3 years is 26–35% (Eddy, 1992). Unfortunately, complete responses do not represent cure in breast cancer. The documentation, both in the laboratory and in the clinic, of a steep dose response curve for a number of drugs in breast cancer and the more acceptable toxicity after the high-dose chemotherapy treatment has promoted a large number of studies with high-dose chemotherapy in patients with metastatic breast cancer. This treatment with high-dose chemotherapy gave about 60% remissions in patients with chemo-therapy-resistant breast carcinoma, but very few patients had a durable survival (Eddy, 1992).

In Groningen we used high-dose chemotherapy in a number of phase I, II and III studies in patients for various stages of breast cancer. Two regimens were developed in phase I studies. The first consisted of cyclophosphamide at a dose of 7 g/m^2 combined with etoposide. For this drug a final dose of 1.2 g/m^2 was used in combination chemotherapy. At this and higher dose levels etoposide was found to be active in breast cancer (Mulder et al., 1984). The second group of regimens was based on mitoxantrone at a dose of 60 mg/m^2 (Mulder et al., 1989a). This drug could be combined with melphalan 180 mg/m^2 or thiotepa 800 mg/m^2. Thiotepa is a drug that can be escalated to a high level with relatively minor toxicity consisting of mucositis and limited hepatotoxicity. Currently in an ongoing protocol with a tandem transplant, thiotepa is administered as a first ablative course followed after recovery from extramedullary toxicity by a second ablative course consisting of melphalan and mitoxantrone. In this setting this first treatment stage can be given partly on an outpatient basis.

Patients with metastatic disease responding to first line chemotherapy were treated in phase I studies and with the cyclophosphamide/etoposide regimen. Out of 13 patients, two remain free of disease after more than 4 years; both patients initially had presented with extensive lung, liver and bone metastases. The others died within 18 months after intensive chemotherapy from disease progression (Mulder et al., 1986). The Dutch

Working Group on ABMT in solid tumors used the mitoxantrone/ melphalan regimen in a phase II study (CKVO-89-07R), in which Maastricht, Utrecht, Rotterdam, Amsterdam and Groningen participated. This trial studied the disease-free survival after high-dose chemotherapy in patients in complete remission of metastatic breast cancer. Thirty women, mean age 42.2 years, with metastatic breast cancer received high-dose chemotherapy. Patients were eligible if they were ≤ 55 years of age, had achieved complete remission within 6 months of the initiation of chemotherapy and had a WHO performance scale of 0 or 1. The high-dose regimen consisted of melphalan 180 mg/m^2 and mitoxantrone 60 mg/m^2 both divided over 3 days. On day 7 bone marrow and/or peripheral stem cells were infused. After bone marrow recovery, external beam radiation was administered to sites of previously metastatic disease in 15 patients. Apart from leuco- and thrombocytopenia, mucositis was the major side effect. One patient died during the bone marrow transplant period due to an aspergillus infection. The median follow-up since high-dose chemotherapy is 25 months (range 13−56 months). The median disease-free survival since high-dose chemotherapy is 27 months and the disease-free survival is still 43% with an overall survival of 53% at 3 years. In two patients tumor relapse occurred only in the brain; in one patient the only relapse sign was a meningeal carcinosis. At the time of writing, 17 patients are disease-free 13−56 months after high-dose chemotherapy. Until now this high-dose regimen in selected patients with complete remission after induction chemotherapy for metastatic breast cancer has resulted in a promising disease-free survival (De Vries et al., 1996a).

In a compilation of phase II studies with high-dose chemotherapy for metastatic breast cancer it was found that high-dose chemotherapy resulted in response durations of 8 months (Eddy, 1992). A number of studies suggest, however, that patients benefit longer from high-dose chemotherapy if they responded on previous induction chemotherapy (Kennedy et al., 1991; Williams et al., 1992; Ayash et al., 1994; Dillman and Barth, 1994). Williams et al. (1992) found that in patients who had received no prior adjuvant chemotherapy, a longer survival after high-dose chemotherapy was observed. In a number of studies with high-dose chemotherapy, long-term disease-free survivors (2−7.3 years) have been reported in percentages of 10−20%. Many investigators are currently performing studies with tandem transplants. It is thus hoped that double treatment results will increase response rate and disease-free survival duration (Ayash et al., 1994). Before firm conclusions can be drawn concerning the role of high-dose chemotherapy in metastatic disease, due to the variable course of the disease, randomized studies will be required. They are currently ongoing in the USA and Europe. Some results of randomized studies are already available. Bezwoda, Seymour and Dansey (1995) randomized 90 patients between two cycles of high-dose cyclophosphamide 2.4 g/m^2, mitoxantrone 35 to 45 mg/ m^2 and etoposide 2.5 g/m^2 versus 6–8 cycles of conventionally dosed cyclophosphamide, mitoxantrone and vincristine. The high-dose regimen had a higher complete remission rate and a longer disease free and overall survival. Peters et al. (1996) presented preliminary results of the ASCO meeting in 1996. A total of 423 hormone-insensitive patients who had not received prior chemotherapy for metastatic disease, received 2–4 cycles induction treatment. Those who obtained complete remission ($n = 98$) were randomized to receive high-dose chemotherapy (cyclo-phosphamide, cisplatin, carmustine) either immediately or at relapse. Those who received the high-dose treatment immediately after induction therapy had the longest disease free survival, but overall survival appeared superior in those who received the high dose at the time of recurrence.

Over the last years a number of groups analyzed whether dose increase of adjuvant chemotherapy without autologous bone marrow reinfusion in patients with multiple positive axillary nodes did improve the out-come. This seemed to be the case. These findings have stimulated high-dose chemotherapy regimens with stem cell support in these patients. Peters reported a study in 85 patients with more than 10 positive axillary lymph nodes who received high-dose chemotherapy with bone marrow reinfusion (Peters et al., 1993b). The disease survival was 72% and was found to be favorable compared to a historical control group. The relatively high mortality in this regimen is probably due to the fact that this regimen also contains BCNU. Gianni et al. treated patients with various regimens of high-dose chemotherapy and peripheral stem cell harvest, which resulted at 21 months in a survival of 93% (Gianni et al., 1992).

We treated patients in the adjuvant setting with the cyclophosphamide/ etoposide regimen (10 patients) or the mitoxantrone/thiotepa regimen (30 patients). The group consisted of women with five or more positive axillary nodes. All of these patients received the same induction treat-ment. Radiotherapy was given in the case of extranodal tumor. All patients received tamoxifen for two years after treatment. The median age of these patients was 43, the median number of lymph nodes involved was nine. In this group there was one toxic death and one death during follow-up possibly related to treatment (cardiac death). Radiation pneumonitis occurred in 50% of patients. Five patients have relapsed after 24, 28, 34, 48 and 66 months. Two of these relapses occurred in the brain. At a median observation of 50 months the disease-free survival is 78%, at 7 years 67% (De Graaf et al., 1994).

Compared to available studies in similar patients, disease free survival seems to be prolonged after this form of treatment at the cost of considerable toxicity that can occasionally be fatal. Of concern are especially the high incidence of radiation pneumonitis, and the signs that seem to point to the role of the sanctuary site of the brain as a site of relapse.

Currently there are no data available from randomized studies comparing standard adjuvant chemotherapy with high-dose chemotherapy in patients with multiple axillary lymph nodes. It cannot be excluded that the positive results in the phase II studies are due to a selection bias. Therefore, randomized studies are mandatory in order to draw firm conclusions and in order to justify the burden of intensive treatment by a better survival. There are ongoing studies in the USA and Europe. In the Netherlands the Dutch Working Group on ABMT in solid tumors, in which all University hospitals and the two cancer hospitals in the Netherlands participate, decided to perform a phase III study in patients with more than three positive axillary lymph nodes and younger than 55 years of age. Rodenhuis et al. (1992) at the Dutch Cancer Institute performed the feasibility study for this regimen. Patients are randomized between either five courses containing cyclophosphamide, epirubicin and 5-fluorouracil as adjuvant therapy or four of these courses followed by peripheral stem cell harvest and high-dose chemotherapy with cyclophosphamide, thiotepa and carboplatin (De Vries et al., 1996b).

Radiotherapy as part of high-dose chemotherapy treatment for breast cancer

In breast cancer studies with high-dose chemotherapy, radiotherapy is currently often part of the treatment regimen. Radiotherapy allows the use of another modality apart from high-dose chemotherapy to attack a resistant population. The concept of relevance of radiotherapy as co-therapy in metastatic disease was recently nicely described by Hellman and Weichselbaum (1995). They propose the clinically significant state of 'oligometastases'. They suggest that for certain tumors the anatomy and physiology may limit or concentrate these metastases to a single or limited number of organs. It is known that there are situations in which resection or radiotherapy of a metastasis can result in cure.

Radiotherapy is added in high-dose chemotherapy breast carcinoma studies for locally advanced as well as metastatic cancer.

In the setting of locally advanced tumors radiotherapy is applied after chemotherapy to chest wall and regional lymph nodes. The study of Marks et al. (1992) suggested that this additive therapy was crucial in preventing a local relapse. This study, in which only nine patients did not receive local radiotherapy, was however too small to draw firm conclusions. They described a higher toxicity of the combined treatment of high-dose chemotherapy and radiotherapy. Refractory thrombocytopenia was observed during radiotherapy and pulmonary toxicity in 31% of the patients during and after radiotherapy. We observed in our adjuvant high-dose chemotherapy phase II study radiation pneumonitis in 50% of patients. Subjective pulmonary dysfunction as a long-term side effect was however rare. It has been suggested that monitoring of the cytokine transforming growth factor β (TGF-β) could help in deciding whether full dose radiotherapy can be administered without side effects. At the moment it is completely unknown whether the best moment to administer radiotherapy is after high-dose chemotherapy. If high-dose chemotherapy plays a real role in increased cure rate in the adjuvant setting then much additional research will be required concerning the value, toxicity and moment of administration of radiotherapy, especially if the patient has had breast-conserving surgery.

In metastatic breast carcinoma, relapses at pretreatment bulky disease have also been reported for patients after high-dose chemotherapy. Therefore, the application of radiotherapy in bulky disease can be of interest. Recently, in 31 patients who achieved a complete response after high-dose chemotherapy for metastatic breast cancer, the pattern of failure and the role of radiotherapy was evaluated (Mudt et al., 1994). The predominant site of relapse was the site of initial failure. Based on these data the authors suggested that patients with less than three sites of disease, bulky disease and locoregional disease should be considered for radiation therapy after high-dose chemotherapy. Depending on the frequency of brain metastases during long-term follow-up, the chemotherapy penetrance in the brain of the drugs used, prophylactic brain irradiation will have to be considered.

Ovarian carcinoma

Although most women with advanced ovarian carcinoma do respond on chemotherapy, after 10 years only around ± 20% of the chemotherapeutically treated patients are still disease-free. This tumor is sensitive for a number of drugs that can easily be executed, such as carboplatin, cyclophosphamide, ifosfamide, etoposide, melphalan, taxol. In addition, 50% of the women in the Netherlands are below the age of 60 years. There is still a debate in the literature concerning dose–response relationship in ovarian cancer without stem cell support. There are studies that do however suggest that there is a dose-response relationship (De Vries et al., 1993).

An increase in dose-intensity may be achieved by administration of higher cytostatic dosages or choosing a shorter time interval between cycles in combination with hematopoietic growth factor support or ablative chemotherapy followed by reinfusion of autologous bone marrow or peripheral stem cell rescue combined with cytokines.

Mulder et al. (1989b) administered cyclophosphamide 7 g/m² and etoposide 1.5 g/m² followed by autologous bone marrow rescue in 11 patients with residual or relapsing ovarian cancer after standard cisplatin-based treatment. In a dose-finding study, the same group treated seven patients with cyclophosphamide 7 g/m² and mitoxantrone 30–60 mg/m² (four patients), or mitoxantrone 60 mg/m² with melphalan 180 mg/m² (two patients) (Mulder et al., 1989a). A peritoneal inspection with biopsies and peritoneal washing was performed prior to and, in those patients with a clinically complete remission, after the high-dose treatment. Patients were considered to have residual microscopic disease when at the prior laparotomy no macroscopic tumor was found, but when biopsies or peritoneal washings revealed tumor cells. Minimal residual disease was defined as when the largest lesion of residual disease after surgery is ≤ 2 cm. In the case of bulky disease the largest lesion is > 2 cm after surgery.

These 18 patients had a median age of 46 (range 29–57) years. One patient received previous monochemotherapy with melphalan; all others had prior-combination chemotherapy: three carboplatin-based, the others cisplatin-based. Before high-dose chemotherapy, 14 patients had lesions < 2 cm; of these 14, three had microscopic evidence of residual tumor only. The other four had bulky residual disease. After ablative chemotherapy there were ten complete remissions; nine were confirmed with biopsies at relaparotomy or laparoscopy. Four patients had progressive disease after recovery from the regimen, three had stable disease. From the ten responding patients, five relapsed within one year, the sixth relapsed after 19 months, the four remaining patients are symptom-free after more than 6–12 years. There was one toxic death due to pulmonary aspergillosis. The four long-term disease-free surviving patients lead a normal life, that does not seem to be compromised by the high-dose chemotherapy regimen.

The application of a high-dose regimen in patients with bulky, larger than 2 cm residual lesions, does not seem to be of value. This conclusion is in agreement with results in a much larger group of patients treated by French investigators (De Vries et al., 1993); 65 patients with macroscopic residual lesions after various forms of first-line therapy relapsed after high-dose chemotherapy over the subsequent years. The same analysis led to better results in a more favorable subset of patients, as in a group of 52 patients with microscopic disease. Five-year progression free survival after high-dose chemotherapy is reported to be 30%.

Shea et al. (1989) reported on a phase I study with carboplatin 375–2400 mg/m^2 over 4 days in 11 patients; from a dose of 1600 mg/m^2 onwards ABMT was added and six patients responded; no follow-up data are available.

Another approach to high-dose treatment is the repeated use of peripheral stem cell reinfusion harvested after stimulation of marrow recovery by a growth factor, administered after marrow depression by an alkylator. Reinfusion after high-dose chemotherapy will result in an enhanced marrow recovery. Tepler et al. (1992) gave intensive therapy as first-line treatment by administering repetitive courses of dose intensive chemotherapy together with peripheral stem cell reinfusion. Shea et al. (1992) have performed a study with three cycles of carboplatin 500 mg/m^2 followed by GM-CSF alone or peripheral stem cell reinfusion with GM-CSF. The latter group did not need dose reduction and the total dose administered was 157% of that in the group treated with GM-CSF without PSCR. Fennelly and coworkers piloted the combination of high-dose carboplatin plus or minus taxol as first-line treatment and showed the remaining capacity to harvest peripheral blood stem cells (Crown et al., 1994; Fennelly et al., 1994).

The recognition of a group of ovarian cancer patients that has a potential for cure with this form of treatment revives the discussion on second look laparotomies, as this form of diagnostics is probably the only method to identify these patients. Currently, there are ongoing phase III studies including high-dose chemotherapy in France and the USA.

Small-cell lung carcinoma

Small-cell lung carcinoma is a very chemosensitive tumor type. However, most patients do relapse with only a low percentage still alive at two years after diagnosis. The fact that it is initially a tumor sensitive for etoposide, carboplatin, anthracyclines and cyclophosphamide, makes it a potentially interesting tumor type for high-dose chemotherapy. A disadvantage is the fact that the performance status of these patients may be low, that there are often other concomitant diseases, and contamination of the bone marrow or peripheral stem cells with tumor cells seems to be very realistic.

In the one randomized study performed in these patients, patients were after response on standard chemotherapy randomized between high-dose and standard chemotherapy. The only difference between the two arms was a slightly longer survival in the high-dose arm (Humblet et al., 1987).

Brugger et al. (1995) piloted high-dose chemotherapy as part of an early intensification strategy in 13 limited small-cell lung cancer patients. After two cycles with etoposide, ifosfamide, carboplatin and epirubicin, the patients got high-dose treatment with the same drugs but cisplatin replaced by carboplatin. Thereafter, the patients received chest radiotherapy and if they were in complete remission, cranial irradiation. The intention is to analyze the design in this patient group in a phase III study.

Probably sensitive assays for tumor cell detection and purging of the hematopoietic stem cells in combination with upcoming new drugs may allow new initiatives in this tumor type.

Tumors of young adults

Small studies are reported on high-dose chemotherapy in patients with metastatic Ewing sarcoma. There seem to be excellent effects initially, but the exact value concerning long-term results is still unknown (Bader, Horowitz and Dewan, 1989; Elias, Ayash and Eder, 1991; Pinkerton, 1991; Dumontet et al., 1992). There might be a potential role in the adjuvant or neo-adjuvant setting.

Glioma and melanoma

These two relatively chemotherapy insensitive tumors have also been analyzed in high-dose chemotherapy regimens. The phase II results of these studies suggest activity but the role of this treatment modality is as yet unclear. Meisenberg et al. (1993) performed a randomized trial in melanoma patients with a low tumor load, namely stage II patients after lymph-node metastases resection. The patients got high-dose cyclophosphamide, BCNU and cisplatin or were observed without treatment. There was no difference in overall survival.

Future

A number of relatively new anticancer drugs, such as paclitaxel and the topoisomerase I inhibitors, have limitedly or not yet been tested in high-dose regimens. Future phase III trials will have to prove whether there is a real survival benefit for patients treated with high-dose regimens. These studies also allow the analysis of effects on quality of life and long-term side effects. Preliminary data from the quality of life analysis as part of a randomized adjuvant breast carcinoma study show that after half year follow-up there was no difference between patients who received or did not receive high-dose chemotherapy and both groups did not differ from healthy individuals (Ten Vergert et al., 1996). Further studies are required to define the role of other modalities to overcome tumor treatment resistance such as radiotherapy, surgery, immuno- and hormonal therapy. Rapid technological progress concerning detection of tumor cells in the peripheral blood, the easier access to peripheral stem cell technology and the potential use of drug resistant genes for tissue protection may allow further extension of this treatment.

References

Ayash, L. J., Elias, A., Wheeler, C. et al. (1994). Double dose-intensive chemotherapy with autologous marrow and peripheral-blood progenitor-cell support for metastatic breast cancer: A feasibility study. J. Clin. Oncol., 12, 37–44.
Bader, J. L., Horowitz, M. E. and Dewan, R. (1989). Intensive combined modality therapy of small round cell and undifferentiated sarcomas in children and young adults. Radiother. Oncol., 16, 187–201.
Bensinger, W., Appelbaum, F., Rowley, S. et al. (1995). Factors that influence collection and engraftment of autologous peripheral blood stem cells. J. Clin. Oncol., 13, 2547–55.

Bezwoda, W. R., Seymour, L. and Dansey, R. D. (1995). High-dose chemotherapy with hematopoietic rescue as primary treatment for metastatic breast cancer: a randomized trial. *J. Clin. Oncol.*, **13**, 2483–9.

Borge, N., Fossa, S. D., Ous, S. et al. (1988). Late recurrence of testicular cancer. *J. Clin. Oncol.*, **6**, 1248–53.

Brandt, S. J., Peters, W. P., Atwater, S. K. et al. (1988) Effect of recombinant human granulocyte–macrophage colony-stimulating factor on hematopoietic reconstitution after high-dose chemotherapy and autologous bone marrow transplantation. *N. Engl. J. Med.*, **318**, 869–76.

Broun, E. R., Nichols, C. R., Kneebone, P. et al. (1992). Longterm outcome of patients with relapsed and refractory germ cell tumors treated with high dose chemotherapy and autologous bone marrow rescue. *Ann. Int. Med.*, **117**, 124–8.

Brugger, W., Bross, K. J., Glatt, M. et al. (1994). Mobilization of tumor cells and hematopoietic progenitor cells into peripheral blood of patients with solid tumors. *Blood*, **83**, 636–40.

Brugger, W., Frommhold, H., Pressler, K. et al. (1995). Use of high-dose etoposide, ifosfamide, carboplatin, epirubicin, and peripheral blood progenitor cell transplantation in limited-disease small cell lung cancer. *Semin. Oncol.*, **22**, 3–8.

Coiffier, B., Philip, T., Burnett, A. K. and Symann, M. L. (1994). Conclusions of a conference on intensive chemotherapy plus hematopoietic stem-cell transplantation in malignancies: Lyon, France, June 4–6, 1993. *J. Clin. Oncol.*, **12**, 226–31.

Crown, J., Fennelly, D., Schneider, J. et al. (1994). Escalating dose taxol high-dose cyclophosphamide/G-CSF as induction and to mobilize peripheral blood progenitors for use as rescue following multiple courses of high-dose carboplatin: a phase I trial in ovarian cancer patients. *Proc. Am. Soc. Clin. Oncol.*, **13**, 262.

Datta, Y. H., Adam, P. T., Drobyski, W. R. et al. (1994). Sensitive detection of occult breast cancer by the reverse-transcriptase polymerase chain reaction. *J. Clin. Oncol.*, **12**, 475–82.

Decottignies, A., Kolaczkowski, M., Balzi, E. and Goffeau, A. (1994a). Complete sequence of PDR5 from *Saccharomyces cerevisiae*. *J. Biol. Chem.*, **269**, 2206–14.

Decottignies, A., Kolaczkowski, M., Balzi, E. and Goffeau, A. (1994b). Solubilization and characterization of the overexpressed PDR5 multidrug resistance nucleotide triphosphatase of yeast. *J. Biol. Chem.*, **269**, 12797–803.

De Graaf, H., Willemse, P. H. B., De Vries, E. G. E. et al. (1994). Intensive chemotherapy with autologous bone marrow transfusion as primary treatment in women with breast cancer and more than 5 involved axillary lymph nodes. *Eur. J. Cancer*, **30A**, 150–3.

De Graaf, H., Mulder, N. H., Willemse, P. H. B. et al. (1995). Additive effect of peripheral blood stem cells, harvested with low-dose cyclophosphamide, to autologous bone marrow reinfusion on hematopoietic reconstitution after ablative chemotherapy in breast cancer patients with localized disease. *Anticancer Res.*, **15**, 2851–6.

De Vries, E. G. E., Hamilton, T. C., Lind, M. et al. (1993). Drug resistance, supportive care and dose intensity in ovarian carcinoma. *Ann. Oncol.*, **4** (suppl. 4), S57–S62.

De Vries, E. G. E., De Graaf, H., Boonstra, A. et al. (1995). High-dose chemotherapy with stem cell reinfusion and growth factor support for solid tumors. *Stem Cells*, **13**, 597–606.

De Vries, E. G. E., Rodenhuis, S., Schouten, H. C. et al. (1996a). Phase II study of intensive chemotherapy with autologous bone marrow transplantation in patients in complete remission of disseminated breast cancer. *Breast Cancer Res. Treat.*, **39**, 307–13.

De Vries, E. G. E., Ten Vergert, E. M., Mastenbroek, C. G. et al. (1996b). Breast cancer studies in the Netherlands. *Lancet*, **348**, 407–8.

Dillman, R. O. and Barth, N. M. (1994). Intensive chemotherapy with autologous peripheral blood stem-cell rescue in metastatic breast cancer. *J. Clin. Oncol.*, **12**, 22–37.

Dumontet, C., Biron, P., Bouffet, E. et al. (1992). High dose chemotherapy with ABMT in soft tissue sarcomas. A report of 22 cases. *Bone Marrow Transplant*, **10**, 405–8.

Eddy, D. M. (1992). High-dose chemotherapy with autologous bone marrow transplantation for the treatment of metastatic breast cancer. *J. Clin. Oncol.*, **10**, 657–70.

Elias, A. D., Ayash, L. and Eder, J. P. (1991). A phase I study of high-dose ifosfamide and escalating doses of carboplatin with autologous bone marrow support. *J. Clin. Oncol.*, **9**, 320–7.

Fennelly, D., Wasserheit, C., Schneider, J. et al. (1994). Simultaneous dose escalation and schedule intensification of carboplatin-based chemotherapy using peripheral blood progenitor cells and filgrastim: a phase I trial. *Cancer Res.*, **54**, 6137–42.

Gianni, A. M., Siena, S., Bregni, M. et al. (1989). Granulocyte–macrophage colony-stimulating factor to harvest circulating haemopoietic stem cells for autotransplantation. *Lancet*, **ii**, 580–5.

Gianni, A. M., Siena, S., Bregni, M. et al. (1992). Growth factor-supported high-dose sequential adjuvant chemotherapy in breast cancer with ≥ 10 positive nodes. *Proc. Am. Soc. Clin. Oncol.*, **11**, 60.

Gisselbrecht, C., Prentice, H. G., Bacigalupo, A. et al. (1994). Placebo-controlled phase III trial of lenograstim in bone-marrow transplantation. *Lancet*, **343**, 696–700.

Gorin, N. C., Coiffer, B., Hayat, M. et al. (1992). Recombinant human granulocyte–macrophage colony-stimulating factor after high dose chemotherapy and autologous bone marrow transplantation with unpurged and purged marrow in non-Hodgkin's lymphoma: a double-blind placebo-controlled trial. *Blood*, **80**, 1149–57.

Gulati, S. C. and Bennett, C. L. (1992). Granulocyte–macrophage colony-stimulating factor (GM-CSF) as an adjunct therapy in relapsed Hodgkin's disease. *Ann. Intern. Med.*, **116**, 177–82.

Hanania, E. G., Giles, R. E., Claxton, D. et al. (1996). Multiple drug resistance (MDR-1) genetic chemoprotection autologous transplants of retroviral vector mediated mdr-1 stomal transduced CD34 selected cells generated posttransplant bone marrow positive for viral mdr-1 sequences. *Proc. Am. Soc. Clin. Oncol.*, **15**, 583.

Hellman, S. and Weichselbaum, R. R. (1995). Oligometastases. *J. Clin. Oncol.*, **13**, 8–10.

Horwich, A., A'Hearn, R., Gildersleve, J. and Dearnaley, D. P. (1993). Prognostic factor analysis of conventional dose salvage therapy of patients with metastatic non-seminomatous germ cells cancer. *Proc. Am. Soc. Clin. Oncol.*, **12**, 232 (abstract 715).

Humblet, Y., Symann, M., Bosly, A. et al. (1987). Late intensification chemotherapy with autologous bone-marrow transplantation in selected small-cell carcinoma of the lung; a randomized study. *J. Clin. Oncol.*, **5**, 1864–73.

Katzmann, D. J., Burnett, P. E., Golin, J. et al. (1994). Transcriptional control of the yeast PDR5 gene by the PDR3 gene product. *Mol. Cell. Biol.*, **14**, 4653–61.

Kennedy, M. J., Beveridge, R. A., Scott, R. D. et al. (1991). High-dose chemotherapy with reinfusion of purged autologous bone marrow following dose-intense induction as initial therapy for metastatic breast cancer. *J. Natl. Cancer Inst.*, **83**, 920–6.

Levi, J. A., Thomson, D., Sandeman, T. et al. (1988). A prospective study of cisplatin based combination chemotherapy in advanced germ cell malignancy: role of maintenance and long-term follow-up. *J. Clin. Oncol.*, **6**, 1154–60.

Link, H., Boogaerts, M. A., Carella, A. M. et al. (1992). A controlled trial of recombinant human granulocyte–macrophage colony-stimulating factor after total body irradiation, high dose chemotherapy, and autologous bone marrow transplantation for acute lymphoblastic leukaemia or malignant lymphomas. *Blood*, **80**, 2188–95.

Marks, L. B., Halperin, E. C., Prosnitz, L. R. et al. (1992). Post-mastectomy radiotherapy following adjuvant chemotherapy and autologous bone marrow transplantation for breast cancer patients with ≥ 10 positive axillary lymph nodes. *Int. J. Rad. Oncol. Biol. Phys.*, **23**, 1021–6.

Meisenberg, B. R., Ross, M., Vredenburg, J. J. et al. (1993). Randomized trial of high-dose chemotherapy with autologous bone marrow support as adjuvant therapy for high-risk multi-node-positive malignant melanoma. *J. Natl. Cancer Inst.*, **85**, 1080–5.

Motzer, R. J. and Bosl, G. J. (1992). High-dose chemotherapy for resistant germ cell tumors: recent advances and future directions. *J. Natl. Cancer Inst.*, **84**, 1703–9.

Motzer, R. J., Geller, N. L., Tan, C. C. Y. et al. (1991). Salvage chemotherapy for patients with germ cell tumors. *Cancer*, **67**, 1305–10.

Motzer, R. J., Gulati, S. C., Crown, J. P. et al. (1992). High-dose chemotherapy and autologous bone marrow rescue for patients with refractory germ cell tumors. Early intervention is better tolerated. *Cancer*, **69**, 550–6.

Mudt, A. J., Sibley, G. S., Williams, S. et al. (1994). Patterns of failure of complete responders following high-dose chemotherapy and autologous bone marrow transplantation for metastatic breast cancer: implications for the use of adjuvant radiation therapy. *Int. J. Rad. Oncol. Biol. Phys.*, **30**, 151–60.

Mulder, N. H., Meinesz, A. F., Sleijfer, D. Th. et al. (1984). High dose etoposide with or without cyclophosphamide and autologous bone marrow transplantation in solid tumors. In *Autologous Bone Marrow Transplantation and Solid Tumours* (ed. J. G. McVie, O. Dalesio and I. E. Smith), pp. 125–30. Raven Press, New York.

Mulder, N. H., Sleijfer, D. Th., Smith Sibinga, C. Th. et al. (1986). High-dose chemotherapy with autologous bone marrow reinfusion in the treatment of patients with solid tumours. *Neth. J. Med.*, **29**, 359–64.

Mulder, P. O. M., De Vries, E. G. E., Schraffordt Koops, H. et al. (1988). Chemotherapy with maximally tolerable doses of VP 16-213 and cyclophosphamide followed by autologous bone marrow transplantation for the treatment of relapsed or refractory germ cell tumors. *Eur. J. Cancer Clin. Oncol.*, **24**, 675–9.

298   *E. G. E. de Vries, W. Dolsma, G. A. P. Hospers & N. H. Mulder*

Mulder, P. O. M., Sleijfer, D. Th., Willemse, P. H. B. et al. (1989a). High-dose cyclophosphamide or melphalan with escalating doses of mitoxantrone and autologous bone marrow transplantation for refractory solid tumors. *Cancer Res.*, **49**, 4654–8.

Mulder, P. O. M., Willemse, P. H. B., Aalders, J. G. et al. (1989b). High-dose chemotherapy with autologous bone marrow transplantation in patients with refractory ovarian cancer. *Eur. J. Cancer Clin. Oncol.*, **25**, 645–9.

Nemunaitis, J., Rabinowe, S. N., Singer, J. W. et al. (1991). Recombinant granulocyte–macrophage colony-stimulating factor after autologous bone marrow transplantation for lymphoid cancer. *N. Engl. J. Med.*, **324**, 1773–8.

Nichols, C. R., Tricot, G., Williams, S. D. et al. (1989). Dose-intensive chemotherapy in refractory germ cell cancer – a phase I/II trial of high-dose carboplatin and etoposide with autologous bone marrow transplantation. *J. Clin. Oncol.*, **7**, 932–9.

O'Slaughnessy, J. A., Cowan, K. H., Cottler-Fox, M. et al. (1994). Autologous transplantation of retrovirally marked CD34-positive bone marrow and peripheral blood cells in patients with multiple myeloma or breast cancer. *Proc. Am. Soc. Clin. Oncol.*, **13**, A963.

Pastan, I., Gottesman, M. M., Ueda, K. et al. (1988). A retrovirus carrying an mdr1 cDNA confers multidrug resistance and polarized expression of P-glycoprotein in MDCK cells. *Proc. Natl. Acad. Sci. USA*, **85**, 4486–90.

Peters, W. P., Rosner, G., Ross, M. et al. (1993a). Comparative effects of granulocyte–macrophage colony-stimulating factor (GM-CSF) and granulocyte colony-stimulating factor (G-CSF) on priming peripheral blood progenitor cells for use with autologous bone marrow after high-dose chemotherapy. *Blood*, **81**, 1709–19.

Peters, W. P., Ross, M., Vredenburgh, J. J. et al. (1993b). High-dose chemotherapy and autologous bone marrow support as consolidation after standard-dose adjuvant therapy for high-risk primary breast cancer. *J. Clin. Oncol.*, **11**, 1132–43.

Peters, W. P., Jones, R. B., Vredenburgh, J. J. et al. (1996). Large prospective randomized trial of high-dose combination alkylating agents with autologous cellular support as consolidation for patients with metastatic breast cancer achieving complete remission after intensive doxorubicin-based induction therapy. *Proc. Am. Soc. Clin. Oncol.*, **15**, 149.

Pinkerton, C. R. (1991). Megatherapy for soft tissue sarcomas. *Bone Marrow Transplant*, **3**, 120–2.

Rabinowe, S. N., Neuberg, D., Bierman, P. J. et al. (1993). Long-term follow up of a phase III study of recombinant human granulocyte–macrophage colony-stimulating factor after autologous bone marrow transplantation for lymphoid malignancies. *Blood*, **81**, 1903–8.

Rodenhuis, S., Baars, J., Schornagel, J. H. et al. (1992). Feasibility and toxicity study of a high-dose chemotherapy regimen incorporating carboplatin, cyclophosphamide and thiotepa. *Ann. Oncol.*, **3**, 855.

Rodenhuis, S., Van der Wall, E., Ten Bokkel Huinink, W. W. et al. (1995). Pilot study of a high-dose carboplatin-based salvage strategy for relapsing or refractory germ cell cancer. *Cancer Invest.*, **13**, 355–62.

Ross, A. A., Cooper, B. W., Lazarus, H. M. et al. (1993). Detection and viability of tumor cells in peripheral blood cell collections from breast cancer patients using immunocytochemical and clonogenic assay techniques. *Blood*, **82**, 2605–10.

Schmitz, N., Linch, D. C., Dreger, P. et al. (1996). Filgrastim-mobilized peripheral blood progenitor cell transplantation versus autologous bone-marrow transplantation in lymphoma patients. *Lancet*, **3**, 47353–7.

Shea, T. C., Flaherty, M., Elias, A. et al. (1989). A phase I clinical and pharmacokinetic study of carboplatin and autologous bone marrow support. *J. Clin. Oncol.*, **7**, 651–61.

Shea, T. C., Mason, J. R., Storniolo, A. M. et al. (1992). Sequential cycles of high-dose carboplatin administered with recombinant human granulocyte–macrophage colony-stimulating factor and repeated infusions of autologous peripheral blood progenitor cells: a novel and effective method for delivering multiple courses of dose-intensive therapy. *J. Clin. Oncol.*, **10**, 464–73.

Sheridan, W. P., Morstyn, G., Wolf, M. et al. (1989). Granulocyte colony-stimulating factor and neutrophil recovery after high-dose chemotherapy and autologous bone marrow transplantation. *Lancet*, **ii**, 891–5.

Sorrentino, B. P., Brandt, S. J., Bodine, D. et al. (1992). Selection of drug-resistant bone marrow cells in vivo after retroviral transfer of human mdr1. *Science*, **257**, 99–103.

Stoter, G., Koopman, A., Vendrik, C. P. J. et al. (1989). Ten-year survival and late sequelae in testicular cancer patients treated with cisplatin, vinblastine, and bleomycin. *J. Clin. Oncol.*, **7**, 1099–104.

Taylor, K. M., Jagannath, S., Spitzer, G. et al. (1989). Recombinant human granulocyte colony-stimulating factor hastens granulocyte recovery after high-dose chemotherapy and autologous bone marrow transplantation. *J. Clin. Oncol.*, **7**, 1791–9.

Ten Vergert, E. M., Rodenhuis, S., Bontenbal, M. et al. (1996). Quality of life in a randomized adjuvant breast carcinoma study with standard versus high-dose chemotherapy. *Proc. Am. Soc. Clin. Oncol.*, **15**, 77.

Tepler, I., Cannistra, S., Anderson, K. et al. (1992). Repetitive dose-intensive chemotherapy made possible by initial collection and repetitive rescue with peripheral blood progenitor cells in previously untreated outpatients with ovarian cancer. *Proc. Am. Soc. Clin. Oncol.*, **11**, A768.

Vanin, E. F., Kaloss, M., Broscius, C. and Nienhuis, A. W. (1994). Rapid progressive T-cell lymphomas were observed in 3 of 10 rhesus monkeys several months after autologous transplantation of enriched bone marrow stem cells that had been transduced with a retroviral vector preparation containing replication competent virus. *J. Virol.*, **86**, 4241–50.

Williams, S. F., Gilewski, T., Mick, R. et al. (1992). High-dose consolidation therapy with autologous stem-cell rescue in stage IV breast cancer: follow-up report. *J. Clin. Oncol.*, **10**, 1743–7.

10

Enhancing drug effectiveness by gene transfer

KAROL SIKORA

Introduction

Despite the development of sophisticated chemotherapy regimens together with new surgical and radiotherapy techniques, little headway has been made in the treatment of patients with common types of cancer. Indeed the overall cancer mortality in the population in the Western world is increasing due to a combination of its increasing age distribution and failure of therapeutic impact (Price and Sikora, 1995). Whilst advances in the local control of cancer will continue, these are unlikely to have a major effect on survival, which depends on our ability to control the growth of metastatic disease. Indeed the benefits of adjuvant chemotherapy in breast, colon and several childhood cancers indicate the need for more effective systemic approaches to cancer (Patel and Loprinzi, 1991). Current chemotherapy has a low therapeutic ratio, leading to significant toxicity, poor quality of life and in some programs, a significant mortality. Furthermore tumor cells have the capacity to evolve sophisticated genetic and biochemical mechanisms to overcome the toxic effects of administered drugs. For many types of cancer — breast, ovary, small cell lung and certain types of non-Hodgkin's lymphoma — the initial complete response rate is high but the majority of patients will die of drug resistant metastases within two years of their response (Thames Cancer Registry, 1994). The effects of chemotherapy can be classified into three groups — tumors in which a high complete response and high cure rate is obtained; those with a low response and cure rate and a group where tumor shrinkage is frequent but patients rapidly relapse with drug resistant disease.

The key to the effectiveness of chemotherapy is selectivity. Our current combinations of drugs have been optimized by trial and error and their true selective mechanisms are unclear. Most anticancer drugs have been discovered through systematic screening of organic chemicals and natural products followed by modification to enhance their therapeutic ratio. Some have been designed to enhance their selective metabolism in tumor cells (Connors, 1991). Cyclophosphamide, for example, is activated by the phosphoramidases found in abundance in many tumors, although it is now clear that many normal cells also possess the necessary activating enzymes (De Neve et al., 1989). Novel methods to increase selectivity empirically have included high-dose therapy, with or without peripheral blood stem cell grafting and the continuous infusion of drugs such as 5-fluorouracil using portable pumps (Lokich, Ahlgren and Gullo, 1989).

The last decade has seen dramatic advances in our understanding of the mechanisms involved in the control of cell growth and their deregulation in cancer. Certain classes of genes encode proteins that play distinct roles in the processing of signals from the outside of the cell to the nucleus. Any changes to the delicate system of control by these oncogenes or tumor suppressor genes may result in the formation of cancer (Sikora, 1994). Increasingly it is becoming clear that a series of molecular changes are necessary for tumor formation. Pre-existing genetic factors and environmental events clearly play a major role in the cancer process. Fundamental genetic differences between normal and tumor cells may be exploited in novel genetically based cancer therapies. The development of effective systemic gene targeting systems is now on the horizon, so making gene therapy for cancer a realistic prospect.

Several strategies for the genetic intervention of cancer have been proposed and over 100 protocols are now active worldwide (Table 10.1). The most promising for the intermediate term are those in which gene transfer can elicit a bystander effect that amplifies the direct effects on transduced cells. These include prodrug activation strategies and those involving immunization by genes expressing tumor-specific epitopes. Another promising strategy is to use gene transfer to reduce selectively the toxicity of chemotherapy on critical tissues. Drug activation and resistance strategies will be considered here.

Genetic prodrug activation systems

There are already a number of genes known to be preferentially expressed in tumors (Pandha, Waxman and Sikora, 1994) (Table 10.2). Furthermore, high throughput analysis of differences in gene expression using techniques such as mRNA differential display and differential

Table 10.1. *Strategies for cancer gene therapy*

- genetic tagging to detect minimal residual disease and to explore the cause of relapse after bone marrow transplantation
- the development of enhanced tumor vaccines by the ex vivo or in vivo transduction of genes encoding immunostimulatory molecules such as IL2, other cytokines, co-stimulatory molecules or foreign class 1 HLA determinants
- the construction of polynucleotide vaccines for classical tumor antigens such as CEA, PSA, and idiotypic determinants
- the vectoring of biologically active drugs such as TNF transduced ex vivo into tumor-infiltrating lymphocytes
- the insertion of drug-activating genes that are linked to specific tumor or tissue transcriptional regulatory sequences (genetically directed enzyme prodrug therapy – GDEPT)
- the insertion of stem cell protection genes during BMT or PBSCG
- the inhibition of mutant oncogene expression by antisense or ribozymes
- the insertion of wild type tumor suppressor genes

Table 10.2. *Genes known to be expressed at higher levels in tumors*

Gene	Tumor-tissue
CEA	GI, lung
AFP	Liver, germ cell
DOPA DC	SCLC, neurectodermal
NSE	SCLC
PSA	Prostate
Tyrosinase	Melanoma
TRP	Melanoma
Calcitonin	Medullary thyroid
Thyroglobulin	Thyroid
MUC-1	Breast, GI, lung
Villin	GI
EGFR	NSCLC, head and neck, others
ERB B2	Breast, pancreas, lung
ERB B3	Breast
ERB B4	Breast
L-plastin	Pancreas
Tissue factor	Pancreas

hybridization of high-density gridded cDNA filters are likely to uncover genes that encode previously undiscovered tumor markers (McKie et al., 1995). Genetically directed enzyme prodrug therapy (GDEPT) exploits the differences in gene expression between different cell types to increase the specificity of cell destruction.

Table 10.3. *Selective transcriptional activation systems*

- ideally tumor specific
- only expressed in non-essential tissues
- no cross-specificity with unusual but essential cell types
- regulatory elements from gene cloned and sequenced
- specific transcription factor binding sites identified
- enhancer and inhibitory factors understood

Viral GDEPT systems use a replication-defective recombinant viral vector to introduce a foreign gene encoding an enzyme capable of converting a harmless prodrug into a cytotoxic compound. The viral vector is capable of infecting both normal and malignant cells, but the system is designed so that significant transcription of the enzyme gene is activated only in tumor cells. This 'molecular switch' is achieved by linking the enzyme gene to transcriptional control elements selective for a particular tumor or tissue type. Success has been achieved in targeting tissue types such as melanocytes using the promoters of the genes encoding tyrosinase and tyrosinase-related protein (Vile and Hart, 1993), the gastrointestinal epithelium using the carcinoembryonic antigen gene promoter (Austin and Huber, 1993) and breast cancer using the *MUC*-1 gene. Such tissue-specific systems, however, suffer from the disadvantage that all background cells in the target tissue may also be susceptible to destruction through activation of the prodrug. Examples of tumor specific transcriptional activation include the use of the alpha fetoprotein promoter in hepatoma and upstream sequences of the c-*erb* B2 oncogene in breast cancer. There are essentially two components required for a successful GDEPT system – the transcriptional regulatory sequence that is to act as the specific switch and the enzyme prodrug combination to generate the selectively toxic drug.

Selective transcriptional activation

The properties of an optimal transcriptional activation system are listed in Table 10.3. There are a number of genes expressed at high levels in tumors and at very low levels, if at all, in normal adult tissue, but absolute tumor specificity may not be essential. In metastatic prostate cancer, for example, the eradication of all prostate tissue, both normal and malignant, would in effect be a 'genetic prostatectomy'. It may be possible to develop such a system using the transcriptional regulatory sequences of the prostate specific antigen (PSA) gene. It is clearly important that there is no cross-specificity with essential normal tissues. Past experience with toxin-conjugated monoclonal antibodies is salutary. In early clinical trials of ricin–anti-leukemia antibody conjugates renal failure developed. This was due to a cross-reactivity of the antibody with a small subset of cells in the renal tubules.

The control of eukaryotic gene transcription is extremely complex and only partially understood (Lewin, 1994). Although there are several model genes for which the temporal and spatial relationships of positive and negative transcription signals are understood for most genes the situation is uncharted. Transcription is controlled by a series of upstream promoters that essentially act as gatekeepers for the binding of RNA polymerase. Some of these are non-specific, such as the TATA and CAAT regions. Others are much more specific, binding to unique transcription factors, which in turn are subject to complex control mechanisms. There may also be inhibitory elements both upstream and within the coding sequences of the gene. Enhancers can also profoundly modulate gene expression. These sequences may be located at large distances from the relevant gene, making their functional analysis extremely complex. To fully optimize a GDEPT system requires a detailed understanding of both positive and negative signals in order to develop vectors that maximize discrimination of expression between tumor and normal cells. The exact nature of these signals may differ in their importance in different tissues. The human genome project will undoubtedly give us a much clearer insight into the process of transcription control and lead to new approaches for tissue-specific pharmacology.

Enzyme–prodrug activation systems

There are many potential prodrug–drug activating systems available. Some were developed on the basis of the natural enzyme expression patterns of tumors resulting in selective drug activation (Connors, 1986). Whilst interesting results have been obtained in several animal tumor systems, none have shown efficacy in human tumors, which are metabolically heterogeneous. The advent of antibody dependent enzyme–prodrug therapy (ADEPT) stimulated further interest in these systems (Bagshawe, Springer and Searle, 1988). The problems of antibody targeting are the relatively low specificity and affinity of even the best targeting reagents. New structures with enhanced affinity are being developed and could well produce improved results (Chester et al., 1994).

Table 10.4. *Optimal drug activation system*

Enzyme
    low K_m and high V_{max}
    simple production pathway
    passes through gap junctions

Drug
    lipid-soluble prodrug
    low molecular weight
    high potency
    freely soluble end metabolites
    not cell cycle specific

The desirable enzyme and drug characteristics for GDEPT are listed in Table 10.4. The enzyme should be able to produce the active drug rapidly at low substrate concentrations – possess a high K_{cat} and low K_m. It should be monomeric, of relatively small size, not require post-translational modification and so be simple to produce. Ideally it should be able to pass through gap junctions easily to enhance the bystander effect.

The prodrug and drug and its end metabolites should be lipid soluble, of low molecular weight and high potency. As the GDEPT enzyme may only be transiently expressed, the active drug should have a long half-life. Ideally the drug should not be cell-cycle specific, enabling it to kill non-proliferating tumor cells.

Viral thymidine kinase

Gancyclovir (GCV) was developed as an antiviral drug (Moolten, 1986). It is phosphorylated by viral thymidine kinase (tk) to the monophosphate and mammalian kinases then convert it to the active triphosphate. Both herpes simplex virus (HSV) and varicella zoster kinase systems are available. The latter is not highly lipid-soluble and therefore not freely diffusable. Despite this, significant bystander killing has been observed. Complete cell killing was observed even when only 10% of a mixed population were HSV *tk* positive in vitro (Freeman et al., 1993; Li et al., 1993). Mouse fibroblasts engineered to produce infecting retrovirus particles carrying the LTR-driven HSV *tk* gene have been directly injected intratumorally into a murine brain tumor. The locally produced virus could transduce the dividing glioma cells, thus making them susceptible to GCV. The proportion of the cells transduced was 10–70% and in some cases total tumor regression was observed after GCV was given intraperitoneally. Clinical studies are underway for human gliomas. GCV–triphosphate will only kill actively cycling cells so may not be optimal for the common more slowly growing human tumors with a low growth fraction.

Cytosine deaminase (CD)

5-fluorocytosine (5-FC) is a currently used antifungal agent. The active drug – 5-fluorouracil – is only effective against proliferating cells but is not cell cycle specific. There is considerable clinical experience in its use in colorectal and to a lesser extent breast cancer (Pinedo and Peters, 1988; Handschumacher and Cheng, 1993). Many different methods of administration – oral, intravenous both by bolus injection or continuous infusion, have been used. Furthermore its effects can be enhanced by agents such as folinic acid and the interferons, which stabilize the interaction of its metabolite 5-FdUMP with the enzyme thymidilate synthase (Van der Wilt et al., 1992). The prodrug has low toxicity (IC_{50} of 200 μM) and the activated drug is potent (IC_{50} of 20 μM). Drug resistance may however develop either due to alterations in metabolism or increased drug export. A remarkable bystander effect has been demonstrated. Recent evidence suggests that even when as low as 2% of a cell population in vivo is expressing cytosine deaminase, significant anti-tumor effects are seen (Huber et al., 1993).

Nitroreductase

Bacterial nitroreductases are able to convert a wide range of substrates into extremely potent drugs. Many different classes of cytotoxic drugs can be activated in this way (Antoniw et al., 1990). CB 1954 is activated into the highly potent and lipid soluble bifunctional alkylating agent dinitrobenzamide (Sunters et al., 1991). Several strategies are being developed using this agent both for ADEPT and GDEPT.

Beta-glucosidase

This enzyme catalyses a wide range of sugar substrates into cyanide and benzaldehyde (Rowlinson-Busza et al., 1992). It has been used in the development of ADEPT systems. The optimal prodrug appears to be the disaccharide amygdalin, which is converted to cyanide, benzalde-hyde and glucose. The sugar prodrug has a very low toxicity and the active drug has high potency, and solubility. No mechanisms of drug resistance are known.

Other enzyme systems

A wide range of enzyme prodrug systems is available (Table 10.5). Many can activate several prodrugs simultaneously. The bystander effect is variable and clearly important. The *E. coli DeoD* purine nucleoside phosphorylase activates nontoxic purine analogs to produce a highly toxic drug that is freely diffusable, killing over 99% of cells in vitro even when only 1% of cells express the gene (Sorscher et al., 1994). An interesting concept is the production of radioresistant cell lines by the insertion of the superoxide dismutase gene whose product protects cells from damage by oxygen radicals. Selective expression of antisense mRNA to this enzyme could increase radiation damage to tumors in vivo. It is also possible to express selectively suicide enzyme genes such as ribonucleases and deoxyribonucleases that have a wide range of destructive effects on cells.

Increasing radiation sensitivity

The selective transcription of specific genes by tumor cells can be har-nessed to enhance radiation sensitivity using several strategies. Modern radiation dosimetry permits the precise localization of high dose radi-ation concisely to the anatomical confines of a tumor. The relationship between tumor regression and dose is sigmoid. A small change in radi-ation sensitivity, especially if not affecting normal tissue, can therefore very significantly enhance the local control rate. One potential strategy is to couple antisense to radiation repair genes to tumor specific regulatory sequences so that cancer cells are less able to repair radiation-induced DNA damage. Another intriguing system is to couple radiation inducible genes such as *Egr* to a potentially toxic gene such as that encoding tumor necrosis factor. Such constructs have been inserted into human leukemia cells and shown to enhance responses to irradiation in both transfected cell lines and in xenografts.

Table 10.5. *Drug activation systems for GDEPT*

Enzyme	Prodrug	Active drug
Viral thymidine kinase	Gancyclovir	Gancyclovir TP
Cytosine deaminase	5-FC	5-FU
Linamarase	Amygdalin	Cyanide
cyp1A2	Paracetamol	Toxic metabolites
Nitroreductase	CB 1954	Nitrobenzamidine
β-lactamase	PD	PD mustard
β-glucuronidase	Adria-glu	Adriamycin
Carboxypeptidase A	MTX-alanine	MTX
Alkaline phosphatase	Adria-P	Adriamycin
Carboxypeptidase G2	Benzoic acid-Glu	Benzoic acid mustard
Glucose oxidase	Glucose	Peroxide
Penicillin amidase	Adria-PA	Adriamycin
DeoD phosphorylase	purines	Toxic purines
gpt	6-TX	6-thioguanine
Superoxide dismutase	XRT	DNA damage
Ribonuclease	RNA	Cleaved products
ScFv	antibody	Intracellular changes
egr/RRE	XRT	XRT

Adria-glu, Adriamycin-glutamic acid; Adria-P, Adriamycin phosphate; egr/RRE, early growth response/radiation response element; PA, phenylalanine; PD, penicillin diamine; 6-TX, 6-thiouracil; XRT, X-irradiation.

Bystander effects

The effective killing of bystander cells is crucial to the efficiency of GDEPT systems. Our current vectors are relatively inefficient at transducing or transfecting cells. Although this may be improved, the problem of limited access to tumor cells in vivo will always remain. These will be affected by the cell type and density, the vascular structure of the tumor and its surrounding tissue together with a range of immunological factors both locally and systemically. Gap junctions between cells can act as conduits for the diffusion of enzyme, active drug, its toxic metabolites as well as apoptotic signals. Low molecular weight enzymes and lipid soluble drugs could diffuse through the extracellular fluid. Local cytokine release following cell death could enhance the zone of cytotoxicity produced by a GDEPT system and systemic immunological effects have also been observed. Clearly a detailed understanding of the bystander effect will be essential in order to optimize the selectivity of tumor destruction.

The *ERBB2*–cytosine deaminase system

We have described a gene therapy strategy that is tumor-specific rather than tissue-specific. The oncogene *ERBB2* is frequently overexpressed in a number of different tumor types, particularly carcinomas of the breast, pancreas and gastrointestinal tract from greatly increased transcription of each copy of the *ERBB2* gene, coupled with gene amplification in some cases (Slamon et al., 1987; Hall et al., 1990; Lemoine et al., 1991). Expression of this oncogene has not been observed in normal and inflammatory conditions at levels comparable to those in tumor cells. The expression of high levels of *ERBB2* is thus a tumor-specific phenomenon and the transcriptional control elements of this gene represent a potential targeting device for drug activation.

Our group has shown that the promoter region of the human *ERBB2* gene contains a binding site for a novel member of the AP-2 transcription factor family, responsible for upregulating transcription in human breast cancer (Hollywood and Hurst, 1993). This has been shown to lie within 500 bp upstream of the transcription start site of the *ERBB2* gene. We have designed a GDEPT strategy against human cancers using expression of the cytosine deaminase gene controlled by the human *ERBB2* proximal promoter. We have delivered the prototype chimeric construct comprising the proximal *ERBB2* promoter driving the cytosine deaminase gene into human breast and pancreatic tumor cells using both a recombinant double copy retrovirus, DC/pTH-CD500, and a simple plasmid vector. Transduced cells were analysed for their ability to deaminate cytosine and their susceptibility to 5-FC induced toxicity.

To assess the expression of cytosine deaminase (CD) in the cell lines tested, we used a thin layer chromatography method. CD activity was not detected in any of the parental cell lines nor in the *ERBB2* cell lines. However, all *ERBB2* cell lines that were transduced with DC/pTH-CD500 or the plasmid construct pERCy showed high levels of CD activity, confirming specific expression of cytosine deaminase in our system.

Cells were grown in medium containing 5-FC and the effects of exposure to the prodrug were assayed after 48 hours. Non-transduced cell lines and cell lines with normal low levels of *ERBB2* expression, were unaffected by the treatment with 5-FC. All the DC/pTH-CD500 transduced *ERBB2* cell lines tested showed evidence of marked cell death. The effect of growth of the cells in the presence of a lower concentration of 5-FC for a longer period of time (7 days) was also assessed. As before, the non-transduced and *ERBB2* cells were unaffected by the treatment. However, *ERBB2* cells transduced with DC/pTH-CD500 were all sensitive to 5-FC. Thus, one could achieve the same cell killing effect by using a lower concentration of 5-FC for longer period of time, which could be a significant advantage for clinical application.

These data demonstrate the utility of a tumor-specific targeting strategy for cancer therapy. We chose this system since both the prodrug and the active metabolite have a long history of successful patient use (5-FC for fungal infections and 5-FU for cancer therapy) and we have the opportunity to monitor metabolism of the drugs in vitro and in vivo by positron emission tomography (PET) scanning technology, making this gene therapy system particularly attractive for clinical trial. The metabolism of 5-FU to its cytotoxic end-products is extremely complex, involving a large number of cellular enzymes, and several determinants associated with the cytotoxicity of 5-FU have been described. This drug is used as the compound of choice for gastric, colorectal and pancreatic cancers and is a component of the most widely used protocols for breast cancer. Recent clinical data suggest that enhanced tumor responses can be obtained by altering the pharmacokinetics of 5-FU delivery and by the use of folinic acid to stabilize the interaction of 5-FU with its target enzyme. These strategies can be developed to enhance the selectivity of GDEPT.

Gene targeting is currently the major problem throughout all gene therapy research. Our clinical trial utilizes naked supercoiled DNA mainly for safety reasons. We have explored in xenografts the use of several liposome preparations without evidence of increased plasmid expression. Our original experiments utilized amphotrophic retroviruses but the present generation of such vectors are inactivated in human serum and only able to transduce replicating cells. We now have adenoviral and adeno-associated viral vectors containing the ERBB2–CD construct and we are planning a comparative study in xenografts examining the kinetics and magnitude of selective CD expression.

Clinical trials of GDEPT

For GDEPT to be effective clinically, systemic strategies for gene delivery will be required. However, in the initial studies it is vital that we obtain as much information as possible from each clinical study to guide future developments. For this reason, genetic manipulation by direct injection of recombinant DNA into subcutaneous nodules provides an excellent model system. As such nodules are usually multiple, it is possible to use a neighbouring similarly sized metastasis as a control.

We are currently extending our laboratory observations into a clinical trial using plasmid DNA containing the CD gene under the control of the *ERBB2* promoter directly injected into metastatic subcutaneous nodules in patients with breast cancer. After 24 hours the patients will receive a 48-hour infusion of 5-FC intravenously. The skin lesions are uniquely accessible through the relatively painless technique of fine needle aspiration. We have demonstrated that fine needle aspirate material is adequate to detect specific gene transcripts by RT-PCR. Although any response obtained would be limited to the single treated nodule, this protocol represents a first step in the development of potentially systemic GDEPT strategies for breast cancer.

The direct injection of DNA is an artificial situation resembling the xenograft model. Until suitable tissue tropic vectors become available, we plan to extend our systems to local organ perfusion. An example is the isolated liver perfusion system currently used in liver transplantation. This allows the transduction of the entire liver within a reasonable time course in a serum-free environment. Metastases and normal liver would be equally exposed to the vector in equal amounts but selective expression would take place in metastases.

The development of targeted systemic vectors is likely within the next two years. We are exploring altered retroviruses and adenoviruses using both scFv's (single chain variable fragments) to tumor specific proteins and ligands to tyrosine kinase growth factor receptors. To target retroviruses to tumors, we are constructing fusion proteins between the viral *env* protein and single-chain antibody fragments of tumor-specific antibodies or ligands to growth factor receptors. The latter receptor–ligand approach has been bedevilled by the complexity of ligand interaction with *ERBB2*. Heregulin appears to be the ligand for *ERBB3* and *ERBB4* but through heterodimer formation also increases *ERBB2* activation. We plan to utilize these phenomena to construct doubly selective vectors that can bind more avidly to tumors and are subsequently selectively expressed.

Protecting normal tissues by gene transfer

For the majority of anticancer drugs in current use, it is the bone marrow that is the dose limiting organ. This leads to occasional catastrophic leucopenias often associated with life-threatening septicaemia. There is good evidence that reducing chemotherapy dosage leads to poorer response rates. The evidence that dose escalation increases the cure rate for patients with solid tumors is somewhat more controversial, but for some cancers such as lymphoma, germ cell tumors and probably breast and ovarian cancer, this certainly seems true.

There are several ways in which the bone marrow can be protected. These include the use of exogenous marrow support factors such as G-CSF, autologous bone marrow transplantation and peripheral blood stem cell grafting (PBSCG). An extension of these approaches is to use genetic intervention to increase the resistance of marrow stem cells to chemotherapy by using either G-CSF gene insertion or the enhanced expression of the multiple drug resistance gene *MDR1*. There are several elegant animal models showing the effectiveness of both systems at increasing tolerance to a range of cytotoxic drugs (Hanania et al., 1995a). Several clinical trials are now in progress to test such approaches in patients with breast and ovarian cancer.

A significant problem is ensuring that stem cells rather than terminally differentiated cells receive the relevant gene in a stable manner. Encouraging results have been obtained (Hanania et al., 1995b) using CD34 stem cells. Monoclonal antibody affinity columns were used to purify populations of such cells from donor human bone marrow. After *MDR1* transduction, cells were plated on methylcellulose and tested for resistance to taxol. Up to 13% of such cells were found to contain the *MDR1* gene by RT-PCR. This was confirmed by flow cytometric analysis using antibodies to CD34 and p-glycoprotein. Furthermore dye exclusion studies confirmed the presence of functional P-glycoprotein. Similar results were obtained using CD34 cells purified from peripheral blood, suggesting that *MDR1* transduction could be used with PBSCG.

There are several potential risks in these approaches. Contaminating tumor cells may also be transduced, so making them more resistant to treatment. Another possible problem is the in vivo transfer of the introduced *MDR1* gene to tumor cells in the bone marrow elsewhere. A third risk is the development of drug-resistant hematological malignancies. These potential problems are receiving detailed consideration in the design of clinical studies.

Clearly the bone marrow is only one critical organ for chemotherapy. If such approaches are successful the genetic protection of other organ systems such as the heart and gastrointestinal tract could be contemplated. At present we lack good in vivo targeting systems, but the remarkable progress being made in vector development bodes well for future tissue-targeting systems. The construction of systemically administered vectors home in on CD34 cells that could well be a realistic strategy for the future.

References

Antoniw, P., Springer, C. J., D., et al. (1990). Disposition of the prodrug 4-(bis(2-chloroethyl)amino)benzoyl-L-glutamic acid and its active parent drug in mice. *Br. J. Cancer*, **62**, 909–14.

Austin, E. A. and Huber, B. E. (1993). A first step in the development of gene-therapy for colorectal carcinoma – cloning, sequencing, and expression of *Escherichia coli* cytosine deaminase. *Mol. Pharmacol.*, **43**, 380–7.

Bagshawe, K., Springer, C. and Searle, F. (1988). A cytotoxic agent can be generated selectively at cancer sites. *Br. J. Cancer*, **58**, 700–3.

Cancer in South East England (1994). Thames Cancer Registry, Sutton.

Chester, K., Begent, R., Robson, L. et al. (1994). Phage libraries for the generation of clinically useful antibodies. *Lancet*, **343**, 455–6.

Connors, T. (1986). Prodrugs in cancer therapy. *Xenobiotica*, **16**, 975–88.

Connors, T. (1991). Alkylating agents. In *Cancer Chemotherapy and Biological Response Modifiers* (ed. H. Pinedo, D. Longo and B. Chabner), pp. 27–42. Elsevier, Amsterdam.

DeNeve, W., Valeriote, F., Edelstein, M. et al. (1989). In vivo DNA cross linking by cyclophosphamide. *Cancer Res.*, **49**, 3452–6.

Freeman, S., Abboud, C., Whartenby, K. et al. (1993). The bystander effect: tumor regression when a fraction of the tumor mass is genetically modified. *Cancer Res.*, **53**, 5274–83.

Hall, P. A., Hughes, C. M., Staddon, S. L. et al. (1990). The c-erbB-2 proto-oncogene in human pancreatic cancer. *J. Pathol.*, **161**, 195–200.

Hanania, E., Fu, S., Roninson, I. et al. (1995a). Resistance to taxol chemotherapy produced in mouse marrow cells by safety modified retroviruses containing a human MDR-1 transcription unit. *Gene Ther.*, **2**, 279–84.

Hanania, E., Fu, S., Hegeswisch, S. et al. (1995b). Chemotherapy resistance to taxol in clonogenic progenitor cells. *Gene Therapy*, **12**, 285–94.

Handschumacher, R. E. and Cheng, Y. C. (1993). Purine and pyrimidine antimetabolites. In *Cancer Medicine*, 3rd edition (ed. J. F. Holland, E. Frei, R. C. Bast, et al.), pp. 712–32. Lea & Febiger, London.

Hollywood, D. and Hurst, H. C. (1993). A novel transcription factor, OB2-1, is required for overexpression of the proto-oncogene c-erbB-2 in mammary tumour lines. *EMBO J.*, **12**, 2369–75.

Huber, B. E., Austin, E. A., Good, S. S. et al. (1993). In vivo antitumor activity of 5-fluorocytosine on human colorectal carcinoma cells genetically modified to express cytosine deaminase. *Cancer Res.*, **53**, 4619–26.

Lemoine, N. R., Jain, S., Silvestre, F. et al. (1991). Amplification and overexpression of the EGF receptor and c-erbB-2 oncogenes in human stomach cancer. *Br. J. Cancer*, **64**, 74–83.

Lewin, B. (1994). *Eucaryotic Transcription and mRNA Processing. Genes V*, pp. 847–901. Oxford University Press.

Li, B. W., Culver, K., Walbridge, S. et al. (1993). In vitro evidence that metabolic co-operation is responsible for the bystander effect observed with HSV tk retroviral gene therapy. *Human gene therapy*, **4**, 725–31.

Lokich, J., Ahlgren, J. and Gullo, J. (1989). A prospective randomised comparison of continuous infusion fluorouracil with conventional bolus schedule in metastatic colorectal carcinoma. *J. Clin. Oncol.*, **7**, 425–32.

McKie, A. B., Bhatia, A., Hurst, H. C. and Lemoine, N. R. (1995). Nucleic acid fingerprinting strategies for the identification of novel genetic events in pancreatic cancer. In *Pancreatic Cancer: Molecular and Clinical Advances* (ed. J. P. Neoptolemos and N. R. Lemoine), pp. 142–51. Blackwell Scientific, Oxford.

Moolten, F. (1986). Tumour chemosensitivity conferred by inserted herpes thymidine kinase genes: paradigm for a prospective cancer control strategy. *Cancer Res.*, **46**, 5276–81.

Pandha, H., Waxman, J. and Sikora, K. (1994). Tumour markers. *Brit. J. Hosp. Med.*, **51**, 297–302.

Patel, S. and Loprinzi, C. (1991). Breast cancer. In *Cancer Chemotherapy and Biological Response Modifiers* (ed. H. Pinedo, D. Longo and B. Chabner), pp. 571–89. Elsevier, Amsterdam.

Pinedo, H. M. and Peters, G. F. J. (1988). Fluorouracil: biochemistry and pharmacology. *J. Clin. Oncol.*, **6**, 1653–44.

Price, P. and Sikora, K. (eds) (1995). *Treatment of Cancer*, 3rd edition. Chapman & Hall, London.

Rowlinson-Busza, G., Bamias, A., Kraus, T. and Epenetos, A. A. (1992). Antibody guided enzyme nitrile therapy. In *Monoclonal Antibodies Applications in Clinical Oncology* (ed. A. Epenetos), pp. 111–18. Chapman & Hall, London.

Sikora, K. (1994). Genes, dreams and cancer. *Br. Med. J.*, **308**, 1217–22.

Slamon, D. J., Clark, G. M., Wong, S. G. et al. (1987). Human breast cancer: correlation of relapse and survival with amplification of the HER-2/neu oncogene. *Science*, **235**, 177–82.

Sorscher, E. J., Peng, S., Bebok, Z. et al. (1994). Tumour bystander killing in colonic carcinoma utilising the *E. coli* DeoD gene to generate toxic purine. *Gene Therapy*, **1**, 233–8.

Sunters, A., Baer, J. and Bagshawe, K. B. (1991). Cytotoxicity and activation of CB1954 in a human tumour cell line. *Biochem. Pharmacol.*, **9**, 1293–8.

Van der Wilt, C. L., Pinedo, H. M., Smid, K. et al. (1992). Effect of folinic acid on fluorouracil activity and expression of thymidylate synthase. *Semin. Oncol.*, **19**, 16–25.

Vile, R. G. and Hart, I. R. (1993). In vitro and in vivo targeting of gene expression to melanoma cells. *Cancer Res.*, **53**, 961–7.

Index